Comprehensive Practical Hepatology

Edited By

Yukihiro Shimizu

Director, Gastroenterology Center
Nanto Municipal Hospital
Toyama
Japan

CONTENTS

FOREWORD

First of all, I am honored to introduce this exciting book. Dr. Shimizu has been involved in hepatology for over 30 years and has studied hepatology in the United States twice. On the first occasion at the age of 30 years old, he joined the Pittsburgh Cancer Institute, where he undertook research for 2 years on tumor immunology in human liver tumors as part of the laboratory of Dr. Theresa L. Whiteside and published 6 papers with her. When he was 36 years old, he joined the Scripps Research Institute, and studied immunology of viral hepatitis under the guidance of Dr. Francis V. Chisari. Since returning to his home university (Toyama Medical and Pharmaceutical University), he has been engaged in clinical and basic research and presented many papers at domestic and international hepatology meetings, that have been published in international journals. Since I became involved in molecular analysis of hepatitis virus, I have had the opportunity to meet him several times at various meetings and discussions on hepatology research.

In 2006, he left the Toyama Medical and Pharmaceutical University, and started a new career as a clinical specialist of hepatology. He is now the Director of Nanto Municipal Hospital at which several general physicians work alongside organ specialists. He believes the role of general physicians in liver disease will become more important as the proportion of elderly in the population increases. Many patients with liver injury will first see their general physician and the role of general physicians will increase in the management of patients with liver diseases. Although there are many books on hepatology most are aimed at hepatologists with few books on liver disease focusing on primary care management performed by general physicians. I believe that this e-Book will be a very helpful and practical guide for general physicians.

Nobuyuki Enomoto
Professor, First Department of Internal Medicine
University of Yamanashi
Japan

PREFACE

More than 500 million people are infected with hepatitis B or hepatitis C virus, and 500,000 patients with hepatocellular carcinoma die every year. Therefore, a provision for those patients is an urgent and important issue worldwide. Although promising therapies have been developed for hepatitis viral infection, management of liver cirrhosis, and hepatocellular carcinoma, many patients may not have received them if they were not examined by hepatologists. As many patients with liver function disorder first consult non-hepatologist clinicians or general physicians, enlightenment of primary care physicians concerning early management of liver disease is important for eradication of viral hepatitis infection and eventually hepatocellular carcinoma. In this eBook, I would like to provide a current standard guideline for primary care or early management of patients with liver function abnormalities, who are often seen in daily practice. This book provides practical advice on management of liver disease to non-hepatologists and general physicians for better treatment and prognosis of patients with liver diseases as achieved by hepatologists

Yukihiro Shimizu
Director, Gastroenterology Center
Nanto Municipal Hospital
Toyama
Japan

CONTRIBUTORS

Masami Minemura   The Third Department of Internal Medicine, University of Toyama, Toyama, Japan

Yasuhiro Nakayama   The First Department of Internal Medicine, University of Yamanashi, Yamanashi, Japan

Yukihiro Shimizu   Gastroenterology Center, Nanto Municipal Hospital, Toyama, Japan

Yoshiharu Tokimitsu   Department of Internal Medicine, Toyama Red Cross Hospital, Toyama, Japan

Kazuto Tajiri   The Third Department of Internal Medicine, University of Toyama, Toyama, Japan

Symptoms and Signs Suggestive of Liver Disease

Masami Minemura[*]

The Third Department of Internal Medicine, University of Toyamam, Japan

Abstract: Patients without advanced or severe liver disease may not display any signs or symptoms specific for liver diseases. Careful record of medical history may play an important role in diagnosing these patients. More advanced liver disease may present with symptoms such as fatigue, pruritus, abdominal fullness, and/or muscle cramps. Jaundice, ascites, hepatomegaly, splenomegaly, dilated abdominal wall veins, asterixis (encephalopathy), spider angiomata, and palmar erythema on physical examination may also suggest advanced liver diseases.

Keywords: Family history, liver disease, medical history, physical findings, signs, symptoms.

KEY POINTS

1. Asymptomatic patients with liver disease may be incidentally diagnosed with liver disease based on tests of liver enzymes and hepatitis viral markers during routine annual physical checkups or screening for employment or blood donation.

2. Most patients with slight or moderate liver dysfunction are asymptomatic, whereas patients with advanced liver diseases frequently have fatigue, pruritus, abdominal fullness, and/or muscle cramps.

3. Taking medical history is very important for the diagnosis of liver diseases; the history should include questions on alcohol consumption, medications, sexual activity, travel and blood transfusion. Taking family history is also useful for the diagnosis of hereditary liver disorders and hepatitis virus infections.

4. Physical examination may be useful in finding signs of liver disorders in asymptomatic patients.

*Corresponding author Masami Minemura: The Third Department of Internal Medicine, University of Toyama, Toyama, Japan; Email: minemura@med.u-toyama.ac.jp

5. Typical physical findings in advanced liver diseases are jaundice, ascites, hepatomegaly, splenomegaly, dilated abdominal wall veins, asterixis (encephalopathy), spider angiomata, and palmar erythema. Encephalopathy, ascites, dilated abdominal wall veins, and spider angiomata may suggest liver cirrhosis.

6. Although jaundice is thought to be a typical sign of hepatobiliary diseases, jaundice may also be caused by non-hepatic disorders such as hemolysis and congestive heart failure.

INTRODUCTION

Several blood tests are available to examine liver functions, allowing physicians to rapidly detect liver abnormalities prior to patients showing symptoms or signs such as jaundice and ascites. Therefore, some physicians may regard careful medical history taking and physical examination as less than important. This may lead to false diagnoses and excessive laboratory testing. This chapter describes common symptoms (Table 1) and signs (Table 2, Fig. 1) in patients with liver diseases. It also presents a diagnostic algorithm for patients suspected of liver diseases (Fig. 2).

HISTORY TAKING

Taking medical history is the first step in patients suspected of liver diseases. Medical history is important in determining liver disease and narrowing the differential diagnosis.

1. History of alcohol intake: Alcohol consumption greater than 33 to 45 g/day in men and greater than 22 to 30 g/day in women is associated with increased rates of alcoholic liver disease [1, 2].

2. Use of drugs: Both prescription medications and non-prescription drugs, including birth control pills, herbal compounds, and dietary supplements, may cause liver dysfunction [3].

3. Hepatitis risk factors: Sexual activity, sexually transmitted diseases (STDs), tattooing, body piercing, and use of injection drugs are risk factors for hepatitis B virus (HBV) and hepatitis C virus (HCV) infections [4, 5]. A family history of hepatitis, liver cirrhosis or liver cancer is also important, because maternal-infant transmission occurs

with both HBV and HCV. Travel to an underdeveloped area of the world is a risk factor for hepatitis A and E infections [6, 7]. Eating raw shellfish, especially oysters, is a risk factor for hepatitis A. Eating raw meat from wild boars, pigs, and deer has also been associated with hepatitis E infection [8].

4. Blood transfusion and use of blood products: Blood transfusion before 1986 is a risk factor for HBV, because donors were not screened for antibody to HB core antigen (anti-HBc) before then. Transfusion before 1992 is also a risk factor for HCV, when sensitive enzyme immunoassays for antibody to HCV (anti-HCV) were introduced [9, 10].

5. Past history of liver diseases: Past history including jaundice and acute viral hepatitis is important, because persistent hepatitis C infection occurs in about 60% to 70 % of patients with acute HCV infection and repeated exacerbations may be seen in patients with chronic HBV infection [4, 5].

6. History of gallstones in the gallbladder and/or the biliary tract: Gallstones may cause obstructive jaundice and abnormalities in liver biochemistry [11].

7. History of non-hepatic diseases: Non-hepatic diseases causing abnormalities in liver biochemistry include heart failure [12, 13], renal disease, nephrotic syndrome, diabetes, collagen diseases, thyroid disorders [14], hemolytic anemia, recent trauma, surgery, organ transplantation, sepsis [15], total parental nutrition (TPN) [16], and acquired immune deficiency syndrome.

8. Family history: Familial causes of liver disease include Wilson disease [17], hemochromatosis [18], α1-antitrypsin deficiency [19], and familial intrahepatic cholestasis [20].

COMMON SYMPTOMS IN PATIENTS WITH LIVER DISEASES

Liver diseases are accompanied by both constitutional and liver-specific symptoms. Constitutional symptoms include fatigue, weakness, poor appetite, and malaise, whereas liver-associated symptoms include jaundice, abdominal fullness, pruritus, and muscle cramps. Primary care physicians should know the common symptoms of liver diseases.

1. **Fatigue** is a subjective sensation and a very common symptom of physical and psychological diseases [21]. Fatigue can be caused by psychogenic diseases (57 %, *e.g.* depression or anxiety) and organic diseases (37 %, *e.g.* infection, cardiovascular, or endocrine diseases). Despite its many causes and non-specificity, fatigue is the most frequent symptom in patients with advanced liver diseases [22]. A clinical history of hepatitis virus infection and/or alcohol abuse and signs of jaundice and/or ascites suggest liver diseases.

2. **Pruritus** is an unpleasant cutaneous sensation, eliciting scratching behavior. It can be caused not only by skin disorders but also by other organic diseases, including liver diseases [23, 24]. Although chronic renal failure is a systemic disorder most commonly associated with secondary pruritus, patients with cholestasis due to drugs, obstructive jaundice, or cirrhosis frequently complain of itching.

3. **Abdominal fullness** is a common symptom of both organic and functional disorders. Abdominal fullness with acute onset should be considered due to obstruction of the gastrointestinal tract. In contrast, abdominal fullness in a patient with liver disease should be considered due to an increasing volume of ascites [25]. Hepatomegaly and splenomegaly may also cause abdominal fullness. Hepatomegaly can occur in patients with acute hepatitis, alcoholic hepatitis and liver tumors (hepatocellular carcinoma and metastatic tumors).

4. **Abdominal pain** is the most common complaint of outpatients, with rapid assessment required to determine whether the pain requires emergency treatment. Differential diagnosis should consider the quality and location of the pain. Epigastric pain may be due to peptic ulcer, pancreatitis, or aneurysm; right upper quadrant pain may be due to cholecystitis, gallstones, choledocholithasis, hepatitis, or liver abscess; and lower abdominal pain may be caused by appendicitis, diverticulitis, or intestinal ischemia. Since patients with chronic liver disease rarely experience severe abdominal pain, severe abdominal pain in these patients may indicate infection or obstruction of the biliary tract, spontaneous bacterial peritonitis (SBP) [26], or rupture of a hepatocellular carcinoma.

5. **Muscle cramps** are painful contractions of skeletal muscles caused by several disorders including hypocalcemia and thyroid disease. Patients with cirrhosis may experience severe muscle cramps [27, 28].

Although the cause is unclear, these cramps may be caused by reductions in effective circulating plasma volume. Muscle cramps and pruritus are major complaints in patients with liver cirrhosis.

Table 1. Common symptoms in patients with advanced liver diseases.

Symptoms	Diagnostic assessment	Possible liver disease
Fatigue	Fatigue is the most common symptom in patients with advanced liver diseases, although it is multicausal and nonspecific. A patient history of hepatitis virus infection or alcohol abuse and signs of jaundice or ascites suggest liver diseases. Psychogenic diseases and other organic diseases should be excluded.	Liver cirrhosis Acute hepatic failure Acute viral hepatitis
Pruritus	Pruritus can be caused not only by skin disorders but by systemic diseases, including liver and renal diseases. Patients with cholestasis caused by drugs, obstructive jaundice, or cirrhosis frequently complain of itching. Systemic disorders such as chronic renal failure frequently cause secondary pruritus.	Cholestasis Obstructive jaundice Liver cirrhosis Primary biliary cirrhosis (PBC) Primary sclerosing cholangitis (PSC)
Abdominal fullness	Abdominal fullness is a common symptom, caused by both organic and functional disorders. Patients with liver diseases having abdominal fullness may have increased volume of ascites.	\<Ascites\> liver cirrhosis \<Hepatomegaly\> Acute hepatitis, Alcoholic hepatitis, Liver tumors (hepatocellular carcinoma or metastatic tumor) \<Splenomegaly\> Liver cirrhosis, Idiopathic portal hypertension (IPH)
Abdominal pain	Abdominal pain is the most common complaint of outpatients. Patients with chronic liver disease rarely have severe abdominal pain. Patients with chronic liver diseases having severe abdominal pain should be suspected of having infection or obstruction of the biliary tract, spontaneous bacterial peritonitis (SBP), or rupture of hepatocellular carcinoma.	\<Colicky pain or severe pain\> Acute biliary tract obstruction by stones, Rupture of hepatocellular carcinoma \<Dull pain\> Acute viral hepatitis, Alcoholic hepatitis, Liver abscess, Spontaneous bacterial peritonitis (SBP)
Muscle cramps	Muscle cramps are painful contractions of skeletal muscles caused by several disorders such as hypocalcemia and thyroid disease. Patients with cirrhosis may often have severe muscle cramps. Hypocalcemia, hypomagnesemia, or thyroid diseases should be excluded in patients with advanced liver diseases having muscle cramps.	Liver cirrhosis

PHYSICAL EXAMINATION AND COMMON CLINICAL SIGNS IN PATIENTS WITH LIVER DISEASES (FIG. 1, TABLE 2)

Typical physical findings in patients with liver diseases include jaundice, ascites, hepatomegaly, splenomegaly, dilated abdominal wall veins, asterixis (encephalopathy), spider angiomata, and palmar erythema; however, most patients with slight or moderate liver dysfunction have no symptoms or signs. Although physical examination rarely detects evidence of liver diseases in asymptomatic patients, it can disclose signs indicative of liver disease. Physical examination is therefore important, especially in patients with portal hypertension or hepatic failure.

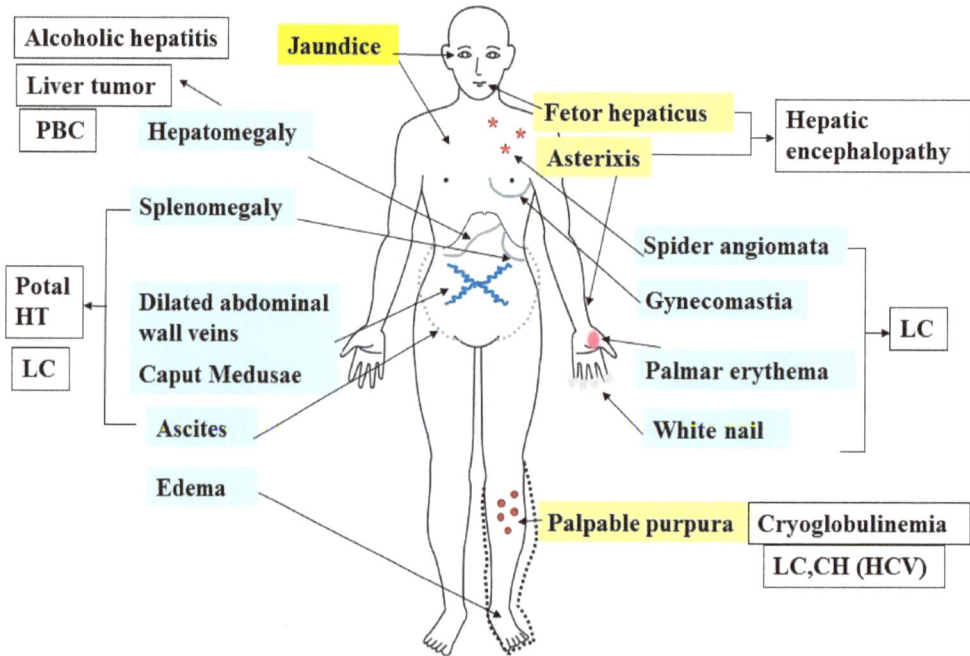

Figure 1: Physical signs in liver diseases.
PBC; primary biliary cirrhosis, HT; hypertension, LC; liver cirrhosis, CH; chronic hepatitis, HCV; hepatitis C virus.

Jaundice

Jaundice is a yellowing of the skin and sclera resulting from the deposition of bilirubin, a byproduct of hemoglobin metabolism that is removed from the bloodstream by the hepatobiliary system [29, 30]. The normal serum bilirubin concentration in children and adults is less than 1 mg/dl (17 μmol/L). Jaundice occurs together with serum hyperbilirubinemia when the hepatobiliary system does not work properly or hemolytic disorder causes bilirubin overproduction.

A careful clinical examination can generally detect jaundice in patients with serum bilirubin >2.5 mg/dl [31]. The yellow discoloration is best detected in the sclerae, which have a particular affinity for bilirubin due to their high elastin contents. Patients usually notice darkening of the urine before sclera icterus is observed. Jaundice without dark urine indicates unconjugated hyperbilirubinemia, which is due to hemolysis or inherited disorders of bilirubin metabolism such as Gilbert's syndrome [32-34].

One of the differential diagnoses for yellowing of the skin is carotenoderma [35], due to the presence of carotene after ingesting excessive amounts of fruits and vegetables. The yellowish discoloration can be seen in the skin, especially the palms, soles, and nasolabial fold, but the conjunctiva are spared, in contrast to jaundice.

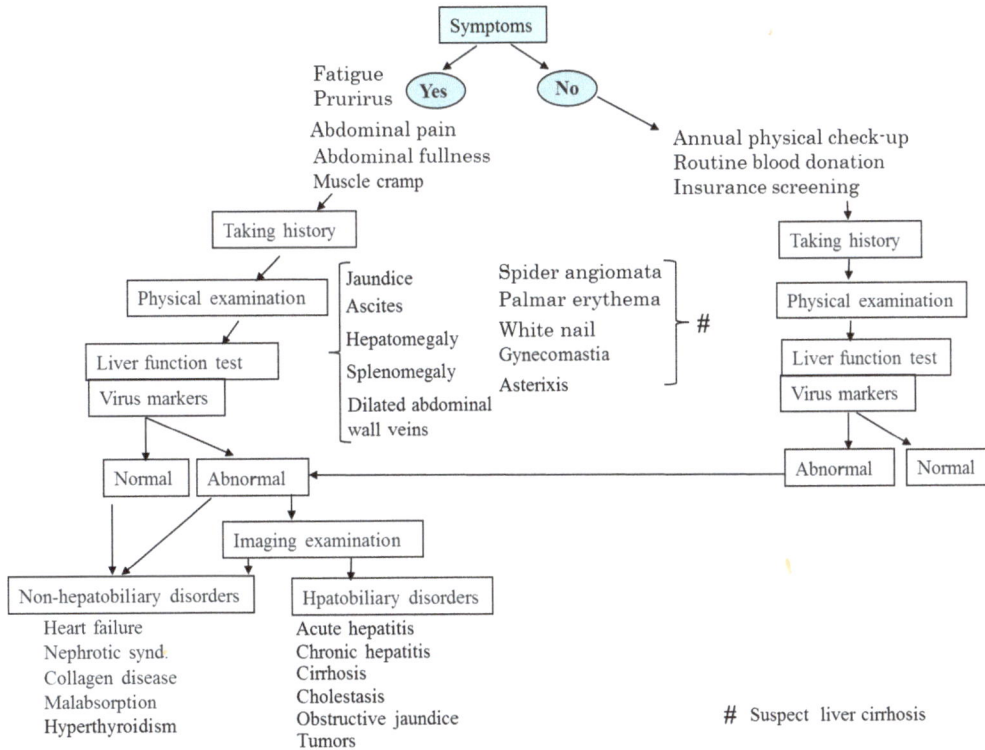

Figure 2: Diagnostic approach to patients with liver disease.

Table 2. Common clinical signs in patients with liver diseases.

Signs	Diagnostic assessment	Possible liver disease
1) Jaundice	1) Jaundice can be detected when serum bilirubin is greater than 2.5 mg/dl (47 μmol/L). 2) Jaundice can be caused not only by hepatobiliary disorders but by several non-hepatic systemic diseases. 3) Hyperbilirubinemia may be predominantly conjugated or unconjugated. 4) Hyperbilirubinemia may be accompanied by other abnormalities on biochemical liver tests. 5) One of the differential diagnoses for yellowing of the skin is carotenoderma. 6) Imaging studies such as US and CT are very useful in revealing biliary obstructions.	<Non-hepatic> Hemolysis, ineffective erythropoiesis <Hepatic> Unconjugated (Indirect): Inherited disorders (Gilbert's synd., Crigler-Najjar synd) Conjugated (Direct): Inherited disorders (Dubin-Johnson synd., Rotor's synd) Cholestasis due to drug injury, decompensated liver cirrhosis (including PBC/PSC), acute hepatitis, or obstructive jaundice.
2) Ascites	1) Does a patient with ascites have a generalized edema (anasarca)? 2) Look for signs of chronic liver disease (jaundice, vascular spiders, palmar erythema, gynecomastia, or caput medusae) in the diagnosis of causes of ascites, because cirrhosis is the most common cause of ascites. 3) A small volume of ascites cannot be detected by physical examination such as shifting dullness. In contrast, ultrasonography can detect as little as 100 ml of ascites. 4) Diagnostic paracentesis should be performed to determine the nature of the ascites. 5) Serum-to ascites albumin gradient (SAAG) is more useful than the concept of protein-based exudates/transudates. SAAG can be calculated by subtracting the albumin concentration in ascitic fluid from serum albumin concentration. An SAAG >1.1 g/dl is indicative of portal hypertension with 97 % accuracy.	<Non-hepatic> Cardiac failure Nephritic syndrome Tuberculous peritonitis, Pancreatic ascites Peritoneal carcinomatosis <Hepatic> Liver cirrhosis IPH Budd-Chiari syndrome Acute liver failure <<SAAG>> >1.1g/dl →portal hypertension(+): Cirrhosis, Heart failure, Alcoholic hepatitis, Budd-Chiari syndrome <1.1g/dl →portal hypertension(-):Peritoneal carcinomatosis, Tuberculous peritonitis, Pancreatic ascites, Nephritic syndrome
3) Hepatomegaly	1) It is important to distinguish whether hepatomegaly results from hepatobiliary disease or a non-hepatic disease. 2) Palpation of the liver 2cm below the costal margin correlates with hepatomegaly (with 50% accuracy). 3) The shape of the liver (smooth or nodular surface) and the presence or absence of tenderness are useful for the differential	<Hepatic> Acute viral hepatitis, Alcoholic hepatitis, Fatty liver, PBC <Secondary> Congestive heart failure, Sarcoidosis, Amyloidosis, Infiltration of lymphoma,

Table 2: contd…

		diagnosis of hepatomegaly.	Liver tumors (HCC or metastatic tumors)
4) Splenomegaly		1) A palpable spleen on physical examination is thought to be abnormal. 2) Ultrasonography is useful to confirm splenomegaly and evaluate liver size. 3) It is important to find signs of liver cirrhosis such as vascular spider in patients with splenomegaly, because the most frequent cause of splenomegaly is liver cirrhosis. 4) Cytopenia often results from hypersplenism.	<Hepatic> Liver cirrhosis Hepatic or portal vein obstruction, Hepatic schistosomiasis <Non-hepatic> Infection Congestive heart failure, Sarcoidosis, Amyloidosis, Hematologic malignancy (*e.g.* Infiltration of lymphoma) Myeloproliferative disorders
5) Skin lesions in liver diseases		1) Spider angiomata is most frequently associated with cirrhosis, but may also occur during pregnancy. Spider angiomata disappears when the central prominence is pressed with a pinhead. 2) Palmar erythema is a bright red color change in the palms, not as in patients with cirrhosis as spider angiomata. 3) White nails are observed in 82 % of patients with cirrhosis.	< Vascular spiders, palmar erythema, and white nail > Liver cirrhosis <Palpable purpura, lichen planus> Chronic HCV infection <Gianotti-Crosti syndrome> Acute HBV infection
6) Gynecomastia		1) Feminization is more frequent in alcoholic than in other types of cirrhosis. 2) Spironolactone therapy may be related to gynecomastia in cirrhotic patients.	Liver cirrhosis, especially alcoholic cirrhosis
7) Dilated abdominal wall veins (*e.g. caput Medusae*)		1) To distinguish vena caval obstruction from portal hypertension, it may be useful to pass the finger along dilated veins located below the umbilicus to strip them of blood and determine the direction of blood flow during refilling.	*<caput Medusae >* Portal hypertension, Liver cirrhosis < Dilated abdominal wall veins> Inferior vena cava syndrome
8) Asterixis (Flapping tremor)		1) Blood ammonia concentrations are usually increased in patients with asterixis. 2) The administration of sedatives, hypokalemia, and hyponatremia may also be associated with asterixis in patients with cirrhosis.	Decompensated liver cirrhosis Portosystemic shunt <Differential diagnosis> Uremia

Diagnostic Points

1) Jaundice can be caused not only by hepatobiliary disorders [36] but also by several non-hepatic systemic diseases including hemolysis [37], congestive heart failure [38], and sepsis [39].

2) In evaluating jaundice, the following are important;

- Whether hyperbilirubinemia is predominantly conjugated or unconjugated

- Whether other biochemical liver tests are normal or not

- The importance of distinguishing hepatocellular jaundice from obstructive jaundice.

3) Imaging modalities such as ultrasonography (US) and computed tomography (CT) scan are very useful in detecting biliary obstructions [40, 41].

Physical Examinations

1) Detection of jaundice: Clinical studies reveal that 70% to 80% of observers detect jaundice when serum bilirubin concentration is greater than 2.5 to 3 mg/dL [31].

2) In patients with jaundice, findings of dilated abdominal veins (likelihood ratio [LR] 17.5), palmar erythema (LR 9.8), spider angiomata (LR 4.7), ascites (LR 4.4), and palpable spleen (LR 2.9) suggest hepatocellular jaundice [42].

3) A nontender, distended palpable gallbladder (Courvoisier's sign) in a patient with jaundice suggests extrahepatic obstruction [43].

4) Disturbed consciousness with asterixis (flapping tremor) in patients with jaundice suggests either acute hepatic failure or decompensated liver cirrhosis [44].

5) Findings of hepatic encephalopathy (LR 8.8), ascites (LR 6.6), dilated abdominal veins (LR 5.4), spider angiomata (LR 3.7), and peripheral edema (LR 3.0) suggest liver cirrhosis [45].

6) Xanthoma suggests hyperlipidemia, a frequent finding in patients with primary biliary cirrhosis (PBC) [46].

7) Kayser-Fleischer rings (copper-colored rings) in the eyes suggest Wilson's disease [47].

Laboratory Tests

Initial laboratory tests include measurements of serum bilirubin (total, conjugated, and unconjugated), aminotransferases (aspartate aminotransferase (AST) and alanine aminotransferase (ALT)), alkaline phosphatase (ALP), gamma-glutamyl transpeptidase (γ-GTP), albumin, and prothrombin time [48]. Plasma elevation of predominantly unconjugated bilirubin is due to the overproduction of bilirubin and may be caused by hemolysis [37], ineffective erythropoiesis [49], reabsorption of hematoma, and transfusion [50], and a reduced ability to conjugate bilirubin. In contrast, elevation of both unconjugated and conjugated bilirubin may result from hepatocellular disease, impaired canalicular excretion, or biliary obstruction [36].

Normal liver enzymes, together with hyperbilirubinemia, suggest that the jaundice was not caused by hepatic injury or biliary tract disorders. Hemolysis or inherited disorders of bilirubin metabolism may be responsible for the hyperbilirubinemia. Serum bilirubin concentration rarely exceeds 5 mg/dl in patients with inherited [51] and acquired [52] hemolysis. In the absence of hemolysis, impaired bilirubin conjugation should be considered due to Crigler-Najjar syndrome type I or II or Gilbert's syndrome [34]. Gilbert's syndrome is common, affecting 3% to 7% of the population with male predominance (2-7:1). Isolated conjugated hyperbilirubinemia may be due to Dubin-Johnson [53] or Roter [54] syndrome, but these syndromes are rare.

Markedly elevated serum aminotransferases suggest that jaundice is caused by a hepatocellular disease, such as alcoholic or acute viral hepatitis. When serum ALP is more elevated than aminotransferases, biliary obstruction or intrahepatic cholestasis should be considered.

Diagnostic Imaging

When initial laboratory studies suggest cholestasis in a patient with jaundice, diagnostic imaging is required to distinguish between biliary obstruction and intrahepatic cholestasis. The sensitivity of abdominal US for the detection of dilated bile ducts and biliary tract obstruction ranges from 55% to 91% [55]. If US cannot identify the suspected biliary tract obstruction, CT scans and magnetic resonance imaging (MRI) are used to examine the liver, pancreas, and bile duct.

Ascites

Ascites is the accumulation of free fluid within the abdominal cavity. The most frequent cause of ascites in the United States is liver cirrhosis, observed in about 80 % of patients [56]. Hypoalbuminemia and portal hypertension are important factors for ascites formation in patients with cirrhosis. Ascites with malignancy (peritonitis carcinomatosa) should be considered in patients without cirrhosis. Cardiac failure, constrictive pericarditis, and peritoneal infection (tuberculosis, chlamydia) lead to ascites in some patients. An obese abdomen with abdominal wall thickening and subcutaneous fat can masquerade as ascites. A description of the onset of symptoms is useful to distinguish obese abdomen from ascites, because ascites usually develops within a few weeks. Patients with ascites and extremely distended abdomen or respiratory compromise require urgent diagnosis.

Points for Diagnosis

1) Does a patient with ascites have generalized edema (anasarca)? Ascites may occur as part of anasarca, which may be very useful in determining the cause of ascites.

2) Because cirrhosis is the most frequent cause of ascites, physicians should look for signs of chronic liver disease (jaundice, spider angiomata, palmar erythema, gynecomastia, and dilated abdominal wall veins) in diagnosing causes of ascites.

3) A small volume of ascites cannot be detected by physical examination such as shifting dullness. In contrast, ultrasonography can detect as little as 100 ml of fluid in the abdomen.

4) Should peritonitis be suspected in a patient with ascites? Ten to 27% of patients admitted with ascites have spontaneous bacterial peritonitis (SBP) [57].

5) Diagnostic paracentesis should be performed to determine the nature of the ascites and the presence of peritonitis, especially in patients with SBP or malignancy [58].

Physical Examination

1) Skin lesions, such as palmar erythema, spider angiomata, and abdominal wall collaterals, can increase the likelihood of cirrhosis. Patients with more advanced liver disease also have jaundice.

2) Generalized edema (anasarca) may indicate hypoalbuminemia or heart failure. Hypoalbuminemia, which decreases oncotic pressure, results from decreased intake (starvation), decreased albumin production

(severe liver disease), or increased loss of albumin (nephrotic syndrome, protein-losing enteropathy).

3) Jugular venous distension, a third heart sound, pulmonary crackles, and peripheral edema suggest that heart failure may be associated with the formation of ascites.

4) Abdominal tenderness can reflect pancreatitis or peritonitis (including SBP).

5) Physical findings, such as shifting dullness, bulging flanks, flank dullness, and fluid wave, are helpful in confirming the presence of ascites. These tests, however, may not be worthwhile in patients with a small volume (<1,000 ml) of ascites. Physical examinations have shown a sensitivity of 50% to 94 % and a specificity of 29% to 82% [59].

Laboratory Tests

Abdominal paracentesis with analysis of ascites is the most efficient method of diagnosing the cause of ascites and of evaluating whether ascitic fluid is infected.

Cell count can be used to evaluate the possibility of SBP, tuberculosis, or malignancy. A polymorphonuclear leukocyte count >250 cells/mm^3 in ascitic fluid indicates infection (SBP). In contrast, mononuclear cells are usually predominant in the ascitic fluid of patients with tuberculous peritonitis. Bacterial cultures of ascitic fluid should be performed if a patient has fever, abdominal pain, azotemia, acidosis, or confusion, because Gram staining of a smear of ascitic fluid stain has low yields.

About two-thirds of patients with malignancy-related ascites have peritoneal carcinomatosis, and viable malignant cells can be seen in most of those patients. The overall sensitivity of cytology for detection of malignant cells has been reported to range from 58% to 75 %.

Serum-to Ascites Albumin Gradient

The serum-to ascites albumin gradient (SAAG) is more useful than the protein-based exudates/transudate concept [60]. The SAAG is calculated by subtracting the concentration of albumin in ascitic fluid from its concentration in serum. An SAAG >1.1 g/dl is indicative of portal hypertension with 97 % accuracy, whereas an SAAG <1.1 g/dl indicates an absence of portal hypertension, suggesting other causes such as peritoneal carcinomatosis, tuberculous peritonitis, pancreas ascites, and nephritic syndrome.

Other tests, including those for amylase, triglycerides, lactate dehydrogenase, and glucose, should be ordered when there is suspicion of something other than simple cirrhotic ascites. The amylase concentration in ascitic fluid of patients with pancreatic ascites is approximately 2,000 IU/L, 6-fold higher than in serum. Milky fluid (chylous ascites) usually has triglyceride concentrations >200mg/dL (often >1,000mg/dL), which may result from lymphatic obstruction. An elevated LDH or low glucose level may indicate tuberculosis or malignancy.

Diagnostic Imaging

To confirm or refute the presence of ascites, cirrhosis, pancreatitis, or malignancy, these patients should be evaluated by imaging modalities such as ultrasonography [61, 62]. Ultrasonography is safe and cost-effective and useful in guiding diagnostic paracentesis. Splenomegaly or recanalization of the umbilical vein can be detected by ultrasonography, providing indirect evidence of portal hypertension.

Hepatomegaly

Hepatomegaly is a physical sign on abdominal examination in patients with both hepatobiliary diseases and non-hepatic diseases such as heart failure [63], amyloidosis [64], and lymphoma [65]. Although the size of normal adult liver size has been estimated at 8 to 12 cm in men and 6 to 10 cm in women, relative to the midclavicular line, accurate determination of liver size diagnostic for hepatomegaly is unclear because of the high variability in liver size [66-69]. Determination of hepatomegaly is important for primary care.

Points for Diagnosis

1) It is important to determine whether hepatomegaly results from hepatobiliary disease or non-hepatic disease (*e.g.*, congestive heart failure, amyloidosis, or lymphoma)

2) The shape of the liver (smooth or nodular surface) and the presence or absence of tenderness are useful for the differential diagnosis of hepatomegaly.

3) Hepatomegaly is often observed in patients with alcoholic cirrhosis and PBC [70]. In contrast, atrophic changes in the right lobe and

compensating enlargement of the left lobe of the liver are commonly observed in patients with HBV or HCV associated cirrhosis.

4) Hepatomegaly is usually observed in patients with acute viral hepatitis [71]. In contrast, fulminant hepatitis should be considered if liver size rapidly decreases or atrophic changes occur [72].

Physical Examination

1) Most clinicians attempt to evaluate the size and shape of the liver by physical examinations (palpation and percussion). The liver span has usually been measured in the right midclavicular line, and palpation at the midline is required to identify an enlarged left lobe. The extent of palpation below the costal margin and the texture and consistency of the liver should be noted during palpation [66-69]. Palpation of the liver 2 cm below the costal margin has been reported to correlate with a 50 % likelihood of hepatomegaly [73]. Palpation of a smooth, nontender liver may suggest hepatomegaly due to fatty infiltration, congestive heart failure, PBC, lymphoma, hepatic venous obstruction, amyloidosis, and schistosomiasis. Palpation revealing an enlarged, smooth-surfaced liver accompanied by tenderness may be due to acute hepatitis [71] or liver abscess [74]. Nodular liver suggests liver cirrhosis caused by hepatitis virus (especially HBV) or metastatic carcinoma.

2) Percussion is useful in detecting the upper margin of the liver. If the lower margin of the liver is not palpated, percussion may be useful in determining liver size.

3) The presence of associated physical findings, including jaundice, vascular spiders, palmar erythema, gynecomastia, ascites, splenomegaly, and peripheral edema, is useful in diagnosing causes of hepatomegaly.

Laboratory Tests

Initial laboratory tests should include a complete blood count, liver enzyme tests (AST, ALT, LDH, ALP, and γ-GTP), and liver function tests (albumin, bilirubin, and prothrombin time). If liver enzymes are elevated, serological tests for hepatitis should be performed. If a patient is negative for hepatitis virus markers, anti-nuclear antibody, anti-mitochondrial antibody, ferritin, ceruloplasmin, and α1-antitrypsin concentrations should be measured.

If lactate dehydrogenase (LDH) is very high compared with ALT, the presence of metastatic liver tumor or lymphoma invasion into the liver should be considered. In such cases, several tumor markers (*e.g.* CEA, CA19-9, sIL-2 receptor) should be measured, since these markers are useful for further diagnostic approaches.

Diagnostic Imaging and Liver Biopsy

Hepatomegaly on ultrasonography or CT scan is defined as a size > 15.5 cm. Liver biopsy is required for patients with unexplained hepatomegaly [75-79].

Splenomegaly

The spleen is a major lymphopoietic organ that participates in the removal of senescent red blood cells and particles (*e.g.* opsonized bacteria, antibody-coated cells). The spleen is also associated with cellular and humoral immunity. A normal spleen measures less than 12cm x 7cm and has a median weight of about 150 g in adults [80]. The spleen is not usually palpable unless it is enlarged. A palpable spleen on physical examination is thought to be abnormal [81]. Among the disorders causing splenomegaly are liver diseases, congestive disorders of the splenic vein, infections, and hematopoietic diseases [82]. The most frequent cause of splenomegaly is liver cirrhosis, making it important to find signs of portal hypertension in patients with splenomegaly.

Points for Diagnosis

1) It is important to distinguish whether splenomegaly results from congestive disorders of the splenic vein (*e.g.* liver cirrhosis, portal vein thrombosis), reactive splenic hyperplasia (*e.g.* mononucleosis), or hematopoietic disorders (*e.g.* myeloproliferative diseases and hemolysis) [83].

2) Splenomegaly is frequently accompanied by hypersplenism, a condition in which the spleen inappropriately removes excess amounts of leukocytes, platelets, and erythrocytes. In contrast, it is very important to measure spleen size in patients with pancytopenia.

3) Several systemic infectious agents such as EB virus can induce a systemic immunologic response and splenomegaly because the spleen is a lymphoid organ. Therefore, symptoms and signs such as fever, lymph node swelling, and eruption are useful in diagnosing the etiology of splenomegaly [84].

4) All patients with hypersplenism have splenomegaly, but only a small percentage of patients with splenomegaly have hypersplenism.

5) Splenomegaly is often associated with liver diseases such as liver cirrhosis. Acute splenomegaly may be caused by traumatic hematoma or acute infections including malaria and mononucleosis.

Physical Examination

Abdominal palpation and percussion of Traube's semilunar space are usually performed in patients suspected of splenomegaly [85-88]. The patient should also be examined for evidence of hepatomegaly, lymphadenopathy, skin rash, and subcutaneous nodules.

1) Palpation method: The sensitivity of palpation may be increased by placing the patient in the right lateral decubitus position with knees and neck flexed. The specificity of direct splenic palpation was 92 %, with a positive predictive value of 92 % [87].

2) Percussion of Traube's semilunar space: Traube's space is the triangular space overlying the stomach bubble in the left lateral hemithorax and is normally tympanic by percussion [89]. Dullness to percussion over Traube's space had a sensitivity and specificity for splenomegaly of 62% and 72%, respectively [90]. Traube's space dullness is less accurate in obese patients and in patients who have recently eaten.

Laboratory Tests

The complete blood count (CBC) with platelets, analysis of peripheral smears and liver biochemistry teats should be performed to determine the cause of an enlarged spleen. Neutropenia, anemia, and/or thrombocytopenia is usually present in patients with splenomegaly, because these cells can be trapped in the enlarged spleen. Cytopenias in patients with hypersplenism do not consist of abnormal white or red blood cells. Increased numbers of abnormal cells in the peripheral blood may indicate a hematologic malignancy or malignant invasion of the bone marrow.

Diagnostic Imaging

Splenic weight and size have been reported closely correlated on external scanning; with splenic weight (g) = 0.43 x length (cm) x width (cm) x thickness (cm).

1) Ultrasonography: Ultrasonography is useful to confirm the presence of splenomegaly and evaluate liver shape and size. The spleen is thought to be enlarged if its length is >13 cm or its thickness is >5 cm on ultrasonography [91].

2) CT scanning: The spleen is thought to be enlarged if its length is >10 cm [92], with a sensitivity, specificity, and accuracy of 81%, 90%, and 88 %, respectively.

Skin Lesions in Liver Diseases

Spider angiomata and palmar erythema are frequently observed skin lesions in patients with liver cirrhosis [93]. Spider angiomata are vascular lesions consisting of a central arteriole surrounded by many smaller vessels. They are frequently seen on the trunk, face, and upper limbs [94, 95]. Palmar erythema is a bright red color change in the palms [96]. It is not specific for liver disease and can be seen in association with pregnancy [97], rheumatoid arthritis, and hyperthyroidism. These skin lesions are thought to be related to estrogen excess, although serum estrogen concentrations may be normal. Nail changes can also be seen in patients with cirrhosis, and white nails may be due to opacity of the nail bed [98]. The exact pathogenesis is unknown, but is thought to be associated with hypoalbuminemia.

Chronic hepatitis virus infection is thought to be associated with various cutaneous lesions, including palpable purpura, porphyria cutanea tarda, lichen planus, pruritus, and urticaria. Palpable purpura is a major finding suggesting some form of vasculitis and may be associated with mixed cryoglobulinemia. Mixed cryoglobulinemia is associated with HCV infection in about 80% of patients [99, 100], and these skin lesions improve as HCV viral load is reduced by treatment with interferon [101].

Gianotti-Crosti syndrome is characterized by a symmetric papular eruption, which is mainly caused by acute HBV infection in infants and young children [102]. The presence of these skin lesions is suggestive of hepatitis virus infection.

Points for Diagnosis

1) Spider angiomata and palmar erythema are most frequently associated with liver cirrhosis, but are not specific for liver diseases.

2) Spider angiomata disappear when the central prominence is pressed with a pinhead, an observation useful for diagnosis.

3) White nails are found in 82% of patients with cirrhosis.

4) If palpable purpura is observed, the patient should be tested for HCV infection.

Gynecomastia

Endocrine changes may occur in patients with cirrhosis. These changes are predominantly feminizing, such as gynecomastia in males [103, 104]. Feminization is more frequent in alcoholic than in other types of cirrhosis. Gynecomastia is defined as a benign proliferation of the glandular tissue of the male breast. Spironolactone therapy may also be associated with gynecomastia in cirrhotic patients [105]. Men with cirrhosis may have other indications of feminization such as loss of chest and axillary hair and testicular atrophy.

Dilated Abdominal Wall Veins (*e.g.* caput Medusae)

Portal hypertension resulting from cirrhosis may cause the umbilical vein to recanalize with blood from the portal venous system shunted through the periumbilical veins into the umbilical and abdominal veins. Prominent collateral veins radiating from the umbilicus are termed *caput Medusae* [106, 107]. A finding of dilated abdominal wall veins can increase the probability of cirrhosis.

In contrast, the collateral venous channels carry blood upwards to the superior vena caval system in patients with inferior vena cava syndrome [108].

Points for Diagnosis

1) To distinguish vena caval obstruction from portal hypertension, it may be useful to pass the finger along dilated veins located below the umbilicus to strip them of blood and determine the direction of blood flow during refilling.

Asterixis (Flapping tremor)

Hepatic encephalopathy is a reversible impairment in brain function occurring in patients with advanced liver failure [109, 110]. The pathogenesis of hepatic encephalopathy is still unclear, but elevated concentrations of ammonia and other toxins may contribute to encephalopathy [111]. Asterixis, or asynchronous flapping motions of outstretched and dorsiflexed hands, is one of the earliest findings in patients with hepatic encephalopathy. Although asterixis is a typical sign in patients with hepatic encephalopathy, it also appears in encephalopathy resulting from hypercapnia, uremia, and other disorders [112].

1) An increase in blood ammonia usually occurs in patients with asterixis.

2) The administration of sedatives, hypokalemia [113], and hyponatremia may also be associated with asterixis in patients with cirrhosis.

MESSAGES FROM HEPATOLOGISTS TO GENERAL PHYSICIANS

1. The symptoms of patients with advanced liver diseases are nonspecific. Jaundice, ascites formation, spider angiomata, gynecomastia, and asterixis are relatively liver-specific signs, but none of these is diagnostic.

2. Leg edema without ascites retention is rare in advanced liver diseases, possibly because of the major contribution of portal hypertension to water retention in these patients.

3. Pleural effusion is found in 5% to 10 % of patients with cirrhosis; this condition is called hepatic hydrothorax and is right sided in 85% of patients. Hepatic hydrothorax is due to the migration of peritoneal fluid through diaphragmatic defects into the pleural cavity [114].

4. Although asterixis is an important sign of hepatic encephalopathy, it may also be observed in uremic patients or subjects with hypercapnia.

ACKNOWLEDGEMENTS

We are very thankful to Ms. Asma Ahmed, manager publications, Bentham Science Publishers, for her patience and long-term assistance.

CONFLICT OF INTEREST

The author confirms that he has no conflict of interest to declare for this publication.

REFERENCES

[1]   Mailliard ME, Sorrell ME. Alcoholic liver disease. In Harrison's Principles of Internal Medicine, 16th Edition: pp1855-1858.
[2]   O'Shea RS, Dasarathy S, McCullough AJ. Alcoholic liver disease. Hepatology 2010;51:307-328.

[3]   Tajiri K, Shimizu Y. Practical guidelines for diagnosis and early management of drug-induced liver injury. World J Gastroenterol 2008;14:6774-6785.
[4]   Yapali S, Talaat N, Lok AS. Management of hepatitis B: our practice and how it relates to the guidelines. Clin Gastroenterol Hepatol 2014;12:16-26.
[5]   Lavanchy D.The global burden of hepatitis C. Liver Int 29 Suppl 2009;1:74-81.
[6]   Wu D, Guo CY. Epidemiology and prevention of hepatitis A in travelers. J Travel Med 2013;20:394-399.
[7]   Tekin R, Yolbas I, Dal T, Demirpence O, Kaya S, Bozkurt F, Deveci O, Celen MK, Tekin A. Evaluation of adults with acute viral hepatitis a and review of the literature. Clin Ter 2013;164:537-541.
[8]   Scobie L, Dalton HR. Hepatitis E: source and route of infection, clinical manifestations and new developments. J Viral Hepat 2013;20:1-11.
[9]   Taira R, Satake M, Momose S, Hino S, Suzuki Y, Murokawa H, Uchida S, Tadokoro K. Residual risk of transfusion-transmitted hepatitis B virus (HBV) infection caused by blood components derived from donors with occult HBV infection in Japan. Transfusion 2013;53:1393-1404.
[10]   Tani Y, Aso H, Matsukura H, Tadokoro K, Tamori A, Nishiguchi S, Yoshizawa H, Shibata H. Significant background rates of HBV and HCV infections in patients and risks of blood transfusion from donors with low anti-HBc titres or high anti-HBc titres with high anti-HBs titres in Japan: a prospective, individual NAT study of transfusion-transmitted HBV, HCV and HIV infections. Vox Sang 2012;102:285-293.
[11]   Al-Jiffry BO, Elfateh A, Chundrigar T, Othman B, Almalki O, Rayza F, Niyaz H, Elmakhzangy H, Hatem M. Non-invasive assessment of choledocholithiasis in patients with gallstones and abnormal liver function. World J Gastroenterol 2013;19:5877-5882.
[12]   Myers RP, Cerini R, Sayegh R, Moreau R, Degott C, Lebrec D, Lee SS.Cardiac hepatopathy: clinical, hemodynamic, and histologic characteristics and correlations. Hepatology 2003;37:393-400.
[13]   Gitlin N, Serio KM. Ischemic hepatitis: widening horizons. Am J Gastroenterol 1992;87:831-836.
[14]   Burra P. Liver abnormalities and endocrine diseases. Best Pract Res Clin Gastroenterol 2013;27:553-563.
[15]   Chand N, Sanyal AJ. Sepsis-induced cholestasis. Hepatology 2007;45:230-241.
[16]   Guglielmi FW, Regano N, Mazzuoli S, Fregnan S, Leogrande G, Guglielmi A, Merli M, Pironi L, Penco JM, Francavilla A. Cholestasis induced by total parenteral nutrition. Clin Liver Dis 2008;12:97-110.
[17]   Bruha R, Marecek Z, Pospisilova L, Nevsimalova S, Vitek L, Martasek P, Nevoral J, Petrtyl J, Urbanek P, Jiraskova A, Ferenci P. Long-term follow-up of Wilson disease: natural history, treatment, mutations analysis and phenotypic correlation. Liver Int 2011;31:83-91.
[18]   Hanson EH, Imperatore G, Burke W.HFE gene and hereditary hemochromatosis: a HuGE review. Human Genome Epidemiology. Am J Epidemiol 2001;154:193-206.
[19]   Stoller JK, Aboussouan LS.A review of alpha1-antitrypsin deficiency. Am J Respir Crit Care Med 2012;185:246-259.
[20]   Strubbe B, Geerts A, Van Vlierberghe H, Colle I. Progressive familial intrahepatic cholestasis and benign recurrent intrahepatic cholestasis: a review. Acta Gastroenterol Belg 2012;75:405-410.
[21]   Kroenke K, Wood DR, Mangelsdorff AD, Meier NJ, Powell JB. Chronic fatigue in primary care. Prevalence, patient characteristics, and outcome. JAMA 1988;260: 929-934.
[22]   Tsai LH, Lin CM, Chiang SC, Chen CL, Lan SJ, See LC. Symptoms and distress among patients with liver cirrhosis but without hepatocellular carcinoma in taiwan. Gastroenterol Nurs 2014;37:49-59.
[23]   Etter L, Myers SA. Pruritus in systemic disease: mechanisms and management. Dermatol Clin 2002;20:459-72.
[24]   Imam MH, Gossard AA, Sinakos E, Lindor KD. Pathogenesis and management of pruritus in cholestatic liver disease. J Gastroenterol Hepatol 2012;27:1150-1158.
[25]   Runyon BA. Introduction to the revised American Association for the Study of Liver Diseases Practice Guideline management of adult patients with ascites due to cirrhosis 2012. Hepatology 2013;57:1651-1653.
[26]   Sheer TA, Runyon BA. Spontaneous bacterial peritonitis. Dig Dis 2005;23:39-46.
[27]   Abrams GA, Concato J, Fallon MB. Muscle cramps in patients with cirrhosis. Am J Gastroenterol 1996;91:1363-1366.

[28]   Chatrath H, Liangpunsakul S, Ghabril M, Otte J, Chalasani N, Vuppalanchi R. Prevalence and morbidity associated with muscle cramps in patients with cirrhosis. Am J Med 2012;125:1019-1025.

[29]   Weiss JS, Gautam A, Lauff JJ, Sundberg MW, Jatlow P, Boyer JL, Seligson D. The clinical importance of a protein-bound fraction of serum bilirubin in patients with hyperbilirubinemia. N Engl J Med 1983;309:147-150.

[30]   Sticova E, Jirsa M. New insights in bilirubin metabolism and their clinical implications. World J Gastroenterol 2013;19:6398-6407.

[31]   Ruiz MA, Saab S, Rickman LS. The clinical detection of scleral icterus: observations of multiple examiners. Mil Med 1997;162:560-563.

[32]   Muraca M, Fevery J, Blanckaert N. Relationships between serum bilirubins and production and conjugation of bilirubin. Studies in Gilbert's syndrome, Crigler-Najjar disease, hemolytic disorders, and rat models. Gastroenterology 1987;92:309-317.

[33]   Bosma PJ, Chowdhury JR, Bakker C, Gantla S, de Boer A, Oostra BA, Lindhout D, Tytgat GN, Jansen PL, Oude Elferink RP, *et al*. The genetic basis of the reduced expression of bilirubin UDP-glucuronosyltransferase 1 in Gilbert's syndrome. N Engl J Med 1995;333:1171-1175.

[34]   Borlak J, Thum T, Landt O, Erb K, Hermann R. Molecular diagnosis of a familial nonhemolytic hyperbilirubinemia (Gilbert's syndrome) in healthy subjects. Hepatology 2000;32:792-795.

[35]   Maharshak N, Shapiro J, Trau H. Carotenoderma--a review of the current literature. Int J Dermatol 2003;42:178-181.

[36]   Reisman Y, Gips CH, Lavelle SM, Wilson JH. Clinical presentation of (subclinical) jaundice--the Euricterus project in The Netherlands. United Dutch Hospitals and Euricterus Project Management Group. Hepatogastroenterology 1996;43:1190-1195.

[37]   Berlin NI, Berk PD. Quantitative aspects of bilirubin metabolism for hematologists. Blood 1981;57:983-999.

[38]   Giallourakis CC, Rosenberg PM, Friedman LS. The liver in heart failure. Clin Liver Dis 2002;6:947-67.

[39]   Bhogal HK, Sanyal AJ. The molecular pathogenesis of cholestasis in sepsis. Front Biosci (Elite Ed) 2013;5:87-96.

[40]   Goldberg BB, Goodman GA, Clearfield HR. Evaluation of ascites by ultrasound. Radiology 1970;96:15-22.

[41]   Levitt RG, Sagel SS, Stanley RJ, Jost RG. Accuracy of computed tomography of the liver and biliary tract. Radiology 1977;124:123-128.

[42]   Schenker S, Balint J, Schiff L. Differential diagnosis of jaundice: report of a prospective study of 61 proved cases. Am J Dig Dis 1962;7:449-463.

[43]   Chen JJ, Changchien CS, Tai DI, Kuo CH. Gallbladder volume in patients with common hepatic duct dilatation. An evaluation of Courvoisier's sign using ultrasonography. Scand J Gastroenterol 1994;29:284-288.

[44]   Schiano TD. Clinical management of hepatic encephalopathy. Pharmacotherapy 2010;30:10S-15S.

[45]   Czaja AJ, Wolf AM, Baggenstoss AH. Clinical assessment of cirrhosis in severe chronic active liver disease: specificity and sensitivity of physical and laboratory findings. Mayo Clin Proc 1980;55:360-364.

[46]   Heathcote J. The clinical expression of primary biliary cirrhosis. Semin Liver Dis 1997;17:23-33.

[47]   Rosencrantz R, Schilsky M. Wilson disease: pathogenesis and clinical considerations in diagnosis and treatment. Semin Liver Dis 2011;31:245-259.

[48]   Green RM, Flamm S. AGA technical review on the evaluation of liver chemistry tests. Gastroenterology 2002;123:1367-1384.

[49]   Alfinito F, Sica M, Luciano L, Pepa RD, Palladino C, Ferrara I, Giani U, Ruggiero G, Terrazzano G. Immune dysregulation and dyserythropoiesis in the myelodysplastic syndromes. Br J Haematol 2010;148:90-98.

[50]   Kim HH, Park TS, Oh SH, Chang CL, Lee EY, Son HC. Delayed hemolytic transfusion reaction due to anti-Fyb caused by a primary immune response: a case study and a review of the literature. Immunohematology 2004;20:184-186.

[51]   Perrotta S, Gallagher PG, Mohandas N. Hereditary spherocytosis. Lancet 2008;372:1411-1426.

[52]   Hoffman PC. Immune hemolytic anemia--selected topics. 10.1182/asheducation-2009.1.80 2009.

[53]   Barve JS, Kelkar SR, Chikhalikar AA, Pimparkar BD. Dubin-Johnson syndrome. (A case report and review of literature). J Postgrad Med 1982;28:46-49.

[54]   van de Steeg E, Stranecky V, Hartmannova H, Noskova L, Hrebicek M, Wagenaar E, van Esch A, de Waart DR, Oude Elferink RP, Kenworthy KE, Sticova E, al-Edreesi M, Knisely AS, Kmoch S, Jirsa M, Schinkel AH. Complete OATP1B1 and OATP1B3 deficiency causes human Rotor syndrome by interrupting conjugated bilirubin reuptake into the liver. J Clin Invest 2012;122:519-528.

[55]   Pedersen OM, Nordgard K, Kvinnsland S. Value of sonography in obstructive jaundice. Limitations of bile duct caliber as an index of obstruction. Scand J Gastroenterol 1987;22:975-981.

[56]   Runyon BA. Care of patients with ascites. N Engl J Med 1994;330:337-342.

[57]   Koulaouzidis A, Bhat S, Saeed AA. Spontaneous bacterial peritonitis. World J Gastroenterol 2009;15:1042-1049.

[58]   Habeeb KS, Herrera JL. Management of ascites. Paracentesis as a guide. Postgrad Med 1997;101:191-2, 195-200.

[59]   Cattau EL Jr, Benjamin SB, Knuff TE, Castell DO. The accuracy of the physical examination in the diagnosis of suspected ascites. JAMA 1982;247:1164-1166.

[60]   Runyon BA, Montano AA, Akriviadis EA, Antillon MR, Irving MA, McHutchison JG. The serum-ascites albumin gradient is superior to the exudate-transudate concept in the differential diagnosis of ascites. Ann Intern Med 1992;117:215-220.

[61]   Goldberg BB, Goodman GA, Clearfield HR. Evaluation of ascites by ultrasound. Radiology 1970;96:15-22.

[62]   Inadomi J, Cello JP, Koch J. Ultrasonographic determination of ascitic volume. Hepatology 1996;24:549-551.

[63]   Kato M, Stevenson LW, Palardy M, Campbell PM, May CW, Lakdawala NK, Stewart G, Nohria A, Rogers JG, Heywood JT, Gheorghiade M, Lewis EF, Mi X, Setoguchi S. The worst symptom as defined by patients during heart failure hospitalization: implications for response to therapy. J Card Fail 2012;18:524-533.

[64]   Park MA, Mueller PS, Kyle RA, Larson DR, Plevak MF, Gertz MA. Primary (AL) hepatic amyloidosis: clinical features and natural history in 98 patients. Medicine (Baltimore) 2003;82:291-298.

[65]   Cooke CB, Krenacs L, Stetler-Stevenson M, Greiner TC, Raffeld M, Kingma DW, Abruzzo L, Frantz C, Kaviani M, Jaffe ES. Hepatosplenic T-cell lymphoma: a distinct clinicopathologic entity of cytotoxic gamma delta T-cell origin. Blood 1996;88:4265-4274.

[66]   Castell DO, O'Brien KD, Muench H, Chalmers TC. Eastimation of liver size by percussion in normal individuals. Ann Intern Med 1969;70:1183-1189.

[67]   Sapira JD, Williamson DL. How big is the normal liver? Arch Intern Med 1979;139:971-973.

[68]   Naylor CD. The rational clinical examination. Physical examination of the liver. JAMA 1994;271:1859-1865.

[69]   Zoli M, Magalotti D, Grimaldi M, Gueli C, Marchesini G, Pisi E. Physical examination of the liver: is it still worth it? Am J Gastroenterol 1995;90:1428-1432.

[70]   Long RG, Scheuer PJ, Sherlock S. Presentation and course of asymptomatic primary biliary cirrhosis. Gastroenterology 1977;72:1204-1207.

[71]   Chau TN, Lai ST, Tse C, Ng TK, Leung VK, Lim W, Ng MH. Epidemiology and clinical features of sporadic hepatitis E as compared with hepatitis A. Am J Gastroenterol 2006;101:292-296.

[72]   Tong C, Xu X, Liu C, Zhang T, Qu K. Assessment of liver volume variation to evaluate liver function. Front Med 2012;6:421-427.

[73]   Rosenfield AT, Laufer I, Schneider PB. The significance of a palpable liver. A correlation of clinical and radioisotope studies. Am J Roentgenol Radium Ther Nucl Med 1974;122:313-317.

[74]   Debnath CR, Debnath MR, Khalid MS, Mahmuduzzaman M. Clinical profile of 250 cases of amoebic liver abscess. Mymensingh Med J 2013;22:712-715.

[75]   Gosink BB, Leymaster CE. Ultrasonic determination of hepatomegaly. J Clin Ultrasound 1981;9:37-44.

[76]   Skrainka B, Stahlhut J, Fulbeck CL, Knight F, Holmes RA, Butt JH. Measuring liver span. Bedside examination *versus* ultrasound and scintiscan. J Clin Gastroenterol 1986;8:267-270.

[77]   Kratzer W, Fritz V, Mason RA, Haenle MM, Kaechele V. Factors affecting liver size: a sonographic survey of 2080 subjects. J Ultrasound Med 2003;22:1155-1161.

[78] Honda H, Onitsuka H, Masuda K, Nishitani H, Nakata H, Watanabe K. Chronic liver disease: value of volumetry of liver and spleen with computed tomography. Radiat Med 1990;8:222-226.

[79] Li WX, Zhao XT, Chai WM, Zhu NY, DU LJ, Huang W, Ling HW, Chen KM, Xie Q. Hepatitis B virus-induced liver fibrosis and cirrhosis: the value of liver and spleen volumetry with multi-detector spiral computed tomography. J Dig Dis 2010;11:215-223.

[80] Picardi M, Martinelli V, Ciancia R, Soscia E, Morante R, Sodano A, Fortunato G, Rotoli B. Measurement of spleen volume by ultrasound scanning in patients with thrombocytosis: a prospective study. Blood 2002;99:4228-4230.

[81] McIntyre OR, Ebaugh FG Jr. Palpable spleens in college freshmen. Ann Intern Med 1967;66:301-306.

[82] O'Reilly RA. Splenomegaly in 2,505 patients at a large university medical center from 1913 to 1995. 1963 to 1995: 449 patients. West J Med 1998;169:88-97.

[83] Michiels JJ, Bernema Z, Van Bockstaele D, De Raeve H, Schroyens W. Current diagnostic criteria for the chronic myeloproliferative disorders (MPD) essential thrombocythemia (ET), polycythemia vera (PV) and chronic idiopathic myelofibrosis (CIMF). Pathol Biol (Paris) 2007;55:92-104.

[84] Chetham MM, Roberts KB. Infectious mononucleosis in adolescents. Pediatr Ann 1991;20:206-213.

[85] Barkun AN, Camus M, Green L, Meagher T, Coupal L, De Stempel J, Grover SA. The bedside assessment of splenic enlargement. Am J Med 1991;91:512-518.

[86] Tamayo SG, Rickman LS, Mathews WC, Fullerton SC, Bartok AE, Warner JT, Feigal DW Jr, Arnstein DG, Callandar NS, Lyche KD, *et al*. Examiner dependence on physical diagnostic tests for the detection of splenomegaly: a prospective study with multiple observers. J Gen Intern Med 1993;8:69-75.

[87] Yang JC, Rickman LS, Bosser SK. The clinical diagnosis of splenomegaly. West J Med 1991;155:47-52.

[88] Chongtham DS, Singh MM, Kalantri SP, Pathak S. Accuracy of palpation and percussion manoeuvres in the diagnosis of splenomegaly. Indian J Med Sci 1997;51:409-416.

[89] Verghese A, Krish G, Karnad A. Ludwig Traube. The man and his space. Arch Intern Med 1992;152:701-703.

[90] Barkun AN, Camus M, Meagher T, Green L, Coupal L, De Stempel J, Grover SA. Splenic enlargement and Traube's space: how useful is percussion? Am J Med 1989;87:562-566.

[91] Doll M, Scholmerich J, Spamer C, Volk BA, Gerok W. [Clinical significance of sonographically detected splenomegaly]. Dtsch Med Wochenschr 1986;111:887-891.

[92] Bezerra AS, D'Ippolito G, Faintuch S, Szejnfeld J, Ahmed M. Determination of splenomegaly by CT: is there a place for a single measurement? AJR Am J Roentgenol 2005;184:1510-1513.

[93] Satapathy SK, Bernstein D. Dermatologic disorders and the liver. Clin Liver Dis 2011;15:165-182.

[94] Foutch PG, Sullivan JA, Gaines JA, Sanowski RA. Cutaneous vascular spiders in cirrhotic patients: correlation with hemorrhage from esophageal varices. Am J Gastroenterol 1988;83:723-726.

[95] Pirovino M, Linder R, Boss C, Kochli HP, Mahler F. Cutaneous spider nevi in liver cirrhosis: capillary microscopical and hormonal investigations. Klin Wochenschr 1988;66:298-302.

[96] Serrao R, Zirwas M, English JC. Palmar erythema. Am J Clin Dermatol 2007;8:347-356.

[97] Winton GB, Lewis CW. Dermatoses of pregnancy. J Am Acad Dermatol 1982;6:977-998.

[98] LloydL CW, Williams RH. Endocrine changes associated with Laennec's cirrhosis of the liver. Am J Med 1948;4:315-330.

[99] Agnello V, Chung RT, Kaplan LM. A role for hepatitis C virus infection in type II cryoglobulinemia. N Engl J Med 1992;327:1490-1495.

[100] Monti G, Galli M, Invernizzi F, Pioltelli P, Saccardo F, Monteverde A, Pietrogrande M, Renoldi P, Bombardieri S, Bordin G, *et al*. Cryoglobulinaemias: a multi-centre study of the early clinical and laboratory manifestations of primary and secondary disease. GISC. Italian Group for the Study of Cryoglobulinaemias. QJM 1995;88:115-126.

[101] Fabrizi F, Dixit V, Messa P. Antiviral therapy of symptomatic HCV-associated mixed cryoglobulinemia: meta-analysis of clinical studies. J Med Virol 2013;85:1019-1027.

[102] Caputo R, Gelmetti C, Ermacora E, Gianni E, Silvestri A. Gianotti-Crosti syndrome: a retrospective analysis of 308 cases. J Am Acad Dermatol 1992;26:207-210.

[103] Cavanaugh J, Niewoehner CB, Nuttall FQ. Gynecomastia and cirrhosis of the liver. Arch Intern Med 1990;150:563-565.

[104] Van Thiel DH. Feminization of chronic alcoholic men: a formulation. Yale J Biol Med 1979;52:219-225.
[105] Overdiek JW, Merkus FW. Spironolactone metabolism and gynaecomastia. Lancet 1986;1:1103.
[106] Bisseru B, Patel JS. Cruveilhier-Baumgarten (C-B) disease. Gut 1989;30:136-137.
[107] Ito K, Mitchell DG. Imaging diagnosis of cirrhosis and chronic hepatitis. Intervirology 2004;47:134-143.
[108] Shrestha SM. Liver cirrhosis and hepatocellular carcinoma in hepatic vena cava disease, a liver disease caused by obstruction of inferior vena cava. Hepatol Int 2009;3:392-402.
[109] Strauss G, Hansen BA, Kirkegaard P, Rasmussen A, Hjortrup A, Larsen FS. Liver function, cerebral blood flow autoregulation, and hepatic encephalopathy in fulminant hepatic failure. Hepatology 1997;25:837-839.
[110] Sundaram V, Shaikh OS. Hepatic encephalopathy: pathophysiology and emerging therapies. Med Clin North Am 2009;93:819-36.
[111] Grippon P, Le Poncin Lafitte M, Boschat M, Wang S, Faure G, Dutertre D, Opolon P. Evidence for the role of ammonia in the intracerebral transfer and metabolism of tryptophan. Hepatology 1986;6:682-686.
[112] Conn HO. Asterixis in non-hepatic disorders. Am J Med 1960;29:647-661.
[113] Artz SA, Paes IC, Faloon WW. Hypokalemia-induced hepatic coma in cirrhosis. Occurrence despite neomycin therapy. Gastroenterology 1966;51:1046-1053.
[114] Lazaridis KN, Frank JW, Krowka MJ, Kamath PS. Hepatic hydrothorax: pathogenesis, diagnosis, and management. Am J Med 1999;107:262-267.

CHAPTER 2

Diagnostic Strategies for Patients with Abnormal Liver Function Tests

Masami Minemura*

The Third Department of Internal Medicine, University of Toyama, Japan

Abstract: Abnormalities in liver function tests (LFTs) may be caused not only by hepatic diseases but also by non-hepatic disorders, while normal values on LFTs do not exclude liver disease. Therefore, LFTs should be interpreted based on all information about the patient. Practically, classification of LFTs into hepatic synthetic function, hepatocellular injury, and cholestasis is important to interpret liver abnormalities and to identify the etiology of liver injury. Liver injuries can be divided into two categories, hepatocellular and cholestatic. These categories are helpful in diagnosing liver diseases and in understanding mechanisms of injury. The hepatocellular pattern is characterized primarily by increased aspartate aminotransferase (AST) and alanine aminotransferase (ALT) levels, whereas the cholestatic pattern is characterized by increased alkaline phosphatase (ALP) and bilirubin levels. Identification of the pattern may narrow the possible causes of liver injury in a patient. Imaging tests, such as ultrasound, CT, and MRI, may be helpful in the final diagnosis of liver diseases.

Keywords: Albumin, aminotransferases, ammonia, bilirubin, cholestasis, hepatocellular injury, liver function tests, prothrombin time.

KEY POINTS

1. Liver function tests (LFTs) include tests of hepatic synthetic (*e.g.* serum albumin, prothrombin time (PT)) and excretory (*e.g.* serum bilirubin, blood ammonia) functions, and tests that indicate hepatocellular injury (*e.g.* aspartate aminotransferase (AST), alanine aminotransferase (ALT)) and cholestasis (*e.g.* bilirubin, alkaline phosphatase (ALP), gamma-glutamyl transpeptidase (γ-GTP)).

2. Abnormalities in LFTs may be caused not only by hepatic diseases but also by non-hepatic disorders such as myocardial infarction and bone diseases.

3. Abnormalities in LFTs are often the first indication of liver disease, because patients with non-advanced liver disease usually have no symptoms.

*Corresponding author **Masami Minemura:** The Third Department of Internal Medicine, University of Toyama, Toyama, Japan; Email: minemura@med.u-toyama.ac.jp

Yukihiro Shimizu (Ed)

4. Normal values in LFTs do not exclude liver disease, because some HCV and HBV carriers have normal LFTs.

5. Medical history and physical examination can be used to select appropriate LFTs and exclude excessive tests.

6. LFTs that distinguish between elevations of a single and multiple liver enzymes are very useful in diagnosing liver diseases, because patients with liver injury usually have multiple abnormalities. Elevations of single liver enzymes are more frequently associated with non-hepatic diseases, such as bone disease.

7. Liver injury can be broadly divided into two categories, a hepatocellular pattern and a cholestatic pattern. These patterns are helpful in diagnosing liver diseases and in understanding their mechanisms.

8. The magnitude of AST and ALT elevations is useful in diagnosing liver disease, although these levels are not related to patient prognosis.

9. The ratio of AST to ALT (AST/ALT ratio) may provide useful information in diagnosing liver diseases.

INTRODUCTION

Liver chemistry tests may be ordered on suspicion of liver disease or for screening. The most common tests used in clinical practice include measurements of serum aminotransferases, bilirubin, ALP, and γ-GTP. Although these tests are usually called "liver function tests", the levels of aminotransferases and ALP indicate liver injury but do not accurately reflect how well the liver is functioning. To evaluate liver function, it is important to measure biosynthetic function (*e.g.* albumin and PT) and excretory function (detoxification) (*e.g.* bilirubin and blood ammonia) (Table **1**).

Patients with one or more abnormalities in LFTs must be carefully evaluated to determine the medical information needed to diagnose a liver disease. Individual LFTs alone rarely suggest a specific diagnosis, but their sensitivity and specificity can be increased by suitable combinations of LFTs.

Clinical history and physical examination can contribute to selecting appropriate LFTs to evaluate abnormalities, as well as excluding excessive or inappropriate tests.

The diagnostic approach generally consists of three steps: 1) LFTs distinguishing elevated levels of single and multiple liver enzymes, 2) categorization of disease into hepatocellular and cholestatic patterns, and 3) evaluation of the magnitude of elevation and the AST/ALT ratio. Imaging modalities such as ultrasound are needed to distinguish intrahepatic from extrahepatic cholestasis.

MARKERS OF HEPATOCELLULAR INJURY

Aminotransferases (AST and ALT)

Aspartate aminotransferase (AST), also known as glutamic oxaloacetic transaminase GOT), is an abundant enzyme in the heart, liver, skeletal muscles, kidneys, and erythrocytes. Two types of AST isoenzymes are located in the cytosol and mitochondria. Alanine aminotransferase (ALT), also known as glutamic pyruvic transaminase (GPT), is a cytosolic enzyme dominantly present in the liver and kidney. These enzymes catalyze the transfer of the alpha-amino groups of aspartate and alanine, respectively, to the alpha-keto groups of oxaloacetate and pyruvate, respectively. These enzymes are released into the blood in greater amounts when liver cells are destroyed and when the permeability of the liver cell membrane is increased. Elevations of serum AST and ALT are sometimes the first clue to the occurrence of liver disease [1, 2]. They are also sensitive indicators of liver cell injury, although the levels of these enzymes do not directly reflect the degree of liver cell damage. Serum concentrations of AST and ALT are normally less than 30 IU/L (Table **1**) [3-5]. The optimal ALT cut offs for men and women have been reported to be 29 IU/L and 22 IU/L, respectively [4]. The cutoff values for serum aminotransferases, especially ALT, should be adjusted for gender and body mass index [3, 6].

The following must be considered:

1) Elevated serum AST is not specific to liver disease. In contrast, elevated ALT is thought to be specific to liver disease, because the proportion of ALT is greater in the liver than in the heart and skeletal muscles.

2) The half-lives of AST and ALT are reported to be 17±5 h and 47±10 h, respectively.

3) The AST/ALT ratio is very useful for differential diagnoses [1, 2, 7].

MARKERS OF CHOLESTASIS

Alkaline Phosphatase (ALP)

The alkaline phosphatase family of enzymes consists of zinc metalloenzymes present on the plasma membranes of many cells. These enzymes have two major primary sources, liver and bone. Several isoenzymes have been identified, each of which is specific to an organ (liver, bone, placenta, and small intestine). ALP is physiologically elevated in children and adolescents undergoing rapid bone growth, and late in normal pregnancies [8-10]. In the liver, ALP is found on the bile canalicular membrane of hepatocytes. The mechanisms of ALP increase are complex, and can include its increased synthesis and release from hepatocyte membranes into the sinusoids [11].

Hepatic ALP is a sensitive marker for biliary tract obstruction. Increased serum ALP is thought to be caused by increased hepatic synthesis and leakage from bile duct cells.

The following must be considered:

1) The range of normal serum ALP levels varies throughout life.

2) Serum ALP from bone in twice as high in adolescents as in normal adults.

3) Elevations of ALP and γ-GTP indicate intrahepatic and/or extrahepatic cholestasis. In the absence of jaundice or elevated aminotransferases, an elevation of liver-origin ALP suggests early cholestasis or hepatic infiltration by a tumor.

4) Isolated elevations of ALP may be caused by bone disorders, Hodgkin's disease, diabetes mellitus [12], chronic kidney disease [9], hyperthyroidism, congestive heart failure, or inflammatory bowel disease.

Gamma- Glutamyl Transpeptidase (γ-GTP)

γ-GTP is a ubiquitous epithelial enzyme that is responsible for catabolism of extracellular glutathione. γ-GTP is located in hepatocytes and biliary epithelial cells. Serum levels of γ-GTP are increased in patients with several disorders, including hepatobiliary disease, alcoholism and drug treatment with barbiturates or phenytoin. Although γ-GTP is useful for detecting hepatobiliary disease, the elevation is not specific for the disease. Measurement of γ-GTP is useful to exclude a bone source of an elevated serum ALP level.

The following must be considered:

1) Parallel elevations in serum γ-GTP and serum ALP indicate hepatobiliary disease, especially cholestasis.

2) An isolated increase in serum γ-GTP is often seen in patients with alcohol abuse [13] and those administered drugs such as barbiturates or phenytoin. Elevated serum γ-GTP has been observed in patients with various clinical conditions, including pancreatic disease, myocardial infarction, renal failure, chronic obstructive pulmonary disease, and diabetes mellitus [14].

3) The half-life of serum γ-GTP is thought to be 2-4 weeks (26 days) [15]. Heavy drinking may increase γ-GTP with a peak at 2-3 days.

Bilirubin

Bilirubin is a breakdown product from the porphyrin ring of heme-containing proteins. The normal serum level is less than 1 mg/dL (17 μmol/L). Total bilirubin can be subdivided into a water-soluble form, called direct/conjugated bilirubin, and an insoluble form, called indirect/unconjugated bilirubin. Conjugated bilirubin can be elevated by disorders in the transport of conjugated bilirubin into the bile canaliculi or obstruction of the bile duct [16, 17]. Both conjugated and unconjugated bilirubin are often elevated in patients with most liver diseases (See Chap. 1. *Symptoms and signs suggestive of liver disease*, *"jaundice"*). Elevated unconjugated serum bilirubin reflects two pathophysiologic mechanisms, bilirubin overproduction and reduced ability to conjugate bilirubin. Isolated elevation of unconjugated bilirubin is seen primarily in patients with hemolytic disorders, but rarely in those with liver diseases. In the absence of hemolysis, isolated unconjugated hyperbilirubinemia may be associated with reduced ability to conjugate bilirubin, such as in Crigler-Najjar syndrome and Gilbert's syndrome [18]. The prevalence of Gilbert's syndrome is 5-10% in Western Europe.

In advanced liver diseases such as cirrhosis, total bilirubin level is useful in evaluating detoxification and excretory function, which are associated with disease severity. Total bilirubin level is a major factor for evaluation of liver function in the modified Child-Pugh classification and in the model for end-stage liver disease (MELD) score [19-22].

The following must be considered:

1) Elevated unconjugated bilirubin is rarely due to liver disease, except for Gilbert's syndrome. Isolated elevation of unconjugated bilirubin is seen primarily in patients with hemolytic disorders.

2) Levels of serum bilirubin are useful for evaluating the severity and prognosis of liver diseases such as advanced cirrhosis and acute hepatic failure. In contrast, levels of serum bilirubin are not well correlated with the severity or prognosis of other liver diseases.

3) Any bilirubin found in the urine is conjugated bilirubin, suggesting the occurrence of liver disease, because unconjugated bilirubin binds to albumin in the serum and is not filtered in the kidney.

4) The half-life of bilirubin is thought to be about 4 h, but the half-life of albumin-bound bilirubin may be as long as 12 to 14 days. Elevated bilirubin level has been reported to decline more slowly than expected during the recovery phase in patients with obstructive jaundice.

5) Patients with bacterial sepsis may have hyperbilirubinemia, although the mechanism is unclear. Multiple factors, including hypotension and bacterial endotoxins, may be responsible for jaundice in these patients.

6) Total parenteral nutrition (TPN) may cause hyperbilirubinemia. Steatosis, lipidosis, and cholestasis are frequently observed in patients receiving TPN for a long time (at least two to three weeks), and TPN itself and biliary sludge may contribute to cholestasis. TPN promotes bacterial overgrowth in the small intestine, which may induce translocation of intestinal endotoxins into the portal system.

MARKERS OF HEPATIC SYNTHETIC FUNCTION

Albumin

About 10 g (6 – 12g) of albumin is synthesized by the liver daily, making it important to maintain oncotic pressure. The half-life of serum albumin is about 15 to 20 days (3 weeks) [23]. Although both prothrombin time and serum albumin level can be used to evaluate hepatic synthetic function in patients with advanced liver diseases, albumin level is not a good indicator of acute or mild hepatic diseases because of its long half-life. Hypoalbuminemia is common in patients with liver cirrhosis [24], but is not specific for liver disease. Excessive loss (protein-losing enteropathy, nephrotic syndrome, burn injury), increased turnover (hormonal dysfunction), and decreased intake (malabsorption, malnutrition) are other causes of hypoalbuminemia [25]. Hypoalbuminemia may also occur in patients with chronic infection, because several inflammatory cytokines (IL-1 and TNF-α) may inhibit albumin synthesis [26-28].

The following must be considered:

1) Serum albumin concentration is a good indicator for hepatic synthetic function only in advanced liver disease.

2) Serum albumin should not be measured in screening for liver disease.

Prothrombin Time (PT)

Blood clotting factors other than factor VIII are synthesized by hepatocytes. Their serum half-lives are much shorter than that of albumin, ranging from 6 h for factor VII to 5 days for fibrinogen. PT reflects the extrinsic clotting pathway involving factors II, V, VII, and X, and is used to assess hepatic synthetic function. PT remains within normal limits until progression to cirrhosis. Moreover, PT is one of the major factors for evaluating liver function in the modified Child-Pugh classification and in the MELD score [19-22]. In addition, monitoring of PT can also be useful in assessing hepatic synthetic dysfunction in patients with acute liver failure [29, 30].

A prolonged PT may also result in vitamin K deficiency, such as obstructive jaundice or fat malabsorption and anticoagulation therapy, because biosynthesis of factors II, VII, IX, and X depends on vitamin K.

The following must be considered:

1) PT is more sensitive and a more rapid reflector of hepatic synthetic function than serum albumin level.

2) Administration of 10 mg vitamin K is useful in patients with prolonged PT to distinguish vitamin K deficiency from hepatic failure.

Table 1. Liver function tests.

Test	Normal range	Value
AST	5-30 IU/L	Indicates hepatocellular damage, but not specific for liver disease, $T_{1/2}$ in serum: about 17 ± 5 h
ALT	5-30 IU/L	Indicates hepatocellular damage, mostly specific for liver disease, $T_{1/2}$ in serum: about 47 ± 10 h
ALP	35-130 IU/L	Indicates cholestasis, biliary obstruction, hepatic infiltration, or bone disease. Not specific for liver disease, isoenzymes are useful for differential diagnosis. $T_{1/2}$ in serum: about 7 h
γ–GTP	10-48 IU/L	Indicates cholestasis, biliary obstruction, or alcoholism, $T_{1/2}$ in serum : < 2-4 weeks
Bilirubin		
Total	0.3-1.0 mg/dL	Indicates jaundice due to cholestasis, biliary obstruction, overproduction of bilirubin, or impaired conjugation $T_{1/2}$ of bilirubin depends on its pathogenesis.
Conjugated	< 0.3 mg/dL	Indicates cholestasis or biliary obstruction
Unconjugated	< 0.7mg/dL	Indicates overproduction of bilirubin (e.g. hemolysis) or impaired conjugation (e.g. Crigler-Najjar syndrome type I and II, or Gilbert's syndrome)
Albumin	35-50 g/L	Synthetic function $T_{1/2}$ in serum: about 15 to 20 days
PT	12-16 sec	Synthetic function PT depends on several coagulation factors. (e.g. $T_{1/2}$ of Factor VII: about 6 h, $T_{1/2}$ of fibrinogen: about 5 days)

DIAGNOSTIC PROCEDURES FOR PATIENTS WITH ABNORMAL LFTs

History Taking and Risk Factors

Clinical history taking and assessment of risk factors are important in interpreting abnormalities on LFTs. Clinical history includes details of alcohol drinking [31], medications (including herbal medicines, birth control pills, and over-the-counter (OTC) medicines) [32], sexual activity [33-35], travel history [36, 37], transfusion with blood and blood products, and familial history of liver disease. Alcohol consumption greater than 33 to 45 g/day in men and greater than 22 to 30 g/day in women has been associated with alcoholic liver disease [31]. Family history can be helpful in diagnosing inherited liver diseases, including Wilson's disease [38], hemochromatosis [39], and α1-antitrypsin deficiency [40]. (See Chapter 1. *Symptoms and signs suggestive of liver disease,* **History taking**)

Evaluation of Abnormalities on LFTs

Effective diagnosis of liver diseases requires suitable combinations of liver chemistry tests. Appropriate LFTs for initial assessment of liver disease include assays of serum AST, ALT, ALP, γ-GTP, and total, conjugated (direct), and unconjugated (indirect) bilirubin (T-Bil, D-Bil, and ID-Bil, respectively). ID-Bil is calculated by subtracting D-Bil from T-Bil concentration. Fig. (**1**) of Chapter 3 shows an algorithm for the evaluation of abnormalities by LFTs (Fig. **1**).

Measurements of serum albumin concentrations and PT (-INR), which reflect liver biosynthetic functions, are initially less useful in diagnosing liver diseases. These measurements, however, can be used to evaluate the severity of liver disease in patients with serious or advanced liver diseases, such as acute liver failure and liver cirrhosis [41, 42].

Distinguish Elevations in Isolated and Multiple Liver Enzymes by LFTs

LFTs showing elevation of isolated liver enzyme may indicate non-hepatic disorders, which should be included in the differential diagnosis of these patients, because multiple abnormalities may be detected in patients with common liver diseases (Fig. **1** and Table **2**). Table **2** summarizes common extrahepatic disorders that could lead to abnormal liver chemistry test results. AST elevation without ALT elevation may suggest non-hepatic disorders, such as myocardial infarction or muscle disease, because AST is an abundant enzyme in heart, liver, skeletal muscle, kidney, and erythrocytes, while ALT predominantly exists in liver [43, 44].

The two major primary sources of ALP are liver and bone. Several isoenzymes of ALP have been identified, each of which is specific to certain organs (*e.g.* liver, bone, placenta, and small intestine). Isolated ALP elevation without γ-GTP elevation may suggest that elevated ALP is caused by non-hepatic diseases, such as bone disease and thyroid dysfunction [45]. On the other hand, isolated ALP elevation can rarely be observed in patients with early stage primary biliary cirrhosis (PBC) or infiltrative diseases of the liver, such as metastatic liver tumors or granulomatous diseases.

While both conjugated (direct) and unconjugated (indirect) bilirubin tend to be elevated in most advanced liver diseases, elevation of indirect bilirubin alone is observed primarily in hemolytic disorders, but rarely in liver diseases, though it has been observed in Gilbert's syndrome [46] and Crigler-Najjar syndrome types I and II. Congenital conjugated hyperbilirubinemia is very rare, and may indicate Dubin-Johnson syndrome [47] or Roter's syndrome [48].

Categorize an Abnormality as Hepatocellular or Cholestatic (Fig. 2)

Liver injury can be broadly divided into two patterns, a hepatocellular and a cholestatic pattern. Categorization is helpful in diagnosing liver diseases and in understanding their mechanisms of abnormalities. The hepatocellular pattern is characterized primarily by increased AST and ALT levels, whereas the cholestatic pattern is characterized by increased ALP and bilirubin levels. In some patients, however, it may be difficult to distinguish between these two patterns, because elevated transaminase levels can occur in both. Disproportionately elevated ALP relative to ALT level suggests a cholestatic pattern, whereas disproportionately elevated ALT relative to ALP suggests a hepatocellular pattern.

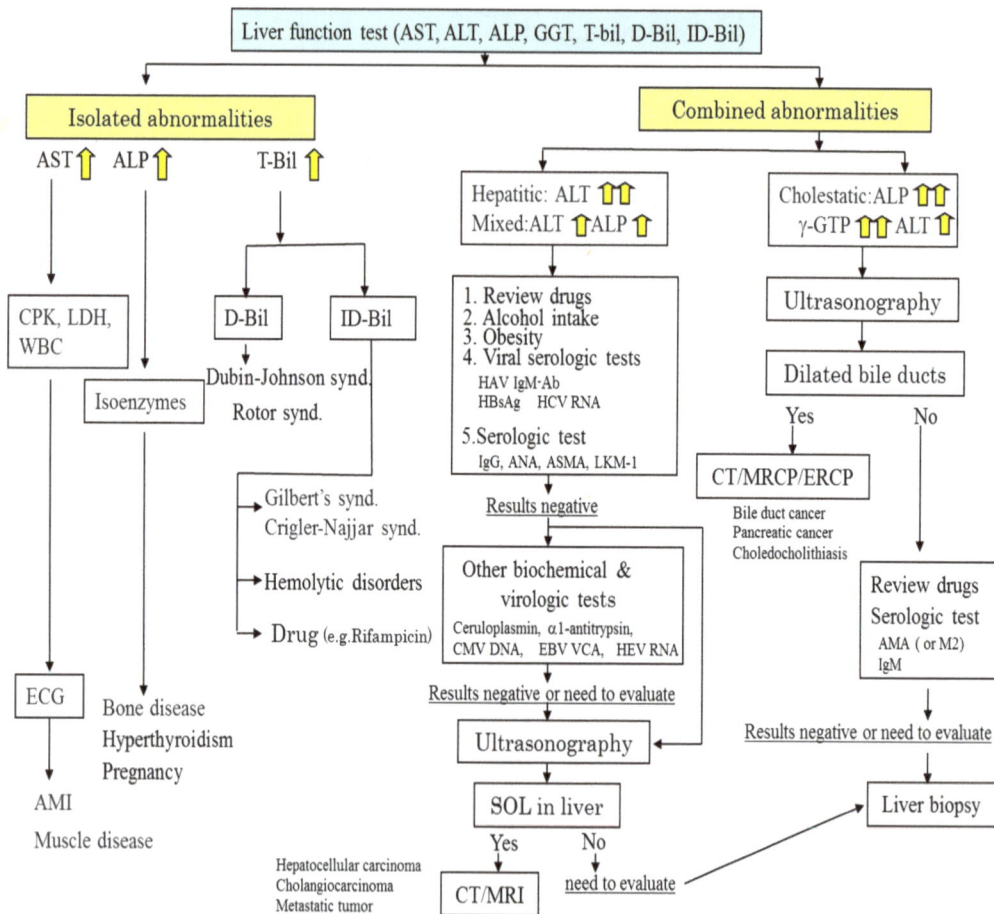

Figure 1: Approach to patients with abnormalities on liver function tests. AMI; acute myocardial infarction, ANA; anti-nuclear antibody, ASMA; anti-smooth muscle antibody, LKM-1; anti-liver kidney microsome type 1, CMV; cutomegalovirus, EBV; Epstein-Barr virus, HEV; hepatitis E virus.

Fig. (1) shows an algorithm for narrowing the differential diagnosis in patients thought to have hepatocellular disorders. Liver diseases with the hepatocellular pattern include viral hepatitis [49-52], alcoholic liver disease [31], non-alcoholic steatohepatitis (NASH) [53], and drug-induced hepatitis [32]. Other less common but important diseases include autoimmune hepatitis (AIH) [54], Wilson disease [38], hemochromatosis [39], and α1-antitrypsin deficiency [43]. To narrow the differential diagnosis, the disease-specific components should be measured.

Table 2. Extrahepatic causes of abnormal liver function test results.

Abnormality	Check points	Potential extrahepatic cause
AST ↑	ALT:N	Myocardial infarction Muscle disorders Hemolysis
ALP↑	γ-GTP:N	Bone disease Pregnancy Hyperthyroidism
Bilirubin ↑	ALP:N	Hemolysis Sepsis TPN
Alb ↓	↑T-Chol	Nephrotic synd.
	↓T-Chol	Malnutrition, Malabsorption Protein-losing enteropathy
PT ↑	Drug	Anticoagulant or antibiotics use Vitamin K deficiency

N; within normal range, TPN; total parenteral nutrition

Patients with the cholestatic pattern (conjugated hyperbilirubinemia in the setting of other liver test abnormalities) are further evaluated by determining whether cholestasis is intra- or extrahepatic. Ultrasound imaging can determine whether the intra- or extrahepatic biliary tree is dilated with high degrees of sensitivity and specificity [55]. The absence of biliary dilation suggests intrahepatic cholestasis, while its presence indicates extrahepatic cholestasis. Although ultrasonography may determine that cholestasis is extrahepatic, it may be difficult to identify the site or cause of obstruction. Further evaluations include computed tomography (CT) [56], magnetic resonance cholangiopancreatography (MRCP) [57], and endoscopic retrograde cholangiopancreatography (ERCP) [58]. In contrast, intrahepatic cholestasis can be caused by drug-induced liver injury and PBC, making measurements of serum anti-mitochondria antibody (AMA) useful in diagnosing PBC [59].

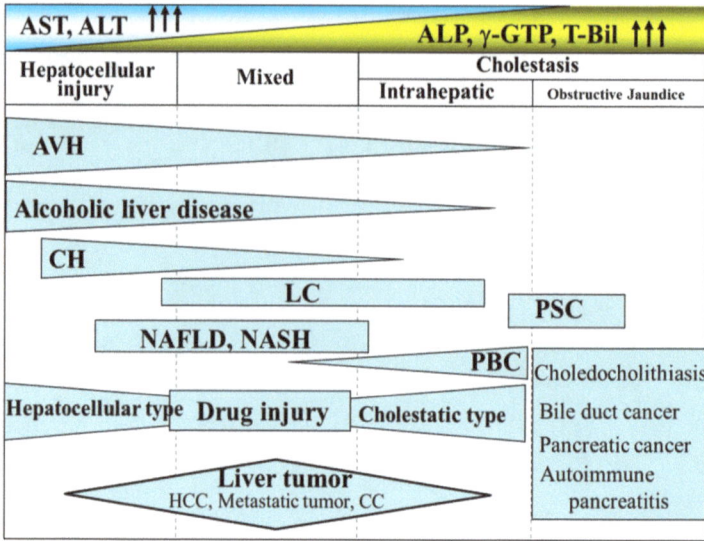

Figure 2: Patterns of liver injury. AVH; acute viral hepatitis, CH; chronic hepatitis, LC; liver cirrhosis, PSC; primary sclerosing cholangitis, PBC; primary biliary cirrhosis, NAFLD; nonalcoholic fatty liver disease, NASH; nonalcoholic steatohepatitis, HCC; hepatocellular carcinoma, CC; cholangiocarcinoma

Evaluation of Abnormalities in Serum ALT and AST Levels

Both the magnitude of AST and ALT concentrations and their ratio (AST/ALT) may be useful in narrowing the differential diagnosis of causes of liver injury [60-62]. The American Gastroenterological Association (AGA) technical review on the evaluation of liver function tests according to the degree of elevated serum ALT and AST ; (1) ALT and AST elevations of less than 5 times the upper limit normal (ULN), with predominant ALT or AST elevation; and (2) ALT and AST elevations greater than 15 times ULN (Figs. **2** and **3**). The AGA review found that ALT and AST elevations in an intermediate range may be caused by numerous disease processes and are less useful for differential diagnosis [63].

ALT and AST Elevations < 5 times ULN

ALT Predominance: Fatty infiltration is the most frequent cause of mild elevated liver enzymes with ALT-predominant. This pattern is frequently associated with obesity and hypertriglyceridemia. An AST/ALT ratio less than 1 can be seen in patients with fatty liver [60, 61].

Chronic viral hepatitis is one of the most frequent causes of abnormal liver tests, and usually presents as mildly elevated transaminases with ALT predominance.

HCV infection is a highly prevalent disease throughout the world, and HBV infection is common in Asia and Africa.

Many medications including OTC and herbal/alternative medicines may cause liver injury, which is usually mild and ALT-predominant [32].

AST Predominance: Alcohol use is a frequent cause of elevated transaminases with ALT-predominant [61, 62]. A more than two-fold elevation of γ-GTP in patients with AST-predominant transaminase elevation strongly suggests alcohol abuse. Patients with alcoholic hepatitis have an AST:ALT ratio of approximately 2:1, with AST rarely exceeding 300 IU/L. Although non-alcoholic steatohepatitis (NASH) is diagnosed only after excluding significant alcohol consumption and other identifiable liver diseases, patients with NASH may have elevated transaminases with AST-predominance [61]. Patients with liver cirrhosis usually have mildly elevated transaminases with AST-predominance [61, 64]. Non-hepatic diseases, including hemolysis and myopathic disorders, can also cause mild elevation of transaminases with AST-predominance.

In patients with liver tumors (primary or metastatic tumors), minimal or mild elevation of AST or ALT can be seen with a mildly or markedly elevated ALP. The initial evaluation using ultrasonography should be perfomed in these cases.

ALT and AST Elevations Greater Than 15 Times ULN

Severe elevations of liver transaminases, to greater than 15 times ULN, usually indicate more marked hepatocellular injury or necrosis, and these etiologies may be relatively limited. Acute viral hepatitis (A-E) can cause marked liver enzyme elevations and can be diagnosed with serologic markers.

Drug-induced hepatotoxicity can also cause marked elevations in liver enzymes [32]. Acetaminophen overdose is the most frequent cause of drug-induced fulminant hepatic failure [65].

Patients with prolonged systemic hypotension due to cardiac arrest or severe heart failure may develop ischemic injury in several organs, including the liver. Ischemic liver diseases such as shock liver can cause marked elevations of aminotransferases (exceeding 1,000 IU/L) and lactic dehydrogenase [66, 67].

Acute bile duct obstruction by gallstones also can cause marked elevations in transaminase levels, along with right upper quadrant pain and nausea. Liver enzyme concentrations usually decline rapidly if a stone passes out of the bile duct [68, 69]. Autoimmune hepatitis [54], Wilson's disease [38, 70], and acute Budd-Chiari syndrome [71] may also cause marked aminotransferase elevations.

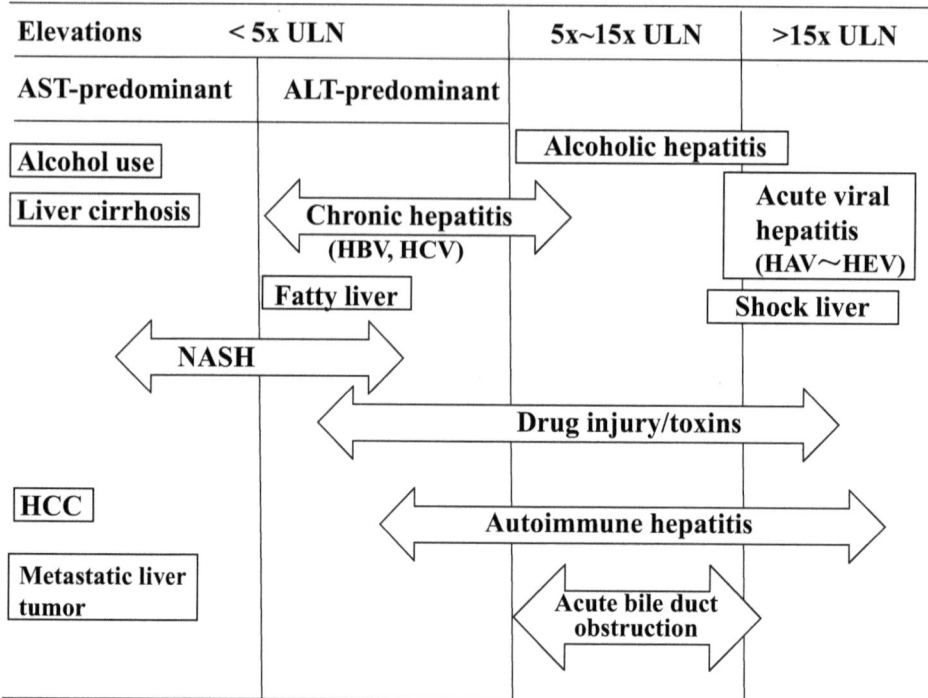

Elevations	< 5x ULN		5x~15x ULN	>15x ULN
AST-predominant		ALT-predominant		

Figure 3: Patterns and etiologies of AST and ALT elevations. ULN; upper limit of normal, NASH; nonalcoholic steatohepatitis, HCC; hepatocellular carcinoma

The figure contains the following labels: Alcohol use, Liver cirrhosis, Alcoholic hepatitis, Chronic hepatitis (HBV, HCV), Acute viral hepatitis (HAV~HEV), Fatty liver, Shock liver, NASH, Drug injury/toxins, HCC, Autoimmune hepatitis, Metastatic liver tumor, Acute bile duct obstruction.

MESSAGES FROM HEPATOLOGISTS TO GENERAL PHYSICIANS

1. Classification of hepatocellular type and cholestatic type of liver injury is essential for diagnosis of the etiology of liver disease.

2. The prevalence of each type of liver disease differs according to country or area, and this information is useful for differential diagnosis. Moreover, the degree of aminotransferase elevation may help in the differential diagnosis.

3. In patients with shock liver (ischemic hepatitis), elevated serum aminotransferase levels normalize a few days after hypotension is corrected. In contrast, normalization takes several weeks in patients with acute viral hepatitis.

4. Hyperbilirubinemia and prolonged prothrombin time may indicate severe liver injury suggesting a possible transition to fulminant hepatic failure. Patients with both signs should be referred to hepatologists irrespective of the etiology.

5. Plasma ammonia level is often elevated in patients with hepatic encephalopathy, but it varies among patients.

6. The most common cause of hyperbilirubinemia is Gilbert's syndrome, and the elevation of unconjugated bilirubin without any other abnormal liver function tests is strongly suggestive of this syndrome.

7. In liver diseases other than Gilbert's syndrome, conjugated bilirubin is exclusively higher than unconjugated bilirubin in jaundiced patients.

8. Since serum AST and ALT levels are very low in patients undergoing dialysis, these levels should be interpreted with caution in diagnosing liver diseases in dialyzed patients [72].

9. Elevated serum ALT may be associated with liver disease mortality. Abnormal ALT (>30 U/L in men and >19 U/L in women) are associated with increased risk of death from liver disease (HR 8.2, 95% CI 2.1-31.9) [73].

10. In liver diseases, serum LDH should be always lower than AST or ALT, except in the hyperacute phase of acute liver injury, and predominant elevation of LDH suggests circulatory disturbances, such as shock or severe dehydration, or hematological malignancy.

11. Due to the differences in half-lives of enzymes, LDH is first decreased at the recovery stage of liver injury followed by AST. The decrease in serum ALT is delayed compared with LDH and AST. Recovery from acute liver injury can therefore be judged from decreases in LDH and AST.

12. The most frequent cause of γ-GTP elevation may be fatty liver, but γ-GTP is often elevated by non-hepatic causes. The causes of mild and solitary elevation of γ-GTP are sometimes difficult to identify. ALP is elevated in cholestasis, but biliary disease may show discordant elevation of γ-GTP and ALP in some cases. ALP is predominantly

elevated not only in bone diseases but also during the period of growth.

13. Patients diagnosed with HBV or HCV infection, autoimmune hepatitis, primary biliary cirrhosis, primary sclerosing cholangitis, Wilson's disease, or hemochromatosis should be referred to hepatologists for proper management. On the other hand, fatty liver disease, alcoholic liver disease, and drug-induced liver injury (DILI) can be managed by general physicians unless the patients show signs of severe liver injury.

14. Abdominal ultrasound should be performed in all patients with liver function abnormalities to obtain information on liver size and morphology, liver mass, fatty deposits, bile duct dilatation, gallstones, spleen size, and ascites retention, which could be helpful in identifying the etiologies of liver diseases.

15. If diagnosis of the etiology of liver disease is difficult based on blood tests and imaging analysis, liver biopsy performed by a hepatologist should be considered. Even when liver biopsy cannot identify the etiology, it can provide important information on the likelihood of progression to cirrhosis.

ACKNOWLEDGEMENTS

We are very thankful to Ms. Asma Ahmed, manager publications, Bentham Science Publishers, for her patience and long-term assistance.

CONFLICT OF INTEREST

The author confirms that he has no conflict of interest to declare for this publication.

REFERENCES

[1]   Dufour DR, Lott JA, Nolte FS, Gretch DR, Koff RS, Seeff LB. Diagnosis and monitoring of hepatic injury. I. Performance characteristics of laboratory tests. Clin Chem 2000;46:2027-2049.
[2]   Dufour DR, Lott JA, Nolte FS, Gretch DR, Koff RS, Seeff LB. Diagnosis and monitoring of hepatic injury. II. Recommendations for use of laboratory tests in screening, diagnosis, and monitoring. Clin Chem 2000;46:2050-2068.
[3]   Prati D, Taioli E, Zanella A, Della Torre E, Butelli S, Del Vecchio E, Vianello L, Zanuso F, Mozzi F, Milani S, Conte D, Colombo M, Sirchia G. Updated definitions of healthy ranges for serum alanine aminotransferase levels. Ann Intern Med 2002;137:1-10.

[4]   Ruhl CE, Everhart JE. Upper limits of normal for alanine aminotransferase activity in the United States population. Hepatology 2012;55:447-454.

[5]   http://mghlabtest.partners.org/MGH_Reference_Intervals_August_2011.pdf (Accessed on March 29, 2013).

[6]   Piton A, Poynard T, Imbert-Bismut F, Khalil L, Delattre J, Pelissier E, Sansonetti N, Opolon P. Factors associated with serum alanine transaminase activity in healthy subjects: consequences for the definition of normal values, for selection of blood donors, and for patients with chronic hepatitis C. MULTIVIRC Group. Hepatology 1998;27:1213-1219.

[7]   Cohen JA, Kaplan MM. The SGOT/SGPT ratio--an indicator of alcoholic liver disease. Dig Dis Sci 1979;24:835-838.

[8]   Gordon T. Factors associated with serum alkaline phosphatase level. Arch Pathol Lab Med 1993;117:187-190.

[9]   Bayer PM, Hotschek H, Knoth E. Intestinal alkaline phosphatase and the ABO blood group system--a new aspect. Clin Chim Acta 1980;108:81-87.

[10]   Wakim-Fleming J, Zein NN. The liver in pregnancy: disease *vs* benign changes. Cleve Clin J Med 2005;72:713-721.

[11]   Seetharam S, Sussman NL, Komoda T, Alpers DH. The mechanism of elevated alkaline phosphatase activity after bile duct ligation in the rat. Hepatology 1986;6:374-380.

[12]   Nannipieri M, Gonzales C, Baldi S, Posadas R, Williams K, Haffner SM, Stern MP, Ferrannini E. Liver enzymes, the metabolic syndrome, and incident diabetes: the Mexico City diabetes study. Diabetes Care 2005;28:1757-1762.

[13]   Moussavian SN, Becker RC, Piepmeyer JL, Mezey E, Bozian RC. Serum gamma-glutamyl transpeptidase and chronic alcoholism. Influence of alcohol ingestion and liver disease. Dig Dis Sci 1985;30:211-214.

[14]   Hedworth-Whitty RB, Whitfield JB, Richardson RW. Serum gamma-glutamyl transpeptidase activity in myocardial ischaemia. Br Heart J 1967;29:432-438.

[15]   Penn R, Worthington DJ. Is serum gamma-glutamyltransferase a misleading test? Br Med J (Clin Res Ed) 1983;286:531-535.

[16]   Zimmerman HJ. Intrahepatic cholestasis. Arch Intern Med 1979;139:1038-1045.

[17]   Scharschmidt BF, Blanckaert N, Farina FA, Kabra PM, Stafford BE, Weisiger RA. Measurement of serum bilirubin and its mono- and diconjugates: application to patients with hepatobiliary disease. Gut 1982;23:643-649.

[18]   Watson KJ, Gollan JL. Gilbert's syndrome. Baillieres Clin Gastroenterol 1989;3:337-355.

[19]   Kim HJ, Lee HW. Important predictor of mortality in patients with end-stage liver disease. Clin Mol Hepatol 2013;19:105-115.

[20]   Kamath PS, Wiesner RH, Malinchoc M, Kremers W, Therneau TM, Kosberg CL, D'Amico G, Dickson ER, Kim WR. A model to predict survival in patients with end-stage liver disease. Hepatology 2001;33:464-470.

[21]   Dunn W, Jamil LH, Brown LS, Wiesner RH, Kim WR, Menon KV, Malinchoc M, Kamath PS, Shah V. MELD accurately predicts mortality in patients with alcoholic hepatitis. Hepatology 2005;41:353-358.

[22]   Wiesner R, Edwards E, Freeman R, Harper A, Kim R, Kamath P, Kremers W, Lake J, Howard T, Merion RM, Wolfe RA, Krom R. Model for end-stage liver disease (MELD) and allocation of donor livers. Gastroenterology 2003;124:91-96.

[23]   Rothschild MA, Oratz M, Schreiber SS. Serum albumin. Hepatology 1988;8:385-401.

[24]   Rothschild MA, Oratz M, Zimmon D, Schreiber SS, Weiner I, Van Caneghem A. Albumin synthesis in cirrhotic subjects with ascites studied with carbonate-14C. J Clin Invest 1969;48:344-350.

[25]   Lieberman FL, Reynolds TB. Plasma volume in cirrhosis of the liver: its relation of portal hypertension, ascites, and renal failure. J Clin Invest 1967;46:1297-1308.

[26]   Moshage HJ, Janssen JA, Franssen JH, Hafkenscheid JC, Yap SH. Study of the molecular mechanism of decreased liver synthesis of albumin in inflammation. J Clin Invest 1987;79:1635-1641.

[27]   Perlmutter DH, Dinarello CA, Punsal PI, Colten HR. Cachectin/tumor necrosis factor regulates hepatic acute-phase gene expression. J Clin Invest 1986;78:1349-1354.

[28]   Dinarello CA. Interleukin-1 and the pathogenesis of the acute-phase response. N Engl J Med 1984;311:1413-1418.

[29] O'Grady JG, Alexander GJ, Hayllar KM, Williams R. Early indicators of prognosis in fulminant hepatic failure. Gastroenterology 1989;97:439-445.

[30] Hoofnagle JH, Carithers RL Jr, Shapiro C, Ascher N. Fulminant hepatic failure: summary of a workshop. Hepatology 1995;21:240-252.

[31] O'Shea RS, Dasarathy S, McCullough AJ. Alcoholic liver disease. Hepatology 2010;51:307-328.

[32] Tajiri K, Shimizu Y. Practical guidelines for diagnosis and early management of drug-induced liver injury.World J Gastroenterol 2008;14:6774-6785.

[33] Matthews GV, Nelson MR. The management of chronic hepatitis B infection. Int J STD AIDS 2001;12:353-357.

[34] Lee HC, Ko NY, Lee NY, Chang CM, Ko WC. Seroprevalence of viral hepatitis and sexually transmitted disease among adults with recently diagnosed HIV infection in Southern Taiwan, 2000-2005: upsurge in hepatitis C virus infections among injection drug users. J Formos Med Assoc 2008;107:404-411.

[35] Tohme RA, Holmberg SD. Is sexual contact a major mode of hepatitis C virus transmission? Hepatology 2010;52:1497-1505.

[36] Wu D, Guo CY. Epidemiology and prevention of hepatitis A in travelers. J Travel Med 2013;20:394-399.

[37] Tekin R, Yolbas I, Dal T, Demirpence O, Kaya S, Bozkurt F, Deveci O, Celen MK, Tekin A. Evaluation of adults with acute viral hepatitis a and review of the literature. Clin Ter2013;164:537-541.

[38] Bruha R, Marecek Z, Pospisilova L, Nevsimalova S, Vitek L, Martasek P, Nevoral J, Petrtyl J, Urbanek P, Jiraskova A, Ferenci P. Long-term follow-up of Wilson disease: natural history, treatment, mutations analysis and phenotypic correlation. Liver Int 2011;31:83-91.

[39] Hanson EH, Imperatore G, Burke W.HFE gene and hereditary hemochromatosis: a HuGE review. Human Genome Epidemiology. Am J Epidemiol 2001;154:193-206.

[40] Stoller JK, Aboussouan LS.A review of alpha1-antitrypsin deficiency. Am J Respir Crit Care Med 2012;185:246-259.

[41] Kamath PS, Wiesner RH, Malinchoc M, Kremers W, Therneau TM, Kosberg CL, D'Amico G, Dickson ER, Kim WR. A model to predict survival in patients with end-stage liver disease. Hepatology 2001;33:464-470.

[42] Hoofnagle JH, Carithers RL Jr, Shapiro C, Ascher N. Fulminant hepatic failure: summary of a workshop. Hepatology 1995;21:240-252.

[43] Giallourakis CC, Rosenberg PM, Friedman LS. The liver in heart failure. Clin Liver Dis 2002;6:947-67, viii-ix.

[44] Berlin NI, Berk PD. Quantitative aspects of bilirubin metabolism for hematologists. Blood 1981;57:983-999.

[45] Pantazi H, Papapetrou PD. Changes in parameters of bone and mineral metabolism during therapy for hyperthyroidism. J Clin Endocrinol Metab 2000;85:1099-1106.

[46] Watson KJ, Gollan JL. Gilbert's syndrome. Baillieres Clin Gastroenterol 1989;3:337-355.

[47] Barve JS, Kelkar SR, Chikhalikar AA, Pimparkar BD. Dubin-Johnson syndrome. (A case report and review of literature). J Postgrad Med 1982;28:46-49.

[48] van de Steeg E, Stranecky V, Hartmannova H, Noskova L, Hrebicek M, Wagenaar E, van Esch A, de Waart DR, Oude Elferink RP, Kenworthy KE, Sticova E, al-Edreesi M, Knisely AS, Kmoch S, Jirsa M, Schinkel AH. Complete OATP1B1 and OATP1B3 deficiency causes human Rotor syndrome by interrupting conjugated bilirubin reuptake into the liver. J Clin Invest 2012;122:519-528.

[49] Wu D, Guo CY. Epidemiology and prevention of hepatitis A in travelers. J Travel Med 2013;20:394-399.

[50] Yapali S, Talaat N, Lok AS. Management of hepatitis B: our practice and how it relates to the guidelines. Clin Gastroenterol Hepatol 2014;12:16-26.

[51] Lavanchy D. The global burden of hepatitis C. Liver Int 29 Suppl 2009;1:74-81.

[52] Scobie L, Dalton HR. Hepatitis E: source and route of infection, clinical manifestations and new developments. J Viral Hepat 2013;20:1-11.

[53] Bacon BR, Farahvash MJ, Janney CG, Neuschwander-Tetri BA. Nonalcoholic steatohepatitis: an expanded clinical entity. Gastroenterology 1994;107:1103-1109.

[54] Gossard AA, Lindor KD. Autoimmune hepatitis: a review. J Gastroenterol 2012;47:498-503.

[55]   Goldberg BB, Goodman GA, Clearfield HR. Evaluation of ascites by ultrasound. Radiology 1970;96:15-22.

[56]   Levitt RG, Sagel SS, Stanley RJ, Jost RG. Accuracy of computed tomography of the liver and biliary tract. Radiology 1977;124:123-128.

[57]   Singh A, Mann HS, Thukral CL, Singh NR. Diagnostic accuracy of MRCP as compared to ultrasound/CT in patients with obstructive jaundice. J Clin Diagn Res 2014;8:103-107.

[58]   Di Cesare E, Puglielli E, Michelini O, Pistoi MA, Lombardi L, Rossi M, Barile A, Masciocchi C. Malignant obstructive jaundice: comparison of MRCP and ERCP in the evaluation of distal lesions. Radiol Med 2003;105:445-453.

[59]   Yamagiwa S, Kamimura H, Takamura M, Aoyagi Y. Autoantibodies in primary biliary cirrhosis: recent progress in research on the pathogenetic and clinical significance. World J Gastroenterol 2014;20:2606-2612.

[60]   Giboney PT. Mildly elevated liver transaminase levels in the asymptomatic patient. Am Fam Physician 2005;71:1105-1110.

[61]   Sorbi D, Boynton J, Lindor KD. The ratio of aspartate aminotransferase to alanine aminotransferase: potential value in differentiating nonalcoholic steatohepatitis from alcoholic liver disease. Am J Gastroenterol 1999;94:1018-1022.

[62]   Nyblom H, Berggren U, Balldin J, Olsson R. High AST/ALT ratio may indicate advanced alcoholic liver disease rather than heavy drinking. Alcohol Alcohol 2004;39:336-339.

[63]   American Gastroenterological Association medical position statement: evaluation of liver chemistry tests. Gastroenterology 2002;123:1364-1366.

[64]   Sheth SG, Flamm SL, Gordon FD, Chopra S. AST/ALT ratio predicts cirrhosis in patients with chronic hepatitis C virus infection. Am J Gastroenterol 1998;93:44-48.

[65]   Bunchorntavakul C, Reddy KR. Acetaminophen-related hepatotoxicity. Clin Liver Dis 2013;17:587-607, viii.

[66]   Myers RP, Cerini R, Sayegh R, Moreau R, Degott C, Lebrec D, Lee SS. Cardiac hepatopathy: clinical, hemodynamic, and histologic characteristics and correlations. Hepatology 2003;37:393-400.

[67]   Gitlin N, Serio KM. Ischemic hepatitis: widening horizons. Am J Gastroenterol 1992;87:831-836.

[68]   Al-Jiffry BO, Elfateh A, Chundrigar T, Othman B, Almalki O, Rayza F, Niyaz H, Elmakhzangy H, Hatem M. Non-invasive assessment of choledocholithiasis in patients with gallstones and abnormal liver function. World J Gastroenterol 2013;19:5877-5882.

[69]   Fortson WC, Tedesco FJ, Starnes EC, Shaw CT. Marked elevation of serum transaminase activity associated with extrahepatic biliary tract disease. J Clin Gastroenterol 1985;7:502-505.

[70]   Berman DH, Leventhal RI, Gavaler JS, Cadoff EM, Van Thiel DH. Clinical differentiation of fulminant Wilsonian hepatitis from other causes of hepatic failure. Gastroenterology 1991;100:1129-1134.

[71]   Ferral H, Behrens G, Lopera J. Budd-Chiari syndrome. AJR Am J Roentgenol 2012;199:737-745.

[72]   Yasuda K, Okuda K, Endo N, Ishiwatari Y, Ikeda R, Hayashi H, Yokozeki K, Kobayashi S, Irie Y. Hypoaminotransferasemia in patients undergoing long-term hemodialysis: clinical and biochemical appraisal. Gastroenterology 1995;109:1295-1300.

[73]   Ruhl CE, Everhart JE. Elevated serum alanine aminotransferase and gamma-glutamyltransferase and mortality in the United States population. Gastroenterology 2009;136:477-85.e11.

CHAPTER 3

Approach to Patients with Acute Liver Injury

Yasuhiro Nakayama[1,*] and Yukihiro Shimizu[2]

[1]First Department of Internal Medicine, Faculty of Medicine, University of Yamanashi, Japan and [2]Gastroenterology Center, Nanto Municipal Hospital, Japan

Abstract: Although acute liver injury shows spontaneous improvement in many patients, some require special treatment and can develop fulminant hepatic failure. The etiology of acute hepatitis and acute hepatic failure varies in different countries, making prompt diagnosis and determination of etiology important for determining prognosis and proper patient management. Liver transplantation should be considered for patients who develop fulminant hepatic failure.

Keywords: Acute liver failure, acute liver injury, cholestatic type, hepatocellular type, liver transplantation, medical history, physical findings, signs, symptoms, viral hepatitis.

KEY POINTS

1. Although acute liver injury shows spontaneous improvement in many patients, some require special treatment, whereas others may develop fulminant hepatic failure. Differential diagnosis of the cause of acute liver injury is important.

2. Signs, symptoms and history taking are important for the differential diagnosis of acute hepatitis. Alcohol- and drug-induced liver injury occur frequently, with history taking important in diagnosing these diseases.

3. The etiology of acute hepatitis and acute hepatic failure varies in different countries. Vaccination has decreased the incidence of hepatitis A and hepatitis B in the USA. Acute hepatitis of undetermined etiology is responsible for the highest incidence worldwide.

4. A PT-INR ≥ 1.8 (<40% activity) in patients with acute hepatitis suggests a possible transition to fulminant hepatitis; transfer of these

*Corresponding author Yasuhiro Nakayama: The First Department of Internal Medicine, University of Yamanashi, Yamanashi, Japan; Email: ynakayama@yamanashi.ac.jp

patients to a transplantation center should be considered before they develop encephalopathy.

5.   Various prognostic criteria have been proposed in fulminant hepatic failure. Because no single criterion is sufficient to predict prognosis, a combination of these criteria may be more useful.

PRIMARY CARE FOR ACUTE LIVER INJURY

Liver injury is defined by damage to hepatocytes or bile duct epithelium. Acute liver injury refers to hepatocyte damage that occurs abruptly and terminates within a short period of time. The term "acute liver injury" usually refers to liver injury lasting <6 months. The most consistent feature of acute liver injury is significant elevation of aminotransferases (usually more than eight times the upper normal limit), often accompanied by increased serum bilirubin concentrations. Alkaline phosphatase (ALP) is generally within the upper normal limit in most patients with acute hepatic injury, but may be elevated in patients with hepatic disorders accompanied by cholestasis. The optimal cutoff values for acute hepatic injury include 200 IU/L for aspartate aminotransferase (AST) (sensitivity 91%, specificity 95%) and 300 IU/L for alanine aminotransferase (ALT) (sensitivity 96%, specificity 94%) [1]. Peak ALT is ten to forty times the upper normal limit in patients with viral hepatitis [1]. Ninety percent of patients with toxic or ischemic acute hepatic injury have AST activity >3000 U/L [2]. In alcoholic hepatitis, AST and ALT concentrations are usually lower than 300 IU/L, and 80% have AST/ALT ratios over 2 [3-7]. Jaundice develops in 70% of adults with alcoholic hepatitis [4, 5], 70% of those with acute hepatitis A [8], 33% to 50% of adults with acute hepatitis B [9, 10] and 20% to 33% of those with acute hepatitis C [11, 12]. Jaundice is rare in children with viral hepatitis, and, when it occurs, is less severe than in adults. Elevated direct bilirubin concentration cannot differentiate severe hepatic injury from obstructive jaundice, but the ratio of D-Bil/T-Bil may be less than 0.7 in the former and around 0.8 in the latter.

It is important to classify patients with acute injury as having cholestatic or hepatocellular type (Fig. **1**). In hepatocellular type, the patient may have viral, drug-induced, ischemic or alcoholic hepatitis. In cholestatic type, the patient may have drug-induced cholestasis or obstructive jaundice. Because obstructive jaundice often requires an immediate therapeutic procedure for mechanical relief of the obstruction, abdominal ultrasound is necessary to determine whether the biliary tract is dilated. Plain CT or MRCP may detect small tumors or stones. Plain CT may also be important in assessing the severity of liver injury, because irregular low density areas (possibly corresponding to necrotic areas) in the liver or ascites retention (usually predominant around the liver) likely indicate severe liver injury.

Patients with hepatocellular type acute liver injury who show no evidence of biliary tract obstruction and are deeply jaundiced (T-Bil >10 mg/dL) may be at risk for fulminant hepatic failure. Decreased consciousness level, prolonged PT, and hyperbilirubinemia may indicate the development of hepatic failure, with the patient requiring immediate transfer to a transplantation center [13]. The etiology of acute liver injury influences the prognosis of the patient [14]. Therefore, the etiology and severity of the liver injury must be explored in parallel. Determination of etiology requires history taking and physical examination before blood and/or imaging tests (Fig. **2**).

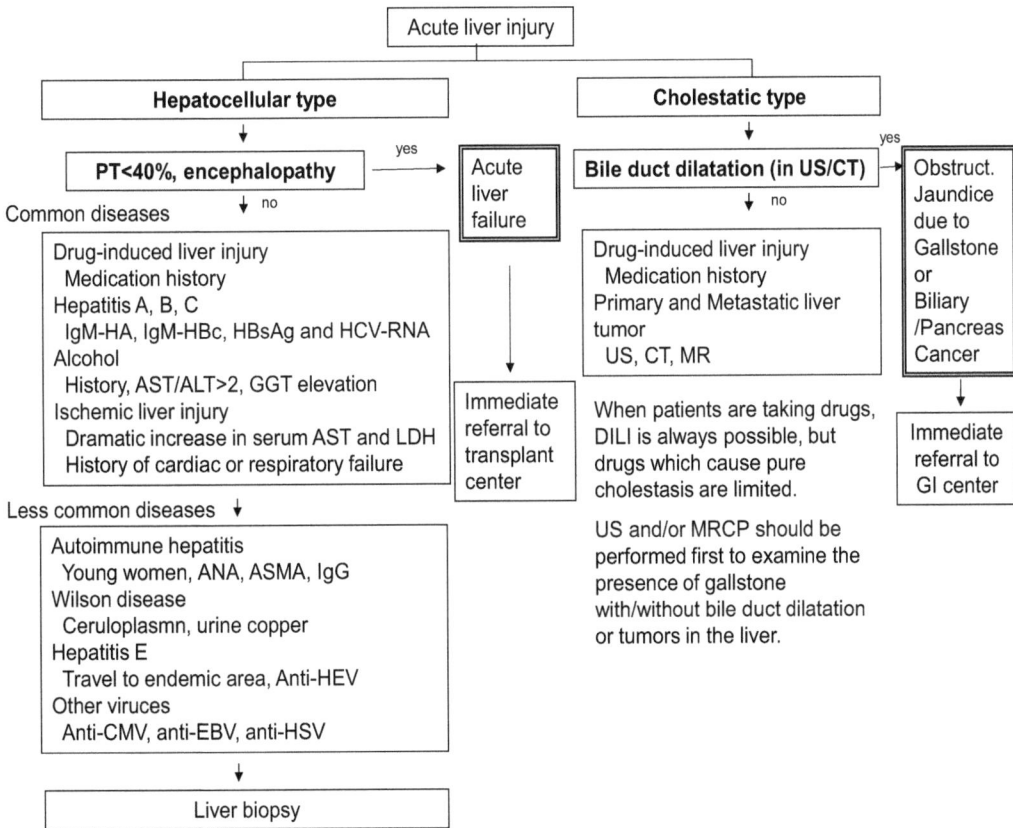

Figure 1: Disorders causing acute abnormal liver function tests and their diagnostic criteria. PT; prothrombin time, GGT; γ-glutamyl transpeptidase, ANA; antinuclear antibody, ASMA; anti-smooth muscle antibody, HEV; hepatitis E virus, CMV; cytomegalovirus, EBV; Epstein-Barr virus, HSV, herpes simplex virus, DILI; drug-induced liver injury, MRCP; MR cholangiopancreatography

A complete medical history is the most important aspect in evaluating patients with elevated LFTs. Past history of liver disease; blood transfusion; a family history of liver disease; visits to Southeast Asia or Africa [15]; intake of raw oysters, raw meat of a wild boar, deer or pig; sex with unspecified partners; tattoos; and history of drug abuse or alcohol consumption should be evaluated.

The presence of any accompanying signs and symptoms, such as jaundice, arthralgia, myalgia, rash, weight loss, anorexia, abdominal pain, fever, and changes in the color of urine or stool may provide information on the etiology, severity and pathophysiology of the disease.

It is sometimes difficult to determine at first presentation whether the injury is acute or chronic. The presence of spider nevi on the anterior chest, palmar erythema, gynecomastia or caput medusae suggests chronic injury, especially liver cirrhosis, but physical signs are not useful for differentiation in most patients. Imaging modalities also have limited value for differentiation. Laboratory examinations to determine etiology should be performed in a step-wise manner, based on the local frequencies of diseases (Table 1).

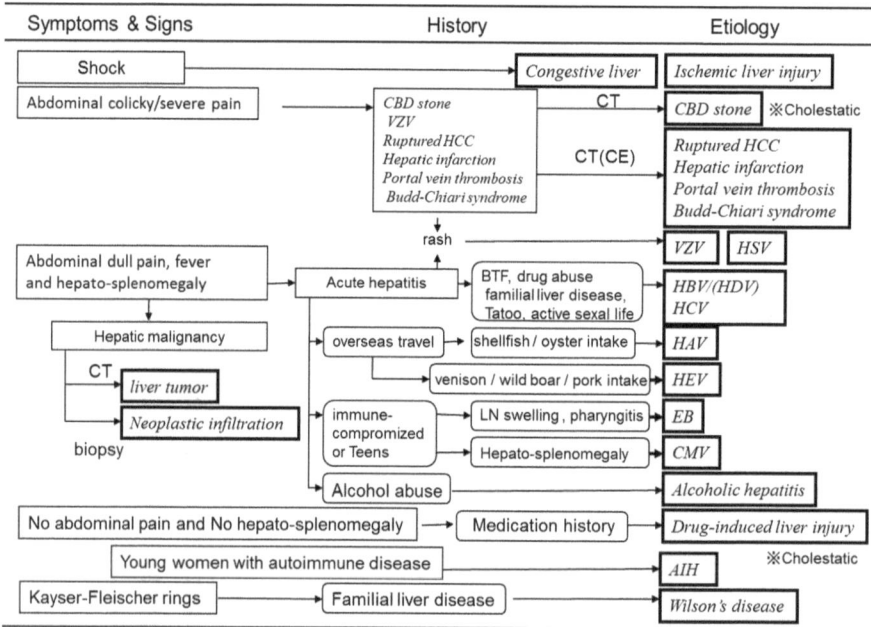

Figure 2: Diagnostic algorithm of acute liver injury from history and signs. CBD; common bile duct, VZV; varicella zoster virus, HCC; hepatocellular carcinoma, BTF; blood transfusion, HSV; herpes simplex virus, HAV, hepatitis A virus, HBV; hepatitis B virus, HCV; hepatitis C virus, HDV, hepatitis D virus, HEV; hepatitis E virus, EBV; Epstein-Barr virus, CMV; cytomegalovirus, LN; lymph node, AIH; autoimmune hepatitis

ETIOLOGY OF ACUTE LIVER INJURY

In 2007, 2,979 patients with acute symptomatic hepatitis A were reported in the USA, or 1.0 per 100,000 population, a 92% decrease from 2005, when the incidence was 12.0 per 100,000 population [16]. The incidence of acute hepatitis B has decreased 82%, from 8.5 per 100,000 population in 1990 to 1.5 per 100,000 population in 2007, with 4,519 cases reported in 2007 [16]. In 2007, 849 cases of acute hepatitis C were reported in the USA, with an overall incidence of 0.3 cases per 100,000 population [16]. HAV, HBV and HCV are the etiologic agents in >95% of patients with acute viral hepatitis in USA.

Table 1. Laboratory tests for determination of causes of acute liver injury.

1st step 【LD】hematological value, LDH, ALT, AST, T-Bil, D-Bil, ALP, GGT, AMY, PT(INR), Alb, NH3, ChE, BS, BUN, CRE, Na, K, Cl, Ca, P, IgG, IgA, IgM, ANA, Anti-HAV IgM, Anti-HBc, Anti-HBc IgM, HbsAg, Anti-HCV, HCV-RNA, Anti-CMV IgM, CMV-DNA, EBV capsid antigen IgM, EBNA 【Image】ultrasonography or plain CT, ECG, chest x-p, SpO2	HAV, HBV, HCV, AIH(type1), EBV, CMV, Obstructive jaundice (due to Cancer or Choledocholithiasis), NASH, Congestive heart failure,
2nd step 【LD】APTT, FIB, FDP, D-dimer, Fe, TIBC, FER, ceruloplasmin, urinary copper, serum copper, p-ANCA, α1-AT, LKM-1, HBV-DNA, IgM HEV-Ab, HEV-RNA, Anti-VZV IgM, VZV-DNA, Anti-HSV IgM, HSV-DNA, anti-HIV, AFP, s-IL2R, HGF, AMA, AMA(m2), TSH, fT3, fT4, HDV-Ab, 【Image】three-phase contrast-enhanced CT	HDV, HEV, VZV, HSV, AIH(type2), Wilson's disease, PBC, PSC, HIV, hypothyroidism, Budd-Chiari syndrome, α1-AT
3rd step 【LD】 parvovirus B19 DNA, anti-parvovirus B19 IgM, anti-parvovirus B19 IgG, anti-leptospira IgM, anti-leptospira IgG, urinary leptospira-DNA, anti-dengue IgM, anti-dengue IgG, 【Image】enhanced MRI(EOB), liver biopsy	Parvovirus B19, Weil disease, Dengue hemorrhagic fever, Neoplastic infiltration of the liver

GGT; γ-glutamyl transpeptidase, FIB; fibrinogen, FER; ferritin, LKM; anti-liver kidney microsomal antibody; VZV; varicella zoster virus, HSV; herpes simplex virus, s-IL2R; soluble IL2 receptor, HGF; hepatocyte growth factor, AMA; anti-mitochondrial antibody, HDV; hepatitis D virus, AIH; autoimmune hepatitis, PBC; primary biliary cirrhosis, AT; antitrypsin

Patients who cannot be diagnosed after history taking and laboratory testing may have steatosis or steatohepatitis. Abdominal ultrasound is often useful for their diagnosis.

However, a significant percentage of individuals with acute viral hepatitis do not have serologic markers of infection with these viruses. Hepatitis E is rare in the USA, with most reported cases associated with travel to countries in which this virus is endemic [17,18]. Other viruses associated with acute hepatitis include Epstein-Barr virus and cytomegalovirus, the etiologic agents of mononucleosis;

and varicella virus, the etiologic agent of chickenpox. Hepatitis also refers to inflammation of the liver caused by drugs and alcohol abuse or toxins in the environment. Other etiologic causes of hepatitis include fat deposition in the liver, called non-alcoholic fatty liver disease (NAFLD), trauma, and autoimmune diseases. A national survey in Japan (2008-2011) examining the causes of acute hepatitis in 2143, found that 7.8% were due to HAV, 30.1% to HBV, 1.8% to *de novo* HBV, 4.9% to HCV, 2.7% to HEV, 3.8% to CMV, 11% to EBV, 13.5% to AIH, and 24.5% to other causes [19].

Acute Hepatitis Caused by Hepatitis Virus

Hepatitis A

Many patients with acute hepatitis A present with fever and gastroenterological symptoms after a one month incubation period. HAV infection is caused by the ingestion of raw shellfishes (especially oysters) and polluted water. Outbreaks have been reported in schools and facilities because the virus is excreted in patient's feces from about ten days before development of hepatitis and extends until more than four weeks after recovery. The risk of fulminant hepatic failure is very low (0.01%–0.1%) [20], but increases with patient age and in those with preexisting liver disease. The mortality rate in patients over age 40 years is 1% [20]. However, most patients recover after one to two months, with no transition to chronic hepatitis or liver cirrhosis, even if acute hepatitis is prolonged >6 months. Acute hepatitis A is diagnosed by the presence in serum of IgM-HA antibody, which can be detected for more than 3 months. Hepatitis A virus can be killed by heating for more than one minute at 85 °C.

Hepatitis B

Seventy to 80% of patients with acute HBV infection show a subclinical course, with clinically overt acute hepatitis developing in 20% to 30% of infected patients. About 1% of these patients may develop fulminant hepatitis, higher than in patients with other types of viral infection [20]. It is important to determine whether hepatitis in a patient is an acute exacerbation of chronic hepatitis or acute hepatitis, because the former has a poorer prognosis following the development of severe hepatitis or fulminant hepatic failure. The differential diagnosis of those two conditions depends on the titers of IgM-HBc and anti-HBc (IgG); patients with acute hepatitis show >10 S/CO (CLIA) of IgM-HBc, and those with acute exacerbation of chronic hepatitis show low or no IgM-HBc and high anti-HBc (>10 S/CO on CLIA or >70% inhibition on EIA).

Hepatitis C

Acute hepatitis C is relatively rare, with few reports of fulminant hepatic failure associated with HCV infection. Acute hepatitis C manifests 4 to 12 weeks after common cold-like symptoms and is diagnosed by the presence of HCV RNA and the absence of anti-HCV. As much as 2 to 3 months are required for the generation of anti-HCV antibodies. Although acute hepatitis C resolves within 12 weeks in 20% to 30% of patients, the remaining 70% to 80% develop chronic hepatitis. Lack of resolution after 12 weeks (serum HCV-RNA remains positive) or the occurrence of multiple ALT flares are indicators of progression to chronic hepatitis, with these patients requiring interferon therapy as soon as possible. The standard interferon-based regimen for acute hepatitis C has not yet been established, but 4 to 6 months of interferon monotherapy has shown to achieve a sustained virological response (viral eradication) rate >90% [20].

Hepatitis E

Although acute hepatitis E has been regarded as a disease of tropical countries, patients with this disease have been identified in developed countries during the last decade. In Japan, 2.7% of patients with acute hepatitis, and 10% of those with non-A, non-B, non-C hepatitis have acute hepatitis E [19]. Population surveys during outbreaks have reported a low mortality rate, of 0.07% to 0.6%, but hepatitis E may become severe in pregnant women, with mortality rates as high as 25% [21]. Four types of hepatitis E virus (HEV) have been identified. Types 1 and 2 are found in developing countries, and usually spread through drinking water; whereas types 3 and 4 are found in developed countries, with infection usually due to eating raw boar, deer or pig meat. The rate of fulminant hepatitis is high in patients infected with types 1 and 2, but not types 3 and 4, HEV, although high rates have been reported in older patients and those with underlying diseases infected with types 3 and 4 HEV [22]. Moreover, chronic infection or development of liver cirrhosis may occur in immunocompromised patients. Although IgA anti-HEV antibody has been reported more sensitive and specific than IgM anti-HEV antibody, HEV infection is diagnosed upon detection of the HEV genome in serum or feces or detection of IgM anti-HEV antibody.

Acute Hepatitis Caused by Non-Hepatitis Virus

Epstein-Barr Virus (EBV)

Patients infected with EBV present with fever, tonsillar swelling, lymph node swelling, and hepatosplenomegaly. White blood cell counts are often elevated, with increases in atypical lymphocytes, most of which are HLA-DR$^+$CD8$^+$ T cells. At least 90% of cases of infectious mononucleosis are caused by primary EBV infection [23]. Serum AST and ALT levels are elevated, to as high as 500 IU/L, and primary EBV infection is diagnosed by the presence of IgM-VCA and/or IgG-VCA and the absence of EBNA. Most patients recover without special therapy.

Cytomegalovirus (CMV)

Adult cases of primary CMV infection have been increasing. The clinical picture of these patients is similar to that of patients infected with EBV, except for lower rates of lymph node swelling and tonsillar swelling. Moreover, ages tend to be higher in patients with primary CMV than EBV infection. CMV infection is diagnosed by the presence of IgM anti-CMV antibody, and the isolation from blood or other clinical samples of CMV (viral culture) or the detection of CMV proteins (pp65) or nucleic acid by polymerase chain reaction (PCR) [24]. Although treatment is unnecessary for mild CMV infection in an immunocompetent adult, antiviral therapy should be considered in immunocompromised patients.

Herpes Simplex Virus

In children, hepatitis caused by human herpes simplex infection is associated with systemic infection. In adults, hepatitis is seen mainly in immunocompromised persons, but fulminant hepatitis in immunocompetent persons (especially pregnant women) has been reported [25, 26]. Hepatitis usually occurs following common cold-like symptoms with high fever. Although there are no specific signs, a decrease in white blood cell count might be a characteristic of HSV infection.

Varicella Zoster Virus (VZV)

The early diagnosis of disseminated VZV hepatitis is usually difficult because of the delay in appearance of characteristic skin lesions, requiring 4–10 days [27]. Disseminated varicella infections in immunocompetent hosts are rare, but the possibility of VZV hepatitis should be considered in examining patients with acute hepatitis accompanying abdominal pain of uncertain etiology. Pain is usually located to the epigastric area, occasionally involving the right upper quadrant or radiating to the back [28]. Acyclovir should be started within 24 h of skin manifestations. Delaying the start of treatment may be fatal, especially in immunosuppressed patients [29].

Parvovirus B19

Parvovirus, which has been found to cause pure red cell aplasia, virus-associated hemophagocytic syndrome and idiopathic thrombocytopenic purpura, can also cause hepatitis, with fulminant hepatitis developing in children. Adults with parvovirus-associated hepatitis usually recover rapidly. Viral DNA can be detected 7 days after infection, but becomes undetectable following the appearance of IgM or IgG antibody against parvovirus B19 [30]. The virus can be transmitted by blood transfusion.

Measles

Measles infection has been reported in adults with decreased antibody titer long after infection or vaccination. Pneumonia and hepatitis are complications frequently observed in infected patients [31]. Skin rash, Koplik spots and an increase in atypical lymphocytes are important in diagnosing this condition.

Adenovirus

Adenovirus often causes hepatitis, which may progress to fulminant hepatic failure especially in immunocompromised patients, such as after liver or bone marrow transplantation or in those infected with HIV [32].

HIV Infection

Liver injury in patients with HIV infection can be caused by HIV itself, by coinfection with hepatitis viruses such as HBV and HCV, or by hepatic involvement of systemic infections including *Mycobacterium tuberculosis, M. avium* complex, *Toxoplasma gondii*, or *Cryptosporidium* [33]. In addition, liver injury in HIV-infected patients may be caused by drugs prescribed to treat HIV [33]. Tuberculosis, *M. avium,* and *Cryptosporidium* have been reported to cause biliary tract injuries [34].

Drugs and Toxins

Drug-Induced Liver Injury

More than 600 drugs causing liver injury have been reported. Nonsteroidal anti-inflammatory drugs, antibiotics, antipsychotic drugs, anticonvulsants and antituberculosis drugs are frequent causes of liver injury, and fulminant hepatic failure can develop in patients taking these drugs (Table **2**) [35].

There is no diagnostic test for DILI, and the relationship between temporal courses of liver injury and administration or discontinuation of a drug is important in identifying the possible causative agent. The development of hepatitis within 90 days after starting a suspected drug and a 50% decrease in serum ALT 8 days after its discontinuation suggest that the drug may be causative. Drug lymphocyte stimulation tests may be helpful, but rechallenge tests are not recommended because of the risk of severe liver injury.

Table 2. Drugs and toxins associated with fulminant hepatic failure.

Acetaminophen
Amiodarone
Carbon tetrachloride
Dideoxyinosine
Gold
Halothane
Isoniazid
Ketoconazole
MAO inhibitors
Methyldopa
NSAIDs
Phenytoin
Poison mushrooms (Amanita phalloides)
Propylthiouracil
Rifampin
Sulfonamides
Tetracycline
Tricyclic antidepressants
Valproic acid

Acetaminophen Overdose (Paracetamol Overdose)

Acetaminophen overdose is a common cause of acute liver failure in both the UK (60.9%) and the USA (46%) [36, 37]. Liver injury develops 24 hours after intake, and treatment should be started before the onset of hepatotoxicity to prevent fetal liver injury. Acetaminophen-associated liver injury is dose-dependent, with massive liver injury occurring after taking more than 7 to 10g. However, intake of only 2 to 6g has been found to cause liver injury in individuals with alcoholism, malnutrition or underlying liver diseases, because of their deficiency of intracellular glutathione [38]. The risk of liver injury after an acetaminophen overdose can be estimated from its concentration in the blood and time after intake using a nomogram [39].

Drug-Induced Hypersensitivity Syndrome (DIHS)/Drug Reaction with Eosinophilia and Systemic Symptom (DRESS)

DIHS, also known as DRESS, presents clinically as an extensive mucocutaneous rash, fever, lymphadenopathy, liver injury, and hematologic abnormalities with eosinophilia and atypical lymphocytes. It may cause damage to several organs such as kidneys, heart, lungs, and pancreas by eosinophilic infiltration [40]. Its pathogenesis is related to specific drugs, altered immune response, and sequential reactivation of human herpes virus 6 and is associated with certain HLA alleles [40]. Drugs associated with DIHS include carbamazepine, phenytoin, phenobarbital, zonisamide, DDS, salazosulfapyridine, mexiletine hydrochloride, allopurinol and minocycline hydrochloride. The drugs associated with DRESS include carbamazepine (47%), allopurinol (11%), salazosulfapyridine (10%), phenobarbital (10%), lamotrigine (10%), and 39 others [41] (Table **3**). Most patients present with fever, skin rash (erythema multiforme, erythroderma), and swelling of head and neck lymph nodes 2 to 6 weeks after starting a drug, with blood tests showing leukocytosis, eosinophilia and elevated numbers of atypical lymphocytes. Liver injury occurs in 90% of these patients. Although the clinical picture of this disease resembles Steven-Johnson syndrome and toxic epidermal necrosis, it can be differentiated from these latter conditions, because DIHS shows fewer mucosal lesions and no epidermal necrotic change. Recognition of this syndrome is of significant importance, since the mortality rate is about 10% to 20%, and a specific treatment may be necessary. DIHS can be diagnosed by a greater than 4-fold elevation of IgG anti-HHV-6 antibody or the presence of serum HHV-6 DNA. Patients are treated with steroids.

Amanita Phalloides Mushroom Poisoning

The typical symptoms of *A. phalloides* mushroom poisoning are nausea, vomiting, abdominal pain, and cholera-like watery diarrhea 6 to 24 hrs after ingestion, symptoms similar to those of infectious gastroenteritis. In the absence of adequate treatment, hepatic and renal failure may progress within several days after ingestion, with the main causes of death in these patients being acute liver failure and acute renal failure. Patients have been reported successfully treated with a Molecular Adsorbent Recirculating System [42].

Alcoholic Hepatitis

The acute form of liver injury caused by alcohol abuse is alcoholic hepatitis, often associated with pre-existing alcoholic fatty liver or cirrhosis. Alcoholic hepatitis is a syndrome with jaundice and liver failure, which generally occurs after decades of heavy alcohol drinking [43]. Patients often present with fever, ascites, and loss of proximal muscle [43, 44]. Blood tests show marked elevation of serum transaminase levels, but these levels rarely exceed 300 IU/ml, and the AST/ALT ratio is usually greater than 2. White blood cell count, neutrophil count, and total serum bilirubin level are elevated, and PT is elongated. The differential diagnosis of alcoholic hepatitis includes nonalcoholic steatohepatitis, acute or chronic viral hepatitis, drug-induced liver injury, fulminant Wilson's disease, autoimmune liver disease, alpha-1 antitrypsin deficiency, pyogenic hepatic abscess, ascending cholangitis, and decompensated liver disease [43]. The prognosis of these patients is poor, with up to 40% of patients with severe alcoholic hepatitis dying within 6 months. The Model for End-Stage Liver Disease (MELD) score can predict 30-day mortality in patients hospitalized with alcoholic hepatitis [45]. Pentoxifylline (Pentoxil, Trental) has been shown to reduce mortality in patients with severe alcoholic hepatitis [46], and corticosteroids may reduce mortality in patients with severe alcoholic hepatitis or encephalopathy [47], but these findings require confirmation.

Table 3. Drugs causing drug-induced hypersensitivity syndrome (DIHS) and drug reaction with eosinophilia and systemic symptom (DRESS).

DIHS	DRESS/DIHS	
Carbamazepine	Abacavir	Imatinib
Phenytoin	Allopurinol	Lamotrigine
Phenobarbital	Amoxicillin	Mexiletine
Zonisamide	plus clavulanic acid	Minocycline
DDS	Amitriptyline	Nevirapine
Salazosulfapyridine	Atorvastatine	Olanzapine
Mexiletine	Aspirin	Oxacarbamazepine
Hydrochroride	Captopril	Phenobarbital
Allopurinol	Carbamazepine	Phenylbutazone
Minocycline	Cafadrodroxil	Phenytoin
Hydrochloride	Celecoxib	Quinine and thiamine
	Chlorambucil	Salazosulfapirydine
	Clomipramine	Sodium meglumine ioxitalamate
	Clopidrogrel	Sodium vaiproate/ethosuximide
	Codein phosphate	Spironolactone
	Cotrimoxazole/Cefixime	Streptomycin
	Cyanamide	Stronium ranelate
	Dapsone	Sulfalazine
	Diaphnylsulfone	Sulfamethoxazole
	Efalizumab	Tribenoside
	Esomeprazole	Vancomycin
	Hydroxichloroquine	Zinosamide
	Ibuprofen	

Autoimmune Liver Disease

Autoimmune liver diseases include autoimmune hepatitis, primary biliary cirrhosis, and primary sclerosing cholangitis. Only autoimmune hepatitis has been reported to present as acute hepatitis.

Autoimmune Hepatitis (AIH)

Ten to 25% of patients with autoimmune hepatitis present with acute hepatitis. Compared with patients with classical AIH, those with acute-onset AIH present with higher serum ALT levels, normal serum IgG levels, and lower AIH scores, making clinical diagnosis difficult [48]. Liver histology often reveals centrilobular necrosis and interface hepatitis in patients with acute-onset AIH. Liver biopsies are necessary if the etiology of acute liver injury is unclear. Two types of acute-onset AIH have been described. One, clinically diagnosed "acute-onset AIH", is characterized pathologically as acute exacerbation of chronic hepatitis; the other is truly "acute-onset AIH", presenting clinically and histologically as acute hepatitis [44]. Liver histology can be used to diagnose the former. In contrast, the latter often do not fulfill the criteria of classical AIH and liver histology may reveal mainly necro-inflammatory reactions around the central vein, but no or mild reactions in the portal area. Moreover, their clinicopathological features resemble those of drug-induced liver injury. The diagnosis of true acute-onset AIH may be determined by its clinical course and response to corticosteroid therapy.

Liver Injury Due to Vascular Causes

Ischemic Hepatitis

Ischemic hepatitis is the most frequent cause of acute liver injury, with a reported prevalence of up to 10% in the intensive care unit [49]. The term ischemic hepatitis is preferable to "shock liver" since the syndrome can occur in the absence of shock. Ischemic hepatitis is usually transient, with AST, ALT and LDH levels returning to normal within 7-10 days if systemic circulation recovers. Ischemic hepatitis has also been described in the setting of severe respiratory failure, systemic hypoxemia, and obstructive sleep apnea [33]. Serum bilirubin and ALP levels are generally normal or only mildly elevated. Mortality rates in patients with ischemic hepatitis are high, up to 50%, but the cause of death is related to the underlying disease, not to liver injury [50].

Hepatic Infarction

Hepatic infarction occurs most frequently after hepatobiliary surgery, transplantation or IVR therapy, but may also be caused by hepatic blood flow insufficiency due to occlusion of the hepatic artery (arteriosclerosis, thrombosis of emboli, hepatic artery aneurysm, polyarteritis nodosa, sickle-cell disease) or without occlusion (shock state, hypercoagulable state, preeclampsia, HELLP syndrome) [51]. Compromising the flow rate of the hepatic artery may also result in focal hepatic infarction, which must be distinguished from a liver abscess or tumor. Ultrasound- or CT-guided needle aspiration of the lesion may be required for a definitive diagnosis. No specific therapy for hepatic infarction is required once infection is ruled out. However, it is important to identify potential sources of emboli, such as infective endocarditis or tumor. In the absence of such a source, hypercoagulable states, including deficiency of protein C or S, abnormal or deficient antithrombin III, factor V Leiden mutation, antiphospholipid syndrome, paroxysmal nocturnal hemoglobinuria, polycythemia vera, and possibly oral contraceptive use should be considered.

Portal Vein Thrombosis (PVT)

Liver cirrhosis is the underlying liver disease in approximately 25% of adult cases with PVT. Other etiologies include pancreatitis; intra-abdominal operation such as splenectomy, cholecystectomy or colectomy; intra-abdominal infection such as appendicitis or diverticulitis; malignant tumors such as hepatocellular carcinoma or pancreatic cancer; and hypercoagulable disorders. Symptom severity depends on the extent and rate of thrombus formation. Therefore, patients with small or slow growing portal thrombi may be asymptomatic, with PVT diagnosed incidentally. Many patients with extended thrombi complain of nausea, postprandial fullness, abdominal pain or fever, and PVT should be suspected if patients with hypercoagulable disorders develop unexplained abdominal pain. Progression of thrombus formation leads to portal hypertension and intestinal ischemia; patients may present with hematochezia, ascites formation, metabolic acidosis or renal failure if intestinal infarction develops.

Early diagnosis is important, because early treatment with anticoagulants has been shown effective for the recanalization of the portal vein, and to inhibit the development of intestinal infarction. Doppler ultrasonography, contrast enhanced ultrasonography or MRI are recommended imaging tests for diagnosis. Patients are recommended to continue anticoagulation for at least 6 months, because recanalization may occur several months after start of treatment [52, 53].

Budd-Chiari Syndrome (Hepatic Vein Thrombosis)

Budd-Chiari syndrome is an uncommon disorder resulting from hepatic vein obstruction, and may be caused by a thrombotic or nonthrombotic mechanism [54]. Patients clinically manifest with the triad of hepatomegaly, ascites and abdominal pain. Most patients with Budd-Chiari syndrome have underlying diseases. In western countries, 50% of patients have a primary myeloproliferative disorder, such as polycythemia vera or chronic myelogenous leukemia. In Asian and African countries, however, most patients have membranous occlusion of the hepatic veins or inferior vena cava. Hepatic manifestations can range from an asymptomatic state to acute hepatic failure in 20% of patients. Since there are no characteristic patterns on liver function tests, Budd-Chiari syndrome should be suspected in patients with acute onset of hepatomegaly, ascites retention, and abdominal pain. Doppler ultrasonography is a noninvasive method for the diagnosis of Budd-Chiari syndrome, but its sensitivity is reported to be around 75%. Contrast enhanced CT, MRI and liver biopsy are also useful for diagnosing this condition.

Hepatic Veno-Occlusive Disease (VOD)

Hepatic veno-occlusive disease (VOD) of the liver is one of the most severe complications following high-dose chemotherapy and hematopoietic stem cell transplantation [55]. Its clinical features are similar to those of Budd-Chiari syndrome, but VOD is characterized by marked elevations of serum bilirubin and AST concentrations. Patients with severe VOD, indicated by a marked elevation of AST or an early elevation of bilirubin, have an extremely poor prognosis, with a mortality rate >80% after stem cell transplantation [56]. CT findings of periportal edema, ascites, and a narrow right hepatic vein suggest VOD [57]. Doppler ultrasonography, MRI and liver biopsy are useful for diagnosis.

Metabolic Diseases

Wilson Disease

Wilson disease (WD) is an inherited autosomal recessive disorder of copper metabolism, leading to hepatic disease and neurological disturbances. WD may present as (1) an asymptomatic elevation of transaminases; (2) chronic active hepatitis; (3) fulminant hepatic failure with hemolysis; or (4) cirrhosis. Because fulminant WD is often, but not invariably, fatal, prompt diagnosis and treatment are important. Although chronic type WD can be screened by measuring serum ceruloplasmin and/or copper concentrations, these markers appear to be less sensitive and specific in patients with fulminant hepatic failure due to WD. Rather, a recent study reported that the combination of the two tests, ALP/T-Bil ratio < 4 [94% sensitivity, 96% specificity] and AST/ALT ratio > 2.2 [94% sensitivity, 86% specificity]), provide a diagnostic sensitivity and specificity of 100% each [58]. Low AST, ALT, and choline esterase activity, high urine copper concentrations and low hemoglobin may help distinguish fulminant WD from acute hepatic failure due to other etiologies [59].

Hepatic Steatosis and Steatohepatitis

Hepatic steatosis and non-alcoholic steatohepatitis (NASH) are often asymptomatic, with patients presenting only with mildly elevated serum aminotransferases, usually less than four fold. NASH is more common in women and is associated with obesity and type 2 diabetes mellitus. In contrast to alcohol related liver disease, the ratio of AST to ALT in patients with NASH is usually less than one. Hepatic steatosis and steatohepatitis usually show chronic courses, but acute drug-induced steatohepatitis, although rare, has been observed in patients treated with amiodarone, steroid hormones, tamoxifen, valproate and perhexiline maleate [60, 61].

Liver Function Disorders Related to Pregnancy

Liver diseases specifically associated with pregnancy are described in Chapter 13.

Acute Liver Injury in Children

Etiologies of acute liver injury in children over 1 month of age include viral hepatitis, acetaminophen toxicity, autoimmune liver disease, and Wilson disease. Viral hepatitis caused by hepatitis viruses A, B and E is common in Latin America and Asia, whereas non-A-E hepatitis is common in western countries. Parvovirus, EBV, and HSV are other viruses that cause acute hepatitis in children. Most patients develop mild hepatitis, but some may develop acute liver failure [62].

Reye's syndrome, a disease exclusively found in children, is characterized by a rapidly enlarging liver due to triglyceride accumulation and hypertrophy of the smooth endoplasmic reticulum. Following common cold-like symptoms, children may present with encephalopathy, elevated concentrations of blood ammonia, and jaundice, with disorientation and coma developing thereafter. There is no specific therapy for this disease and patients with this disease die after 4 to 60 hrs, even with supportive treatment [62].

Other Infectious Diseases [33]

Weil Disease (Leptospirosis)

Leptospirosis is a major health problem in China, Brazil and other developing countries [63]. Its clinical symptoms may be mild and self-limiting, or severe, with jaundice, renal failure, and bleeding manifestations. The more severe type of leptospirosis is called Weil disease. Transmission occurs by contact with urine from infected animals, with incubation periods ranging from 4 days to 4 weeks [64]. There are two clinical phases, the first often marked by jaundice, which lasts for weeks; and the second characterized by jaundice and marked elevation of serum transaminases. Serum bilirubin concentrations may be as high as 30 mg/dl, but elevations of serum transaminases and ALP are usually moderate.

Thrombocytopenia occurs frequently and is associated with poor prognosis. Renal failure, cardiac arrhythmia and hemorrhagic pneumonitis are common complications during the second phase. Mortality rates of patients with severe forms of this disease have been reported high, even when optimally treated. Early clinical suspicion and prompt diagnosis of leptospirosis is important, since delays in diagnosis may increase mortality [64]. Diagnosis is based on the detection of IgM antibody to leptospira by ELISA during the first week of the disease. Leptospiral DNA can also be detected by PCR, but this method has limited availability in developing countries. Patients with mild disease are treated with doxycycline, and those with severe disease treated with intravenous penicillin [65].

Dengue Fever(DF) / Dengue Hemorrhagic Fever(DHF)

Dengue is the most important arthropod-borne viral disease of public health significance, and is present in more than 100 countries worldwide [66]. Dengue fever (DF) is caused by four different serotypes of dengue viruses. The disease ranges from a relatively minor febrile illness to a life-threatening condition characterized by extensive capillary leak, leading to hemorrhage and shock called dengue hemorrhagic fever (DHF) [67]. DF is endemic in Southeast Asia, Africa and South America. Dengue virus has been estimated to cause over 100 million infections worldwide per year, with 250 thousand of these patients developing DHF. Dengue virus-induced liver injury is thought to be mediated by direct viral infection of hepatocytes and Kupffer cells. Mild to moderate elevations of serum transaminases (ALT and AST < 5x normal) with hepatomegaly are common in dengue virus infection, with liver failure rarely developing [68]. Other laboratory findings include decreased white blood cells and platelets. Diagnosis is based on the elevation of IgM antibody against Dengue NS-1 antigen or positivity for reverse transcriptase-PCR.

Typhoid Fever

Typhoid fever remains endemic in Southeast Asia, India, Eastern Europe, Africa and South America. Although marked elevation of serum ALT is rare, jaundice has been observed in 33% of these patients. The clinical features of *Salmonella* hepatitis are similar to those of acute viral hepatitis [33]. However, these diseases may be distinguished by the ALT/LDH ratio, which is < 4.0 in *Salmonella* hepatitis and >5.0 ratio in patients with acute viral hepatitis [69].

Malaria

Malaria is endemic in Southeast Asia, India, and Africa, and may infect travelers to these areas as well as being transmitted through blood transfusions. About 37% of patients with malaria show increased bilirubin, transaminase, ALP and γ-GTP levels. Liver histology revealed the activation of Kupffer cells, with granules of brown-black malarial pigment and iron deposits [70]. Some patients may develop encephalopathy with elevated blood ammonia. Liver dysfunction usually recovers after malarian infection improves, but some patients may progress to multiple organ dysfunctions.

Clostridium Perfringens Infection

C. perfringens may directly affect the liver, in which the pathogen forms an abscess or causes necrotizing massive gas gangrene of the liver, may leading to fulminant hepatic failure [71].

Other infections which involve the liver are Lyme Disease, Q fever, *syphilis*, *Campylobacter* infection, *Clamidya* or *Neisseria* infection, *Mycobacteria* infection, and fungal infection, and liver dysfunctions caused by these infections. Moreover, liver is often involved in hematological malignancies, heat stroke, and metabolic diseases. Clinical features of liver dysfunction are summarized in our previous review [33].

FULMINANT HEPATIC FAILURE AND THE PREDICTION OF PROGNOSIS

Fulminant hepatic failure refers to the rapid development of severe acute liver injury with impaired synthetic function and the development of encephalopathy in patients with previously normal livers or well-compensated liver disease (Fig. **3**).

Three types of fulminant liver failure have been described [13]. (1) Hyperacute liver failure refers to an interval <7 days from the onset of jaundice to the development of encephalopathy; (2) Acute liver failure refers to an interval of 8 to 28 days. (3) Subacute liver failure refers to an interval of 4 to 12 weeks. Patient prognosis correlated inversely with the duration of the interval, with patients with shorter intervals having a better prognosis [72].

Many causes of fulminant liver failure have been described (Table **4**), but their frequency differs geographically (Fig. **4**) [73-80]. Although hepatitis A is the most common cause of acute hepatitis, progression to FHF is relatively rare (<1%). Hepatitis B is probably the most common viral cause of FHF [81], with patient prognosis differing by etiology. Therefore, etiology should be determined, not only to choose appropriate treatment, but also for early prediction of patient prognosis.

A.
> Acute onset of progressive jaundice, decrease in the size of the liver, fetor hepaticus and hepatiic coma:
>
> 1. Within 8 weeks of symptoms
> 2. Patients with no previous liver disease

B.

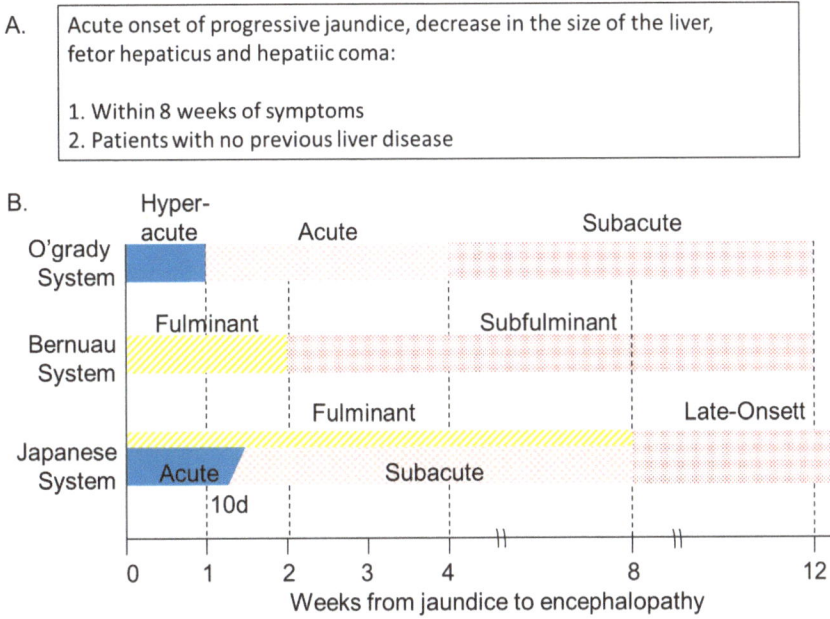

Figure 3: Classic definition and classification systems of acute liver failure **A:** Classic definition **B:** Classification systems for acute liver failure [13, 71, 72].

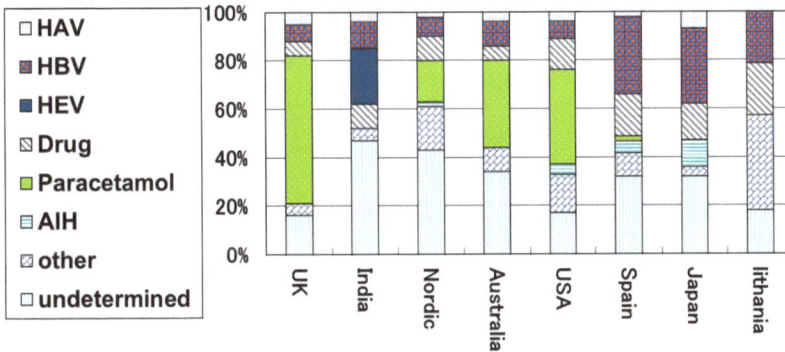

Figure 4: Causes of fulminant hepatic failure in various countries [73-80].

Symptoms suggesting progression to fulminant hepatic failure include severe and longstanding malaise, nausea, vomiting and anorexia, whereas signs suggesting FHF include liver atrophy and ascites retention, both of which should be confirmed by ultrasonography or CT imaging. Liver volume is associated with patient prognosis, with severe liver atrophy strongly linked to poor prognosis. However, liver size usually increases in patients with alcoholic hepatitis, even those with severe disease CT findings in patients with fulminant hepatitis are decreased liver size, diffuse or localized (solitary or multiple) areas of hypoattenuation in the liver, dilatation of the portal vein, and narrow or nondepicted hepatic veins [82]. Moreover, ascites retention around the liver often indicates acute portal hypertension caused by massive hepatic necrosis.

Laboratory data suggesting FHF include prolongation of PT, elevation of T-Bil with decreased D-Bil/T-Bil ratio, decreased BUN, decreased ratio of BCAA/AAA, and elevation of blood ammonia. High HGF concentration and low AFP level may indicate poor liver regeneration, suggesting poor patient prognosis. Continuously elevated T-Bil with prolongation of PT are important in identifying patients at high risk of developing FHF.

Table 4. Mnemonics for causes of fulminant hepatic failure: The ABCs.

A	Acetaminophen, hepatitis A, autoimmune hepatitis
B	Hepatitis B
C	Cryptogenic, hepatitis C
D	Hepatitis D, drugs
E	Esoteric causes - Wilson's disease, Budd-Chiari syndrome
F	Fatty Infiltration - acute fatty liver of pregnancy, Reye's syndrome

Table 5. Prognostic criteria for all patients (non-paracetamol) with fulminant hepatic failure for transplantation [13, 71, 72].

King's College Hospital criteria

INR > 6.5 or any three of the following:
(1) indeterminate cause of acute liver failure
(2) age < 10 or > 40 years
(3) jaundice to coma interval > 7 days
(4) bilirubin > 300 µM/L
(5) INR > 3.5

Clichy's Criteria

Age<30
Encephalopathy stages 3-4 and factor V < 20%
Age>30
or encephalopathy stages 3-4 and factor V < 30%

Japanese Criteria

Grade II or more severe hepatic encephalopathy and any 2 of the following:
(1) age ≥45 years
(2) Interval from the initial symptoms to hepatic encephalopathy ≥11 days
(3) Prothrombin time <10 % of the standardized value
(4) Serum bilirubin concentration ≥18.0 mg/dL
(5) Ratio of the direct to total bilirubin concentration <0.67

Factors predicting the prognosis of patients with FHF are summarized in Table **5** [13, 71, 72]. Because liver transplantation shows good results in patients with FHF, with a 5-year survival rate >70%, early identification of patients with poor prognosis and risk of FHF is needed for prompt transfer to a liver transplant center. Although the King's College and Clichy's criteria are frequently utilized to assess prognosis in patients with FHF, MELD and PELD scores have proven superior in assessing prognosis in patients with FHF [83]. Details are described in Chapter 15.

TREATMENT OF ACUTE HEPATITIS

Supportive therapy with fluid and nutrition is considered only for patients with nausea, vomiting and anorexia. There is no specific therapy for acute hepatitis caused by hepatitis viruses A, D and E. Because acute viral hepatitis is a physiologic reaction designed to eliminate the infective virus, any therapy attempting to suppress acute hepatitis may lead to retardation of viral elimination, leading to prolonged liver injury.

Specific therapies should be considered for the following acute liver injuries (Table **6**).

Table 6. Etiology-specific therapies for acute hepatic failure.

Acetaminophen toxicity: N- acetylcysteine
Drug-induced hypersensitivity syndrome(DIHS) : corticosteroid
Adult-onset Still's disease (AOSD): corticosteroid
Autoimmune hepatitis: corticosteroid
Hepatitis B: lamivudine, entecavir, tenofovir
Hepatitis C: interferon? Direct-acting antiviral agents?
Cytomegalovirus: sometimes gancyclovir
Wilson's disease: D-penicillamine
Varicella zoster and herpes zoster virus: acyclovir
Portal vein thrombosis : emergency operation, urokinase, tPA, heparin
Pregnancy: delivery of fetus
Weil disease(Leptospirosis): doxycycline or penicillin G
Relapsing fever : tetracycline or streptomycin
Malaria: anti-malaria drug

Acetaminophen Poisoning

The initial treatment for paracetamol overdose is gastrointestinal decontamination. Activated charcoal is the most common agent as it adsorbs paracetamol, reducing its gastrointestinal absorption [84]. Benefits from activated charcoal are optimal if given within 30 minutes to two hours of ingestion. Acetylcysteine, also called N-acetylcysteine (NAC), reduces paracetamol toxicity by replenishing body stores of the antioxidant glutathione. NAC is usually administered according to a treatment nomogram. Intravenous acetylcysteine is continuously infused over 20 hours for a total dose of 300 mg/kg. The recommended protocol involves infusion of a 150 mg/kg loading dose over 15 to 60 minutes, followed by a 50 mg/kg infusion over four hours; with the last 100 mg/kg infused over 16 hours [85].

Acute Hepatitis B

Antiviral treatment should be considered for patients with severe acute hepatitis B to inhibit progression to fulminant hepatitis. Early treatment with lamivudine has been shown to have clinical benefits and to reduce mortality rate [86]. Patients with prolonged PT-INR ($\geq$1.6), encephalopathy or elevated T-Bil (>10 mg/dl) may be candidates for therapy [87]. However, since seroconversion rates to anti-HBs may be reduced by antiviral treatment, and there are no standard guidelines for dose and duration of therapy, indications for treatment should be carefully determined. Anti-viral agents to consider include lamivudine, telbivudine, adefovir, entecavir, and tenofovir.

Acute Hepatitis C

About 80% of patients with acute hepatitis C develop chronic infection. Thus, 20% of patients spontaneously recover without treatment, whereas the remainder require treatment with interferon. Peg-IFN treatment has been shown to achieve a high (>90%) sustained virological response rate. Optimal treatment duration has not been determined, but 8 to 12 weeks has been reported effective in patients infected with HCV genotypes 2, 3, and 4, and 24 weeks in patients infected with HCV genotype 1 [88, 89]. Patients positive for serum HCV-RNA at week 8 are likely to develop a persistent infection.

Cytomegalovirus Hepatitis

Most patients primarily infected with cytomegalovirus show self-limiting disease course and require no specific therapy. However, infants and immunocompromized individuals may progress to severe acute hepatitis and should therefore be treated with ganciclovir.

Acute Onset Autoimmune Hepatitis

Ten to 25% of patients with AIH present with acute hepatitis, and some may progress to FHF. The most common forms of FHF associated with AIH are subacute and late-onset hepatic failure, with acute hepatic failure being relatively rare. Treatment of AIH associated acute hepatitis or FHF is the same as that for chronic autoimmune hepatitis, but patients with FHF often show resistance to corticosteroid therapy including pulse therapy, resulting in low survival rates without liver transplantation (20-46%) [90].

Wilson Disease

Many patients with fulminant Wilsonian hepatic failure require orthotopic liver transplantation. Although the diagnosis of fulminant form of Wilson disease is difficult because the patients show unique clinical features and sometimes lack Kayser-Fleisher rings, patients suspected of fulminant Wilsonian hepatic failure should be promptly transferred to a liver transplantation center.

INITIAL AND COMMON TREATMENT OF FULMINANT HEPATIC FAILURE

Treatment of acute hepatic failure has been improving, but the only therapy proven to significantly improve patient outcome in FHF is orthotopic liver transplantation (OLT). Indications for OLT should be analyzed and determined by hepatologists. Thus, patients with liver failure should be transferred as early as possible to a transplant center, since transportation may be hazardous if complications develop, such as severe coagulopathy or increased intracranial pressure. Before transfer to a transplantation center, blood glucose level, brain edema, encephalopathy, coagulopathy, infection and renal injury should be evaluated, and appropriate treatments administered.

MESSAGES FROM HEPATOLOGISTS TO GENERAL PHYSICIANS

1. The most important point for management of acute liver injury is to determine whether the patient has the potential to develop fulminant hepatic failure. Prothrombin time and serum bilirubin levels are key tests for making this judgment. In acute hepatitis, prothrombin activity (%) usually remains over 60% throughout the clinical course, and a decrease to below 60% suggests severe liver injury with possible transition to fulminant hepatic failure.

2. The levels of serum transaminases are not well correlated with the severity of liver injury, and patients with subacute type fulminant hepatic failure usually show only moderate, but sustained, elevation of serum transaminase levels.

3. In most cases of acute viral hepatitis, the patient recovers without specific treatment. However, in patients with acute hepatitis C, early administration of antiviral agents should be performed to inhibit transition to chronic hepatitis. In acute hepatitis B, nucleot(s)ide analogs may be required in patients with severe injury to inhibit the transition to fulminant hepatitis. Therefore, these patients should be referred to a hepatologist.

4. Acute hepatitis C cannot be diagnosed by positivity for anti-HCV antibody, because the antibody becomes positive 2 – 3 months after acute infection. HCV RNA must be examined to diagnose acute hepatitis due to HCV infection.

5. In daily clinical practice, common causes of mild to moderate acute liver injury are DILI and liver injury caused by viral (either hepatitis virus or non-hepatitis virus) or bacterial infection. The common pattern of DILI is a hepatocellular or mixed type (hepatocellular and cholestatic).

6. Uncommon but important causes of acute liver injury include acute onset autoimmune hepatitis or Wilsonian fulminant hepatitis, both of which require prompt treatment after diagnosis.

7. Abdominal ultrasound imaging should be performed in all patients with acute liver injury and the following findings should be explored: fatty deposits in the liver, abnormal liver size, ascites retention, splenomegaly, bile duct dilatation, and gallstones. It should be noted that the presence of stones in the common bile duct cannot be excluded by ultrasound alone, because the lower part of the duct cannot be observed by ultrasound. On the other hand, gallbladder stones can be invisible on plain computed tomography (CT) if the stones are composed of pure cholesterol.

8. Liver enlargement without ascites is common in acute hepatitis, and atrophic liver, irregular areas of low density in the parenchyma of the liver on plain CT, or ascites retention indicate severe liver injury, and may suggest transition to fulminant hepatic failure.

9. Splenomegaly is commonly observed in acute viral hepatitis, whereas DILI rarely shows splenomegaly, which could help in the differential diagnosis.

ACKNOWLEDGEMENTS

We are very thankful to Ms. Asma Ahmed, manager publications, Bentham Science Publishers, for her patience and long-term assistance.

CONFLICT OF INTEREST

The author confirms that he has no conflict of interest to declare for this publication.

REFERENCES

[1]   Rozen P, Korn RJ, Zimmerman HJ. Computer analysis of liver function tests and their interrelationships in 347 cases of viral hepatitis. Isr J Med Sci 1970;6:67-79.
[2]   Dufour DR, Lott JA, Nolte FS, Gretch DR, Koff RS, Seeff LB. Diagnosis and monitoring of hepatic injury. II. Recommendations for use of laboratory tests in screening, diagnosis, and monitoring. Clin Chem 2000;46:2050-2068.
[3]   Mendenhall CL. Alcoholic hepatitis. The VA Cooperative Study Group on Alcoholic Hepatitis. Clin Gastroenterol 1981;10:417-41.
[4]   Mihas AA, Doos WG, Spenney JG. Alcoholic hepatitis—a clinical and pathological study of 142 cases. J Chronic Dis 1978;31:461-72.
[5]   Goldberg S, Mendenhall C, Anderson S, *et al*. VA cooperative study on alcoholic hepatitis. IV. The significance of clinically mild alcoholic hepatitis—describing the population with minimal hyperbilirubinemia. Am J Gastroenterol 1986;81:1029-1034.
[6]   Nissenbaum M, Chedid A, Mendenhall C, Gartside P. Prognostic significance of cholestatic alcoholic hepatitis. Dig Dis Sci 1990;35:891-896.
[7]   Cohen JA, Kaplan MM. The SGOT/SGPT ratio—an indicator of alcoholic liver disease. Dig Dis Sci 1979;24:835-838.
[8]   Lednar WM, Lemon SM, Kirkpatrick JW, Redfield RR, Fields ML, Kelley PW. Frequency of illness associated with epidemic hepatitis A virus infections in adults. Am J Epidemiol 1985;122:226-233.
[9]   Gitlin N. Hepatitis B: diagnosis, prevention, and treatment. Clin Chem 1997;43:1500-1506.
[10]   McMahon BJ, Alward WL, Hall DB, Heyward WL, Bender TR, Francis DP, *et al*. Acute hepatitis B virus infection: relation of age to the clinical expression of disease and subsequent development of the carrier state. J Infect Dis 1985;151:599-603.
[11]   Hoofnagel JH. Hepatitis C: the clinical spectrum of disease. Hepatology 1997;26(Suppl 1):15-20.
[12]   Seeff LB, Wright EC, Zimmerman HJ, McCollum VA. Cooperative study of post-transfusion hepatitis, 1969–1974: incidence and characteristics of hepatitis and responsible risk factors. Am J Med Sci 1975;270:355-362.
[13]   O'Grady JG, Schalm SW, Williams R. Acute liver failure: redefining the syndromes. Lancet 1993;342:273-275.
[14]   O'Grady JG. Acute liver failure. Postgrad Med J 2005;81:148-54.
[15]   Julie Polson, William M. Lee. Etiologies of acute liver failure: Location, location, location 2007;13:1362–1363.
[16]   Danni Daniels, MS, Scott Grytdal, MPH, Annemarie Wasley, ScD. Surveillance for acute viral hepatitis --- United States, 2007. CDC Surveillance Summaries. May 22, 2009 / 58(SS03);1-2.
[17]   Centers for Disease Control and Prevention (CDC).Hepatitis E among U.S. travelers, 1989-1992.MMWR Morb Mortal Wkly Rep 1993;42:1-4.
[18]   Kwo PY, Schlauder GG, Carpenter HA *et al*. Acute Hepatitis E by a new isolate acquired in the United States. Mayo Clinic Proceeding 1997;72:1133-1136.
[19]   K Noso, M Kouda, K Yamamoto, Acute hepatitis national survey results, Current status of acute hepatitis in Japan. K Yamamoto, M Kouda, K Noso (Edt);2012 Cyuugai igakusya:1-12.
[20]   J. Heathcote. Management of acute viral hepatitis. World Gastroenterology Organisation Practice Guidelines 2003

[21]   Aggarwal R, Krawczynski K. Hepatitis E: an overview and recent advances in clinical and laboratory research. J Gastroenterol Hepatol 2000;15:9-20.

[22]   R Aggarwal, K Krawczynski, Chapter 80 Hepatitis E, M Feldman, L S. Friedmaan, L J. Brandt (Edt), Sleisenger and Fordtran's Gastrointestinal and Liver Disease 9th edition:2010 Saunders Elesevier:1337-1342.

[23]   Gershburg E, Pagano JS. Epstein-Barr virus infections: prospects for treatment. J Antimicrob Chemother 2005;56:277-281.

[24]   Ljungman P, Griffiths P, Paya C. Definitions of cytomegalovirus infection and disease in transplant recipients. Clin Infect Dis 2002;34:1094-1097.

[25]   Kang AH, Graves CR.Herpes simplex hepatitis in pregnancy: a case report and review of the literature.Obstet Gynecol Surv 1999;54:463-468.

[26]   Pellisé M, Miquel R. Liver failure due to herpes simplex virus. J Hepatol 2000;32:170.

[27]   Grant RM, Weitzman SS, Sherman CG, Sirkin WL, Petric M, Tellier R. Fulminant disseminated Varicella Zoster virus infection without skin involvement. J Clin Virol 2002;24:7-12.

[28]   Mizoguchi F, Nakamura S, Iwai H, Kubota T, Miyasaka N. Varicella-zoster virus hepatitis in polymyositis. Mod Rheumatol 2008;18:301-305.

[29]   Arvin AM. Varicella-zoster virus. Clin Microbiol Rev 1996;9:361-381.

[30]   Bihari C, Rastogi A, Saxena P, Rangegowda D, Chowdhury A, Gupta N, Sarin SK. Parvovirus B19 Associated Hepatitis. Hepat Res Treat 2013;2013:472027.

[31]   Dinh A, Fleuret V, Hanslik T. Liver involvement in adults with measles. Int J Infect Dis 2013;17:e1243-1244.

[32]   Ronan BA, Agrwal N, Carey EJ, De Petris G, Kusne S, Seville MT, Blair JE, Vikram HR. Fulminant hepatitis due to human adenovirus. Infection 2014;42:105-111.

[33]   Shimizu Y.Liver in systemic disease.World J Gastroenterol 2008;14:4111-4119.

[34]   Gordon SC. Bacterial and systemic infections. In: Schiff ER, Sorrell MF, Maddrey WC, editors. Schiff's Diseases of the Liver. 9th ed. Tokyo: Lippincott William & Wilkins, 2003:1529-1545.

[35]   Murray KF1, Hadzic N, Wirth S, Bassett M, Kelly D.J. Drug-related hepatotoxicity and acute liver failure. Pediatr Gastroenterol Nutr 2008;47:395-405.

[36]   Williams R, Wendon J. Indications for orthotopic liver transplantation in fulminant liver failure. Hepatology 1994;20:S5-10S.

[37]   Lee WM, Squires RH Jr, Nyberg SL, Doo E, Hoofnagle JH. Acute liver failure: Summary of a workshop.Hepatology 2008;47:1401-1415.

[38]   N C. Teon, S Chitturi, G C.Farrell. Chapter 86 Liver disease caused by drugs. M Feldman, L S. Friedmaan, L J. Brandt (Eds), Sleisenger and Fordtran's Gastrointestinal and Liver Disease, 9th edition, 2010 Saunders Elesevier, 1413-1446.

[39]   Chomchai S, Lawattanatrakul N, Chomchai C. Acetaminophen Psi Nomogram: a sensitive and specific clinical tool to predict hepatotoxicity secondary to acute acetaminophen overdose. J Med Assoc Thai 2014;97:165-172.

[40]   Criado PR, Criado RF, Avancini Jde M, Santi CG.Drug reaction with Eosinophilia and Systemic Symptoms (DRESS) / Drug-induced hypersensitivity syndrome (DIHS): a review of current concepts. An Bras Dermatol 2012 ;87:435-449.

[41]   Cacoub P, Musette P, Descamps V, Meyer O, Speirs C, Finzi L, *et al*. The DRESS syndrome: a literature review. Am J Med 2011;124:588-597.

[42]   Covic A, Goldsmith DJ, Gusbeth-Tatomir P, Volovat C, Dimitriu AG, Cristogel F, Bizo A. Successful use of molecular absorbent regenerating system (MARS) dialysis for the treatment of fulminant hepatic failure in children accidentally poisoned by toxic mushroom ingestion. Liver Int 2003;23 Suppl 3:21-27.

[43]   Lucey MR, Mathurin P, Morgan TR. Alcoholic hepatitis. N Engl J Med 2009; 360: 2758–2769.

[44]   Lieber CS. Biochemical and molecular basis of alcohol-induced injury to liver and other tissues. N Engl J Med 1988;319:1639-1650.

[45]   Monsanto P, Almeida N, Lrias C, Pina JE, Sofia C. Evaluation of MELD score and Maddrey discriminant function for mortality prediction in patients with alcoholic hepatitis. Hepatogastroenterology 2013; 60:1089-1094.

[46]   Akriviadis E, Botla R, Briggs W, *et al*. Pentoxifylline improves short term survival in severe alcoholic hepatitis: a double blind, placebo controlled trial. Gastroenterology 2000;119:1637-1648.

[47]   Mathurin P, O'Grady J, Carithers RL, *et al.* Corticosteroids improve short-term survival in patients with severe alcoholic hepatitis: meta-analysis of individual patient data. Gut 2011;60:255-260.

[48]   Tokumoto Y, Onji M. Acute-onset autoimmune hepatitis. Intern Med. 2007;46:1-2.

[49]   Fuhrmann V, Jäger B, Zubkova A, Drolz A. Hypoxic hepatitis - epidemiology, pathophysiology and clinical management. Wien Klin Wochenschr 2010;122:129-139.

[50]   Henrion J. Hypoxic hepatitis. Liver Int 2012;32:1039-1052.

[51]   Francque S, Condat B, Asselah T, Vilgrain V, Durand F, Moreau R, Valla D. Multifactorial aetiology of hepatic infarction: a case report with literature review. Eur J Gastroenterol Hepatol 2004;16:411-415.

[52]   Sheen CL, Lamparelli H, Milne A, Green I, Ramage JK. Clinical features, diagnosis and outcome of acute portal vein thrombosis. QJM 2000;93:531-534.

[53]   Condat B, Valla D. Nonmalignant portal vein thrombosis in adults. Nat Clin Pract Gastroenterol Hepatol 2006;3:505-515.

[54]   Brancatelli G, Vilgrain V, Federle MP, Hakime A, Lagalla R, Iannaccone R, Valla D. Budd-Chiari syndrome: spectrum of imaging findings. AJR Am J Roentgenol 2007;188:W168-176.

[55]   Kumar S, DeLeve LD, Kamath PS, Tefferi A. Hepatic veno-occlusive disease (sinusoidal obstruction syndrome) after hematopoietic stem cell transplantation. Mayo Clin Proc 2003;78:589-598.

[56]   Wadleigh M, Ho V, Momtaz P, Richardson P. Hepatic veno-occlusive disease: pathogenesis, diagnosis and treatment. Curr Opin Hematol 2003;10:451-462.

[57]   Erturk SM, Mortelé KJ, Binkert CA, Glickman JN, Oliva MR, Ros PR, Silverman SG. CT features of hepatic venoocclusive disease and hepatic graft-*versus*-host disease in patients after hematopoietic stem cell transplantation. AJR Am J Roentgenol 2006;186:1497-501.

[58]   Jessica D. Korman *et al.* Hepatology 2008;48:1167-1174.

[59]   Christoph Eisenbach, *et al.* World J Gastroenterol 2007;13:1711-1714

[60]   Farrell GC. Drugs and steatohepatitis. Semin Liver Dis 2002;22:185-194.

[61]   Stravitz RT, Sanyal AJ. Drug-induced steatohepatitis. Clin Liver Dis 2003;7:435-451.

[62]   Rodés J, Benhaumou JP, Blei AT, Reichen J, Rizzetto M, editors. Textbook of Hepatology. 3rd ed. Oxford: Blackwell Publishing, 2007, pp1845-1869.

[63]   World Health Organization, Weekly Epidemiological Record, 1999;74:237–44

[64]   Gancheva G, Karcheva M. Icterohaemorrhagic leptospirosis in patients with history of alcohol abuse - report of two cases. Turk J Gastroenterol 2013;24:549-555.

[65]   Forbes AE, Zochowski WJ, Dubrey SW, Sivaprakasam V. Leptospirosis and Weil's disease in the UK. QJM 2012;105:1151-1162.

[66]   Tantawichien T. Dengue fever and dengue haemorrhagic fever in adolescents and adults. Paediatr Int Child Health 2012;32 Suppl 1:22-27.

[67]   Shah I. Dengue and liver disease. Scand J Infect Dis 2008;40(11-12):993-994.

[68]   Ling LM, Wilder-Smith A, Leo YS. Fulminant hepatitis in dengue haemorrhagic fever. J Clin Virol 2007;38:265-268.

[69]   Gitlin N. Liver involvement in systemic infection. In: Gitlin N editor. The Liver and Systemic Disease. Hong Kong: Pearson Professional Limited,1997:229-236.

[70]   Goljan J, Nahorski W, Felczak-Korzybska I, Górski J, Myjak P. Liver injury in the course of malaria. Int Marit Health 2000;51:30-39.

[71]   Bernuau J, Rueff B, Benhamou JP. Fulminant and subfulminant liver failure:definitions and causes. Semin Liver Dis1986;6:97-106.

[72]   Mochida S, Nakayama N, Matsui A,Nagoshi S, Fujiwara K. Re-evaluation of the Guideline published by the Acute Liver Failure Study Group of Japan in 1996 to determine the indications of liver transplantation in patients with fulminant hepatitis. Hepatol Res 2008;38:970-979.

[73]   Roger Williams, Julia Wendon.Indications for orthotopic liver transplantation in fulminant liver failure. hepatology 1994;20 Suppl 7:S5-S10

[74]   Acharya SK1, Panda SK, Saxena A, Gupta SD.Acute hepatic failure in India: a perspective from the East.J Gastroenterol Hepatol 2000;15:473-479.

[75]   Brandsaeter B1, Höckerstedt K, Friman S, Ericzon BG, Kirkegaard P, Isoniemi H, Olausson M, Broome U, Schmidt L, Foss A, Bjøro K.Fulminant hepatic failure: outcome after listing for highly urgent liver transplantation-12 years experience in the nordic countries.Liver Transpl 2002;8:1055-1062.

[76]   Gow PJ1, Jones RM, Dobson JL, Angus PW.Etiology and outcome of fulminant hepatic failure managed at an Australian liver transplant unit.J Gastroenterol Hepatol 2004;19:154-159.

[77]   Ostapowicz G, Fontana RJ, Schiodt FV, Larson A, Davern TJ, Han SH, McCashland TM, Shakil AO, Hay JE, Hynan L, Crippin JS, Blei AT, Samuel G, Reisch J, Lee WM; U.S. Acute Liver Failure Study Group.Results of a prospective study of acute liver failure at 17 tertiary care centers in the United States. Ann Intern Med 2002;137:947-954.

[78]   Escorsell A, Mas A, de la Mata M; Spanish Group for the Study of Acute Liver Failure. Acute liver failure in Spain: analysis of 267 cases. Liver Transpl 2007;13:1389-1395.

[79]   Miyake Y1, Iwasaki Y, Makino Y, Kobashi H, Takaguchi K, Ando M, Sakaguchi K, Shiratori Y.Prognostic factors for fatal outcomes prior to receiving liver transplantation in patients with non-acetaminophen-related fulminant hepatic failure. J Gastroenterol Hepatol 2007;22:855-861.

[80]   Adukauskiene D, Dockiene I, Naginiene R, Kevelaitis E, Pundzius J, Kupcinskas L. Acute liver failure in Lithuania. Medicina (Kaunas) 2008;44:536-540.

[81]   Lee WM, Squires RH Jr, Nyberg SL, Doo E, Hoofnagle JH. Acute liver failure: Summary of a workshop. Hepatology 2008 47:1401-415.

[82]   Itai Y. CT findings of fulminant hepatitis: terminology and distribution of massive necrosis. Radiology 1996;200:872.

[83]   Yantorno SE1, Kremers WK, Ruf AE, Trentadue JJ, Podestá LG, Villamil FG.MELD is superior to King's college and Clichy's criteria to assess prognosis in fulminant hepatic failure.Liver Transpl 2007;13:822-828.

[84]   Spiller HA, Sawyer TS.Impact of activated charcoal after acute acetaminophen overdoses treated with N-acetylcysteine. J Emerg Med 2007;33:141-144.

[85]   Daly FF1, Fountain JS, Murray L, Graudins A, Buckley NA; Panel of Australian and New Zealand clinical toxicologists.Guidelines for the management of paracetamol poisoning in Australia and New Zealand--explanation and elaboration. A consensus statement from clinical toxicologists consulting to the Australasian poisons information centres. Med J Aust 2008;188:296-301.

[86]   Yu JW, Sun LJ, Zhao YH, Kang P, Li SC. The study of efficacy of lamivudine in patients with severe acute hepatitis B. Dig Dis Sci 2010;55:775-783.

[87]   Kumar M, Satapathy S, Monga R, Das K, Hissar S, Pande C, Sharma BC, Sarin SK. A randomized controlled trial of lamivudine to treat acute hepatitis B. Hepatology 2007;45:97-101.

[88]   Kamal SM, Moustafa KN, Chen J, Fehr J, Abdel Moneim A, Khalifa KE, El Gohary LA, Ramy AH, Madwar MA, Rasenack J, Afdhal NH. Duration of peginterferon therapy in acute hepatitis C: a randomized trial. Hepatology 2006;43:923-931.

[89]   Kamal SM, Fouly AE, Kamel RR, Hockenjos B, Al Tawil A, Khalifa KE, He Q, Koziel MJ, El Naggar KM, Rasenack J, Afdhal NH. Peginterferon alfa-2b therapy in acute hepatitis C: impact of onset of therapy on sustained virologic response. Gastroenterology 2006;130:632-638.

[90]   Ichai P, Duclos-Vallée JC, Guettier C, Hamida SB, Antonini T, Delvart V, Saliba F, Azoulay D, Castaing D, Samuel D. Usefulness of corticosteroids for the treatment of severe and fulminant forms of autoimmune hepatitis. Liver Transpl 2007;13:996-1003.

CHAPTER 4

Approach to Patients with Chronic Liver Injury

Yukihiro Shimizu*

Gastroenterology Center, Nanto Municipal Hospital, Japan

Abstract: Patients presenting with chronic liver injury should be classified as having hepatocellular, cholestatic or mixed injury, because classification can narrow the causes of injury, making history taking and physical examination more effective. Diagnosis of drug- and alcohol-induced liver injury depends on careful history taking. Most patients with chronic liver diseases are asymptomatic, and key examinations for the diagnosis of each disease should be performed in an effective order. Severity of liver injury is estimated by PT-INR and T-Bil. Patients at risk for transition to hepatic failure should likely be transferred to a transplantation center.

Keywords: Autoimmune liver disease, cholestatic type, chronic liver injury, hepatocellular carcinoma, hepatocellular type, hereditary liver disease, liver cirrhosis, medical history, physical examination, viral hepatitis.

KEY POINTS

1. History taking and physical examination are important in the differential diagnosis of chronic liver injury, with history of alcohol or drug taking essential in diagnosing liver disease caused by these materials.

2. Type of liver injury should be classified as hepatocellular, cholestatic or mixed, because classification can help narrow the causes of liver injuries and suggest additional and effective history taking or physical examination.

3. Symptoms in patients with chronic liver diseases are nonspecific, with the most common being fatigue. Although patients with advanced liver cirrhosis often complain of pruritus, anorexia, leg edema and/or abdominal distension due to ascites retention, most patients with chronic hepatitis and early stage cirrhosis are asymptomatic.

*Corresponding author Yukihiro Shimiizu: Gastroenterology Center, Nanto Municipal Hospital, Toyama, Japan; E-mail: rsf14240@nifty.com

4. Differential diagnosis can be a step-by-step process in the absence of severe or advanced liver injury. Elevated T-Bil (>2.0 mg/dl) or elongation of prothrombin time (PT) may suggest severe injury. Although marked elevation of serum aspartate aminotransferase (AST) and/or alanine aminotransferase (ALT) is also an indicator of severe liver injury, there is no clear threshold.

5. Frequency of etiologies of chronic liver injury may differ geographically or ethnically, with the order of blood tests based on the prevalence of each disease in that area.

6. Primary care providers should be aware of the diagnostic criteria for common chronic liver diseases. These providers should also be familiar with methods used to initially assess liver injury, as well as when to refer patients to specialists.

7. Liver biopsy is useful not only to identify etiology, but to determine the grading and staging of liver disease and to assess the likelihood of progression to cirrhosis or liver failure.

8. Cirrhosis is often diagnosed by a combination of laboratory data and patient signs and symptoms. In particular, AST/ALT>1, hypergammaglobulinemia and low platelet count (<100,000/μL) support a diagnosis of cirrhosis. Imaging modalities are also helpful diagnostically, and the presence of portal hypertension (suggested by splenomegaly, enlarged portal vein or esophageal varices) strongly supports a diagnosis of cirrhosis.

9. Patients with advanced chronic liver diseases are at high risk for the development of hepatocellular carcinoma (HCC), and should be assessed by imaging modalities such as ultrasound (US), CT, and MRI, or by measuring serum concentrations of tumor markers, such as alpha-fetoprotein and des-γ-carboxy prothrombin at regular intervals.

INTRODUCTION

The term "chronic liver injury" usually refers to liver injury lasting longer than 6 months. Practically, however, patients who show mild to moderate abnormalities on liver function tests (LFTs) at two different time points should be suspected of having chronic liver disease. Since second tests have been reported to show resolution of initially elevated levels of bilirubin, AST, ALT, alkaline phosphatase (ALP), and γ-GTP in 12% to 38% of patients, these patients should again be checked after 2-3 months [1]. The frequency of abnormal LFTs in asymptomatic subjects depends on the population studied, and has been found to vary from 0.5% to 8.9%. The causes are shown in Fig. (**1**).

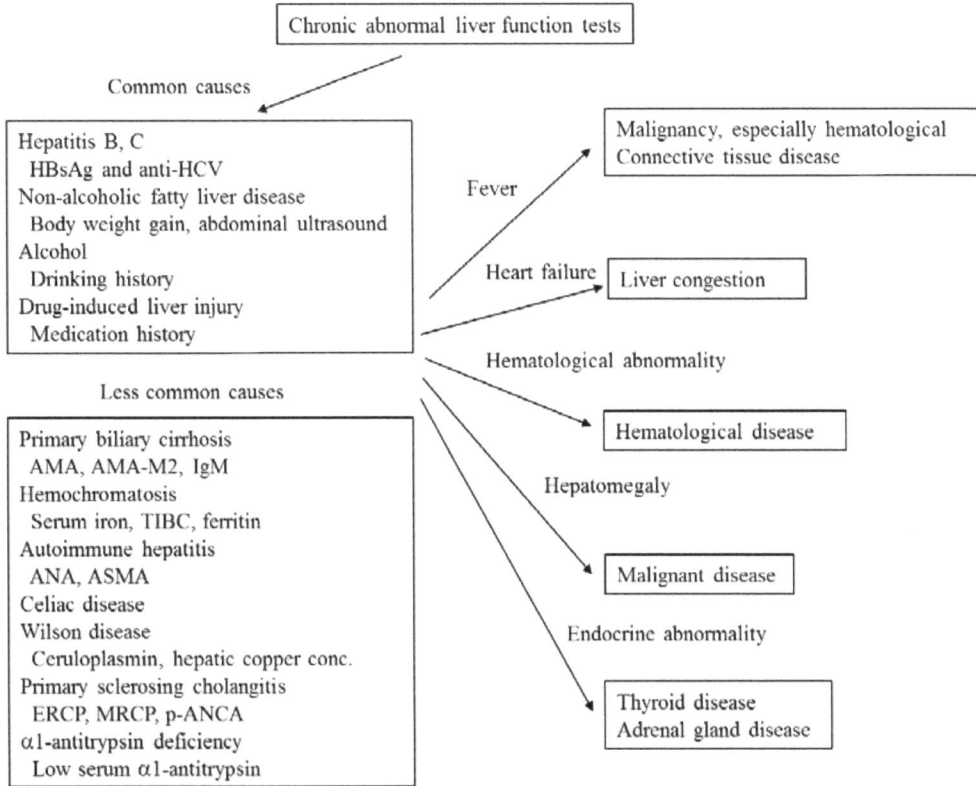

Figure 1: Disorders causing chronic abnormal liver function tests and their methods of diagnosis. Abbreviations: AMA, anti-mitochondrial antibody; ANA, anti-nuclear antibody; ASMA, anti-smooth muscle antibody; ERCP, endoscopic retrograde cholangiopancreatography; MRCP, magnetic resonance cholangiopancreatography; p-ANCA, anti-neutrophilic cytoplasmic antibody.

HISTORY TAKING

History taking should focus on the following points:

1) Use or exposure to medications or chemicals.

    An acute form of drug-induced liver injury (DILI) should be particularly suspected in patients who: 1) started taking a new drug within the past 3 months, 2) have a rash, or 3) have symptoms such as fever, general malaise, and skin itching. However, these signs and symptoms may be absent in patients with the chronic form of DILI. Diagnosis may be difficult in some patients because of the long interval between starting a suspected drug and presentation with liver injury.

2) Family history of liver disease.

Especially important are family history of hepatitis B and inherited diseases.

3) History of hepatitis.

History of acute hepatitis of unknown etiology or after receiving blood transfusion before 1991 may suggest acute hepatitis C, with most of these patients developing chronic hepatitis C. Persistent HBV infection may be present in 5% to 10% of patients with acute hepatitis B, depending on HBV genotype. Of the eight genotypes identified to date, one, genotype A, shows a high rate of chronic hepatitis after acute infection. Patients with resolved acute hepatitis B may have a persistent but low level of HBV replication for a long period of time [2].

4) Alcohol consumption.

Alcoholic hepatitis should be suspected in women who consume 30-40 g/day alcohol and men who consume 60-150 g/day. Long term consumption of lower amounts of alcohol can cause alcoholic fatty liver or liver fibrosis.

5) History of blood transfusion.

Blood transfusion before 1991 could cause posttransfusion hepatitis.

6) History of abdominal operation.

History of jejunoileal bypass surgery may suggest non-alcoholic steatohepatitis (NASH). Operation for gallstones may indicate recurrence of the disease.

7) Presence of autoimmune disease.

Because autoimmune diseases are likely to overlap or occur together, the presence of an autoimmune disease may suggest complication with another autoimmune disease, including autoimmune liver disease.

8) Accompanying symptoms such as fatigue, pruritus, arthralgia, myalgias, rash, anorexia, fever, shaking chills, nausea, and right upper quadrant pain.

Fatigue and pruritus are most often experienced by patients with liver diseases, although neither is specific for liver disease. Liver dysfunction in patients with shaking, chills and fever may be due to bacteremia following biliary tract infection or urinary tract infection. Moreover, many bacterial and viral infections are known to cause abnormal LFT results.

9) Change in body weight.

A recent increase in body weight, usually over 3 kg, suggests nonalcoholic fatty liver disease (NAFLD). Nonalcoholic steatohepatitis (NASH) is also suggested in patients with type 2 diabetes mellitus, hypertension, or hyperlipidemia.

10) Sexual behavior.

Homosexual individuals are at high risk of HIV infection and may be co-infected with HBV.

Use of medications, increased body weight and alcohol consumption, in particular, may often provide clues in identifying causes of liver disease.

PHYSICAL EXAMINATION

Physical examination should focus on the following:

1. Jaundice may suggest advanced liver disease or cholestasis.

2. Brown skin color may suggest hemochromatosis.

3. Skin eruption may suggest drug allergy or cholestasis.

4. Xanthelasmata or xanthomata may suggest chronic cholestasis, usually in patients with primary biliary cirrhosis.

5. Struma may suggest complicating thyroiditis in patients with autoimmune liver diseases.

6. Spider nevi, palmar erythema, gynecomastia, caput medusae, testicular atrophy or muscle wasting may suggest liver cirrhosis.

7. Jugular vein dilatation may suggest right-sided heart failure, which could lead to liver congestion.

8. Dilated superficial veins of the abdominal wall may represent portal hypertension.

9. Hepatomegaly

    The size, shape and consistency of the liver should be determined. Most patients with chronic or alcoholic hepatitis show enlarged tender liver palpable below the right costal margin. In contrast, cirrhotic liver can be palpable only around the middle line. A very large liver with consistency may indicate HCC, metastatic liver tumor, or infiltrative liver disease such as amyloidosis.

10. Splenomegaly

    A palpable spleen usually indicates moderate to marked splenomegaly, which is less sensitive to ultrasound. Splenomegaly is often observed in patients with acute viral hepatitis, especially EB virus infection, and also indicates the presence of portal hypertension or hematological disease. Dullness in Traube's space is an indication of a moderately enlarged spleen.

11. Ascites

    Ascites, one of the common symptoms observed in patients with advanced liver disease, may be caused by hypoalbuminemia and portal hypertension.

12. Leg edema

    Leg edema is rarely the first indication of liver disease. However, this symptom may represent hypoalbuminemia due to advanced liver disease. Patients with advanced liver disease having leg edema often have ascites.

LABORATORY TESTS (FIG. 2)

The order of laboratory tests should be based on the pattern and degree of liver injury and on pretest probability determined by history taking and physical examination. Moreover, the time course of liver injury may be a clue in diagnosing the etiology of liver injury.

The first step in evaluating abnormal LFT results is to divide them into two categories. Hepatocellular injury is characterized by elevated aminotransferases, and cholestatic injury by elevated biliary enzymes.

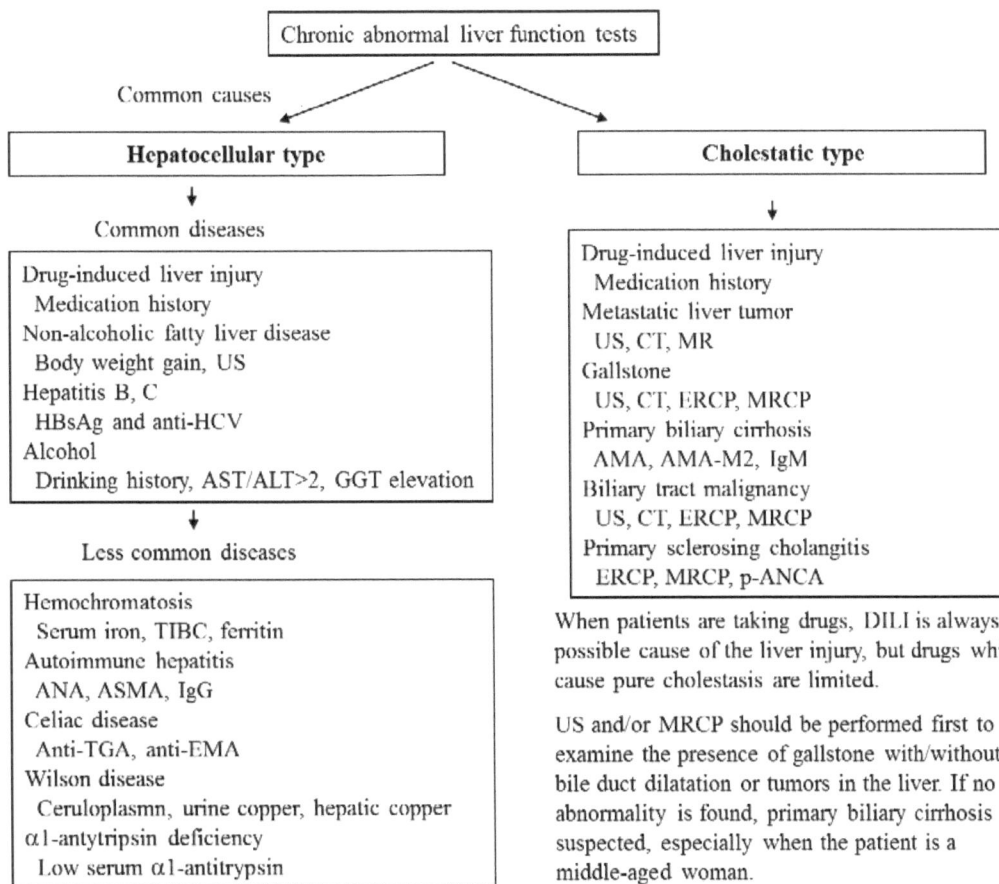

```
                    ┌─────────────────────────────────────┐
                    │ Chronic abnormal liver function tests │
                    └─────────────────────────────────────┘
        Common causes              ╱            ╲
              ┌──────────────────────────┐   ┌──────────────────────────┐
              │    Hepatocellular type   │   │     Cholestatic type     │
              └──────────────────────────┘   └──────────────────────────┘
                          ↓                              ↓
                  Common diseases
```

Hepatocellular type — Common diseases

Drug-induced liver injury
  Medication history
Non-alcoholic fatty liver disease
  Body weight gain, US
Hepatitis B, C
  HBsAg and anti-HCV
Alcohol
  Drinking history, AST/ALT>2, GGT elevation

↓ Less common diseases

Hemochromatosis
  Serum iron, TIBC, ferritin
Autoimmune hepatitis
  ANA, ASMA, IgG
Celiac disease
  Anti-TGA, anti-EMA
Wilson disease
  Ceruloplasmn, urine copper, hepatic copper
α1-antytripsin deficiency
  Low serum α1-antitrypsin

Cholestatic type

Drug-induced liver injury
  Medication history
Metastatic liver tumor
  US, CT, MR
Gallstone
  US, CT, ERCP, MRCP
Primary biliary cirrhosis
  AMA, AMA-M2, IgM
Biliary tract malignancy
  US, CT, ERCP, MRCP
Primary sclerosing cholangitis
  ERCP, MRCP, p-ANCA

When patients are taking drugs, DILI is always a possible cause of the liver injury, but drugs which cause pure cholestasis are limited.

US and/or MRCP should be performed first to examine the presence of gallstone with/without bile duct dilatation or tumors in the liver. If no abnormality is found, primary biliary cirrhosis is suspected, especially when the patient is a middle-aged woman.

Figure 2: Causes and methods of diagnosis of chronic abnormal liver function tests according to type of liver injury. Abbreviations: GGT, γ-glutamyl transpeptidase; AMA, anti-mitochondrial antibody; ANA, anti-nuclear antibody, ASMA; anti-smooth muscle antibody; ERCP, endoscopic retrograde cholangiopancreatography; MRCP, magnetic resonance cholangiopancreatography; p-ANCA, anti-neutrophilic cytoplasmic antibody; DILI, drug-induced liver injury

Hepatocellular Injury

Most chronic liver diseases due to hepatocellular injury show mild elevation of aminotransferases, defined as less than four to five times the upper limit of the normal (ULN) range. Stepwise testing of these patients is recommended to avoid unnecessary testing.

First;

1. Identify medications and supplements

    Most drugs cause acute type of liver injury, but some may cause chronic type.

2. Alcohol consumption

    Although history of alcohol drinking is important, some patients may conceal the true information.

3. Hepatitis B and C

    The prevalence of hepatitis virus carriers varies, depending on the geographic location and ethnicity. However, all patients with chronic liver injury should be tested for HBsAg and anti-HCV antibody. If HBsAg is positive, tests for anti-HBc antibody, HBeAg, anti-HBe antibody, and HBV DNA should be performed. Almost 30% of subjects positive for anti-HCV Ab are negative for HCV RNA, especially those with low antibody titer. Therefore, detection of serum HCV RNA is essential for the diagnosis of chronic HCV infection.

4. Non-alcoholic fatty liver disease

    Hepatic steatosis is suggested in subjects with obesity, high BMI, large waist circumference, or type 2 diabetes mellitus. Fat deposits in the liver are initially evaluated by radiographic imaging. Although ultrasound may not have high sensitivity in detecting steatosis, it is easy to perform and less expensive than CT or MRI. Therefore, ultrasound is recommended as the first test for subjects suspected of steatosis.

If all of the above are negative, the following should be evaluated.

5. Hereditary hemochromatosis

    Hereditary hemochromatosis (HHC) is a common genetic disorder in the United States and Western Europe, with 0.5% of the general population being homozygotic for the C282Y mutation. However, not every patient homozygotic for this mutation has hemochromatosis, and not every patient with HHC has the mutation. The initial screening tests for HHC include those for serum iron concentration and total iron binding capacity. Individuals with iron saturation greater than 45% should undergo testing for serum ferritin concentration. Serum ferritin levels greater than 400 ng/ml in men and 300 ng/ml in women suggest HHC. Iron overload is confirmed by liver biopsy, and a hepatic iron index, calculated as hepatic iron level (mmol/g dry weight) divided by patient age, greater than 1.9 is consistent with HHC homozygotes [3].

6. Autoimmune hepatitis

    Young to middle-aged women with mild to moderate elevation of ALT and shown to be negative for medications, alcohol, and hepatitis virus infection, should be suspected of having autoimmune liver disease, especially autoimmune hepatitis.

7. Wilson disease (WD)

    WD is an autosomal recessive inherited disorder of copper metabolism, resulting in excessive accumulation of copper in virtually all organs, especially in the liver. Patients usually present at age 5 to 25 years, but some may be over 40 years old. WD should therefore be suspected in young patients with chronic hepatitis of unknown etiology. These patients often present with chronic active hepatitis and liver cirrhosis, but may also show only mild biochemical abnormalities or fulminant hepatic failure. The initial screening test is for serum ceruloplasmin, which is reduced in 95% of these patients. Subsequently, 24-hour urine copper excretion should be tested, with excretion of more than 100 µg/day suggestive of WD.

Cholestatic Liver Injury

Chronic cholestatic liver disease is infrequent, but primary biliary cirrhosis is not a rare disease.

1. Malignancy in the liver or biliary tract

   Elderly patients presenting with abnormal liver function tests should be suspected of malignancy. Primary liver tumors, including HCC, cholangiocarcinoma, and cholangiocellular carcinoma, metastatic liver tumors, and bile duct cancer could cause cholestasis by various mechanisms. These conditions, however, are relatively easy to diagnose by imaging modalities.

2. Primary biliary cirrhosis (PBC)

   Middle aged women presenting with chronically elevated ALP and/or γ-GTP without biliary dilatation on ultrasound or CT, should be suspected of having primary biliary cirrhosis. Positivity for antimitochondrial and/or M2 antibody and elevated serum IgM concentrations support this diagnosis. Analysis of liver histology is often helpful for diagnosis and determination of clinical stage (Scheuer's staging).

3. Primary sclerosing cholangitis (PSC)

   In contrast to PBC, PSC predominantly affects men of mean age 40 years. These patients show abnormal LFTs of cholestatic type, and are usually diagnosed by ERCP or MRCP. Liver biopsy is supportive of this diagnosis, and periductal fibrosis with inflammation is characteristic of PSC.

4. LFT abnormalities in systemic disease.

   LFTs often show abnormal results due to non-hepatic causes, with the pattern of these abnormalities depending on etiology. Abnormal cholestatic LFTs may be caused by cardiopulmonary, endocrine, and connective tissue diseases and by infiltration of the liver by malignant cells. Details are described in Chapter 6.

Management of patients with chronic abnormal LFTs

1. Identification of patients needing prompt and extensive management.

   Measurements of serum bilirubin concentrations and PT can be used to assess liver functional reserve capacity and the necessity of prompt treatment.

1) Serum bilirubin levels

   Patients with high serum bilirubin levels (above 2 mg/dl) should be assessed by abdominal ultrasound as soon as possible to determine whether they show biliary dilatation, liver atrophy or ascites. Biliary dilatation is indicative of extrahepatic biliary obstruction, with patients requiring biliary drainage as soon as possible regardless of the underlining abnormality (stone or tumor). Patients with chills or fever may be in shock due to supparative cholangitis and therefore need prompt biliary drainage. Liver atrophy and/or ascites represent advanced liver disease (liver cirrhosis), which should be managed by specialists.

2) Prothrombin time (PT) or international normalized ratio

   PT depends on the production of coagulation factors II, V, VII and X in the liver; thus, measuring PT indicates the protein synthesis ability of the liver. This time is prolonged by a decrease in liver reserve capacity and/or a vitamin K deficiency. The latter may be due to treatment with warfarin or antibiotics (*e.g.* cephalosporin). Although the administration of vitamin K can reverse prolonged PT in patients deficient in vitamin K, patients with prolonged PT should be referred to a specialist due to the possibility of severe liver disease.

2. Identification of advanced chronic liver disease

   Advanced chronic liver diseases are suggested by low serum albumin concentrations, although the latter may also be caused by inflammation or malnutrition. Morphologic indicators of advanced chronic liver disease may include a dull edged, coarse parenchymal pattern, atrophy of the right lobe with compensating left lobe hypertrophy, and ascites retention predominantly around the liver.

3. Steps to perform before referral to a specialist in patients with abnormal LFT results.

1) Careful history taking including medications, alcohol consumption, concomitant systemic diseases and family history of liver disease.

2) Complete blood count and liver biochemistry blood tests including bilirubin. If total bilirubin is elevated, conjugated bilirubin should be also measured.

3)   Screen for viral hepatitis infection (HBsAg and HCV antibody)

4)   Protein electrophoresis

5)   Ultrasound of the liver

MANAGEMENT OF CHRONIC LIVER INJURY IN THE PRIMARY CARE SETTING

Drug-Induced Liver Injury

Chronic forms of DILI include chronic hepatitis (methyldopa, nitrofurantoin), cholestasis (chlorpromazine), granulomas (phenylbutazone), fatty change (amiodarone, tamoxifen), and vascular disease [4].

Diagnostic Considerations

1.   History of intake of causative drugs. Limited numbers of drugs to date have been found to cause chronic liver injury.

2.   Exclusion of other etiologies of chronic liver injury.

3.   Criteria of the Council for International Organizations of Medical Sciences are useful.

Management

1.   Cessation of the causative drug is essential.

2.   Patients with severe liver injury are often treated with corticosteroids or ursodeoxycholic acid.

The most common form of DILI is acute liver injury, with most patients improving after withdrawal of the causative drugs. However chronic liver injury or cirrhosis may occur in some patients even after stopping the suspected causative drugs. Recent studies from Spain and Sweden have shown that about 6% of patients with DILI show a chronic course of disease, despite stopping the causative drug [5]. A diagnosis of chronic DILI requires exclusion of chronic viral hepatitis, alcoholic liver disease, metabolic liver disease and autoimmune liver disease. Thus, serological tests should be performed for hepatitis B and C viruses; concentrations of copper, ferritin, and ceruloplasmin; total iron binding capacity; and the presence of antinuclear antibody (ANA), anti-smooth muscle antibody

(SMA), and anti-mitochondrial antibody (AMA). Ultrasonography of the abdomen should be performed to assess the presence of fatty liver, obstructive jaundice and other biliary diseases.

The criteria of the Council for International Organizations of Medical Sciences (the CIOMS/RUCAM scale) are useful in diagnosing chronic DILI [6]. Similar to acute DILI, most chronic DILI is of hepatocellular type, with liver injury at onset usually severe, including markedly elevated serum ALT and jaundice. Histologic examination may also be helpful in diagnosing chronic DILI. Moreover, centrilobular necrosis (hepatocellular type) or ductopenia or vanishing bile duct syndrome (cholestatic/mixed type) often occur in patients with chronic DILI.

Drugs shown to cause chronic DILI include herbal medicines, antibiotics (ethambutol, isoniazid, rifampicin, pyrazinamide, cefradine, roxithromycin, cephalexin, metronidazole, norfloxacin, amoxicillin), cardiovascular drugs (simvastatin, lovastatin, bezafibrate, fosinopri, levamlodipine besylate), aciclovir, aminophenazone, gliquidone, diethylstilbestrol and propylthiouracil.

Alcoholic Liver Disease (ALD)

Diagnostic Criteria

1. History of excess alcohol consumption

2. Serum AST:ALT>2

3. Thrombocytopenia, hypertriglyceridemia, and/or elevated serum IgA are often observed.

Management

1. Cessation of alcohol consumption and nutritional therapy are essential.

2. The efficacy of corticosterids in patients with severe acute alcoholic hepatitis is unclear.

Although history of alcohol overconsumption is diagnostic for alcoholic liver injury, some patients strongly deny excess alcohol consumption. The occurrence of ALD is gender dependent. In men, consumption of 40-80 g/day alcohol may cause fatty liver, and consumption of 160 g/day for more than 10-20 years may cause liver cirrhosis. In contrast, ALD in women may be caused by drinking 20 g/day alcohol.

Pathologically, ALD is characterized by fatty liver, alcoholic hepatitis and liver cirrhosis. Risk factors for the development of cirrhosis include not only excess alcohol and female gender, but concomitant chronic HCV infection. Biochemical data suggesting alcoholic liver injury, especially alcoholic hepatitis, are an AST/ALT ratio ≥2.0 and elevated concentrations of triglycerides, γ-GTP and serum IgA. In contrast, patients with alcoholic fatty liver have an AST/ALT ratio <1.0. Serum IgA remains elevated for a relatively long period after cessation of alcohol intake. Management of ALD largely depends on nutritional therapy and cessation of alcohol consumption. If these are successful, patients may show significant recovery, even those with livers showing early stage cirrhosis.

Alcoholic hepatitis is a severe form of alcoholic liver injury and the fourth leading cause of death of individuals aged 33-55 years in the USA. Alcoholic hepatitis usually occurs in patients with chronic alcoholic liver injury, with excessive amounts of alcohol consumption triggering severe hepatitis. Low grade fever, delirium (encephalopathy), and jaundice occur in 60% to 80% of patients. Patients may also experience anorexia, fatigue or upper abdominal discomfort. Almost all patients with alcoholic hepatitis demonstrate hepatomegaly, with half showing epigastric/liver tenderness, ascites or splenomegaly. Blood tests show two to seven fold increases in both AST and ALT, which usually does not exceed 300 IU/ml. Leukocytosis; elevated γ-GTP, ALP and T-Bil concentrations; and anemia may occur. Prolongation of PT suggests severe hepatitis, indicating the need for intensive treatment. Although corticosteroid therapy has been reported to improve short-term survival in patients with severe acute alcoholic hepatitis, its efficacy remains unclear.

Diagnosis of alcoholic liver cirrhosis may be confusing in livers showing diffuse hypertrophy and a fine parenchymal US pattern, reflecting fine fibrosis and small node formation.

Nonalcoholic Fatty Liver Disease (NAFLD)

About 10% of patients with hepatic steatosis have NASH, with 10% to 20% of the latter developing liver cirrhosis and even HCC [7]. Several serum markers have been used to assess fibrotic liver changes, attempting to diagnose NASH without liver biopsy. However, liver biopsy remains the gold standard for the diagnosis of NASH and should be performed if NASH is highly suspected.

Diagnostic Criteria (Fig. 3) [8]

1. Presence of fatty liver on imaging modalities.

2. Exclusion of other etiologies causing fatty changes in the liver.

3. Concomitant presence of NAFLD and liver disease of other etiology should always be considered.

4. Identification of NASH is important, because it is progressive and patient prognosis may be poor.

5. Scoring systems have been developed to evaluate fibrosis in NAFLD, but the gold standard for the diagnosis of NASH remains liver biopsy.

Management

1. Dietary restriction is essential.

2. Some drugs that improve insulin sensitivity have been reported to show efficacy in patients with NASH.

NAFLD is one of the most frequent causes of chronic LFT abnormalities in the USA and other western countries, affecting 20% to 40% of the general population with male predominance. Because the clinical picture of NAFLD is similar to that of alcoholic fatty liver disease, except for history of alcohol consumption, it may be difficult to distinguish these two diseases if patients conceal their history of alcohol consumption. Most patients with NAFLD are asymptomatic and the disease is usually incidentally detected during a regular check-up or screening ultrasound. Patients suspected of NAFLD should be tested for hepatitis virus infection, autoantibodies, ferritin and ceruloplasmin (young patients) to exclude other etiologies of liver injury. More importantly, NAFLD may coexist with other chronic liver diseases, such as chronic hepatitis B, chronic hepatitis C and autoimmune liver disease, complicating the pathophysiology of the liver. Elevated serum autoantibodies are common in patients with NAFLD, with 23% reported to have serum anti-nuclear antibodies of low to moderate titers [9]. Low titers of anti-smooth muscle and anti-mitochondrial antibodies have also been detected in patients with NAFLD. The significance of these autoantibodies is unknown, but liver biopsy may be required to exclude the possibility of a co-existing autoimmune liver disease and select the optimal treatment. NAFLD is closely associated with metabolic syndrome, with many of these patients having obesity, type 2 diabetes mellitus and/or hyperlipidemia. Reduction of body weight by dietary restriction may be sufficient to improve NAFLD, but complicating abnormalities, including type 2 diabetes mellitus or hyperlipidemia, may require specific treatments.

Elevated liver enzymes
Fatty liver suspected

↓

Viral serology to exclude hepatitis B and C
(anti-HBc, HBsAg, anti-HCV)

↓

Assess alcohol intake

Alcohol intake less than
two drinks per day

Alcohol intake of two or
more drinks per day

↓

↓

Imaging study (e.g.,
ultrasonography or CT)
showing fatty infiltrate

Alcohol fatty liver
disease likely

↓

Nonalcoholic fatty liver disease likely

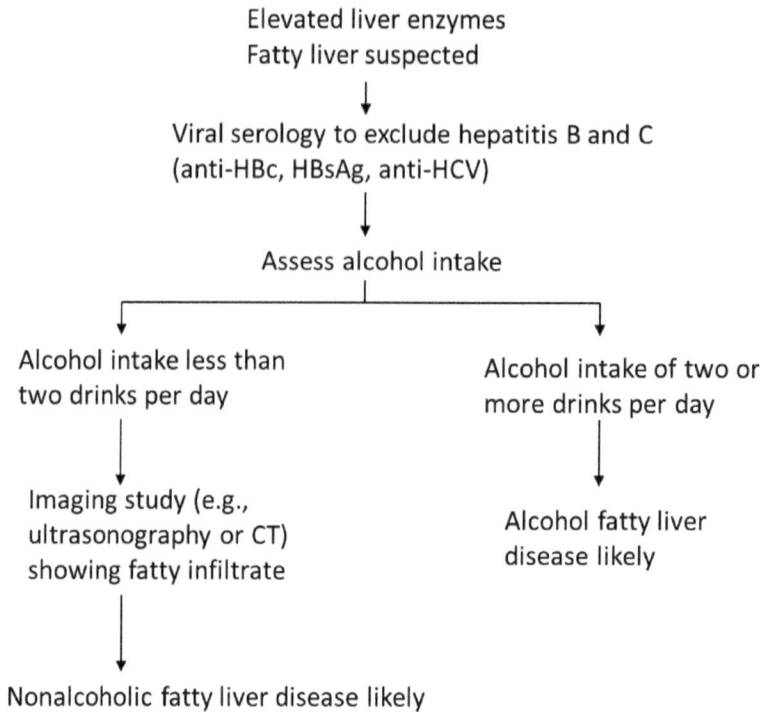

Figure 3: Diagnostic algorithm for nonalcoholic fatty liver disease [8].

NAFLD can be classified as simple fatty liver and NASH, with about 10% of patients with NAFLD having NASH. NASH is thought to affect 3% to 5% of the general population in the USA and may lead to liver cirrhosis and even HCC. Since many drugs can cause both NAFLD and NASH [5], patients who are not obese, glucose intolerant or hyperlipidemic should be asked about drugs they are currently taking.

Several attempts have been made to distinguish NASH from NAFLD by non-invasive methods, although liver biopsy remains the gold standard method for their differentiation. Currently, three systems are used to diagnose, but they require future validation:

i) NAFLD fibrosis score [10]

$-1.675 + 0.037$ x age (years) $+0.094$ x BMI (kg/m^2) $+1.13$ x impaired glucose tolerance/diabetes (yes=1, no=0) $+0.99$ x AST/ALT ratio-0.013 x platelets (x10^9/L) -0.66 x albumin (g/dL). A low cutoff point (score <-1.455) is indicative of the absence of advanced fibrosis, whereas a high cutoff point (score >0.676) is indicative of advanced fibrosis.

ii) A single biomarker, the terminal peptide of procollagen III, has been reported to distinguish between patients with simple steatosis and NASH [11].

iii) BARD score [12].

The BARD score is a weighted sum of three easily measured variables (BMI > 28 kg/m^2 [1 point], AST/ALT $\geq$ 0.8 [2 points], and diabetes [1 point]). Scores of 2 to 4 were associated with an odds ratio [OR] of 17 (95% confidence interval [CI]: 9.2-31.9) for predicting advanced fibrosis. Recently, an improved score BARDI (BARD plus PT-INR), was shown to have higher positive predictive values than the original BARD score [13]. If any one of these scores strongly suggests NASH, liver biopsy should be performed to establish its diagnosis and to exclude other etiologies of liver disease including alcoholic liver disease.

Once NASH is diagnosed, patients should be educated and carefully monitored. Emerging evidence suggests that NAFLD is the most common cause of cryptogenic cirrhosis in western countries. Moreover, HCC is the leading cause of death in NASH patients, and a prospective cohort study from Japan showed that the 5-year cumulative incidence of HCC was 7.6% [14], with most of these patients having liver cirrhosis as the underlining liver disease.

To date, no treatment has proven effective for NASH, but the following regimen is considered the treatment of choice:

i)   Weight control

ii)   Vitamins E and C

iii) Metformin

iv)   Pioglitazone

v)   Ursodeoxycholic acid

Of these five, weight control is most important and necessary even in patients who have progressed to cirrhosis.

Chronic Hepatitis B

Diagnostic Criteria

1. Positivity for HBsAg and anti-HBc Ab

2. Positivity for HBV DNA irrespective of the presence/absence of other markers

Management

1. Measure HBeAg/Ab, ALT, and HBsAg titers, and HBV DNA concentration.

2. Select patients who require antiviral therapy based on ALT and HBV DNA levels.

3. Nucleot(s)ide analogs and peg-interferon are the main drugs used to suppress HBV replication.

4. Estimate disease stability and prognosis and the risk of HCC development in HBV carriers by measuring HBeAg/Ab, ALT, HBsAg and HBV DNA levels.

5. Imaging, including ultrasonography, CT or MRI, should be performed at regular intervals to assess patients for complications of chronic HBV infection and/or the development of HCC.

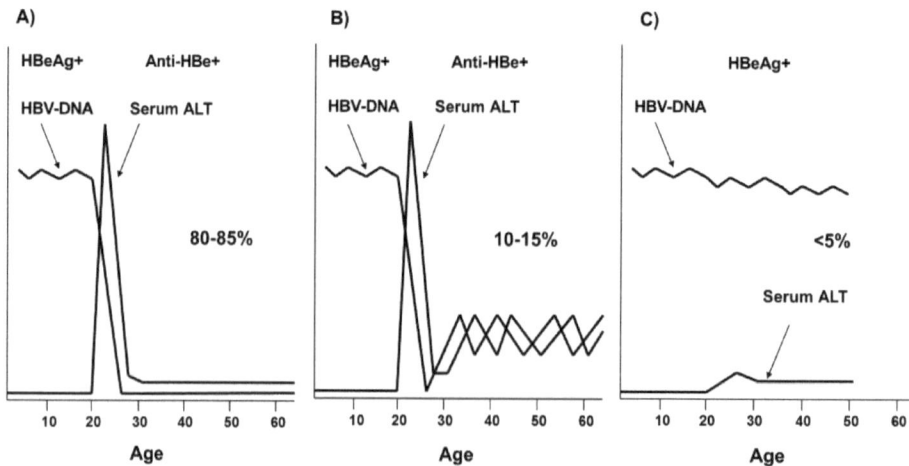

Figure 4: Natural clinical courses of HBV carriers. **A)** Most HBV carriers become inactive after liver inflammation and do not require any treatment. **B)** About 10% of HBV carriers show persistent (chronic) hepatitis after an immunotolerant phase. **C)** In fewer than 5% of HBV carriers, the immunotolerant phase persists for several decades.

A diagnosis of chronic HBV infection requires positivity for both HBsAg and anti-HBc antibody. HBV carriers usually have high titers (above 10 IU/ml) of anti-HBc antibody, but may have low titers or even no antibody.

Latent or occult HBV is a condition defined as low level HBV DNA in the blood or the liver without serum HBsAg [15]. The natural course of this condition remains unclear. Although not likely associated with progressive liver disease, it may be the cause of HCC in patients with non-B (HBsAg negative), non-C (anti-HCV negative) cirrhosis [16].

The natural history of chronic HBV infection is shown in Fig. (**4**). In diagnosing patients, it is important to determine the point at which the patient is located. Therefore, serum concentrations of ALT, HBeAg, and anti-HBe antibody should be determined, and quantitative PCR for HBV DNA performed. Most patients (80-85%) become inactive HBV carriers after hepatitis (immune-active phase) requiring no further treatment. The remaining 10-15% of patients will show persistent hepatitis and require anti-HBV treatment. Strong predictors of progression to cirrhosis and HCC include high serum HBV DNA and ALT. Importantly, patients with active HBV replication and high ALT often progress to cirrhosis rapidly [17]. Therefore, those patients require careful and frequent follow-up, and should start antiviral treatment if they show high hepatitis activity.

Although the presence of HBeAg usually represents high levels of serum HBV DNA, and may be closely associated with the progression of liver disease, the absence of HBeAg, which is related to a mutation in the basic core promoter or precore region of HBV DNA, does not always indicate a stable state if HBV is actively replicating. Thus, serum levels of HBV DNA and ALT are the factors that determine the necessity of antiviral therapy. The incidence of HCC has been reported to vary according to serum HBV DNA levels, even in patients with normal ALT and without cirrhosis. Recently, normal ALT, low HBsAg (<1,000U/ml), and low HBV DNA were found to be markers of minimal HCC risk in HBV carriers [17], indicating that measurement of these three markers can be used to estimate the stability of HBV infection and prognosis of patients with chronic HBV infection.

The goals of treatment are suppression of HBV replication and inhibition of liver disease progression and the development of HCC. However, indications for antiviral treatment in patients with high serum HBV DNA and normal ALT are undetermined. Loss of HBsAg may be the ultimate end point, because it may reduce the likelihood of progression to cirrhosis and HCC. However, loss of HBsAg is usually difficult to achieve, due to the presence of covalently closed circular DNA in the nuclei of infected hepatocytes.

To date, seven agents have been approved by the U.S. Food and Drug Administration to treat patients with HBV infection: interferons (conventional interferon and peginterferon-α2a) and nucleoside and nucleotide analogs (lamivudine, adefovir, entecavir, tenofovir and telbivudine). These agents are used as monotherapy or in combination. Nucleoside and nucleotide analogs have shown potent antiviral activity, have improved hepatitis activity and fibrosis, and have significantly inhibited the development of HCC [18]. Drawbacks to their use include high rates of hepatitis relapse after treatment cessation, emergence of drug-resistant mutants during long-term treatment, low rates of HBeAg and HBsAg loss, and the absence of universal guidelines for timing of treatment cessation. General management of HBsAg-positive patients is shown in Fig. (5).

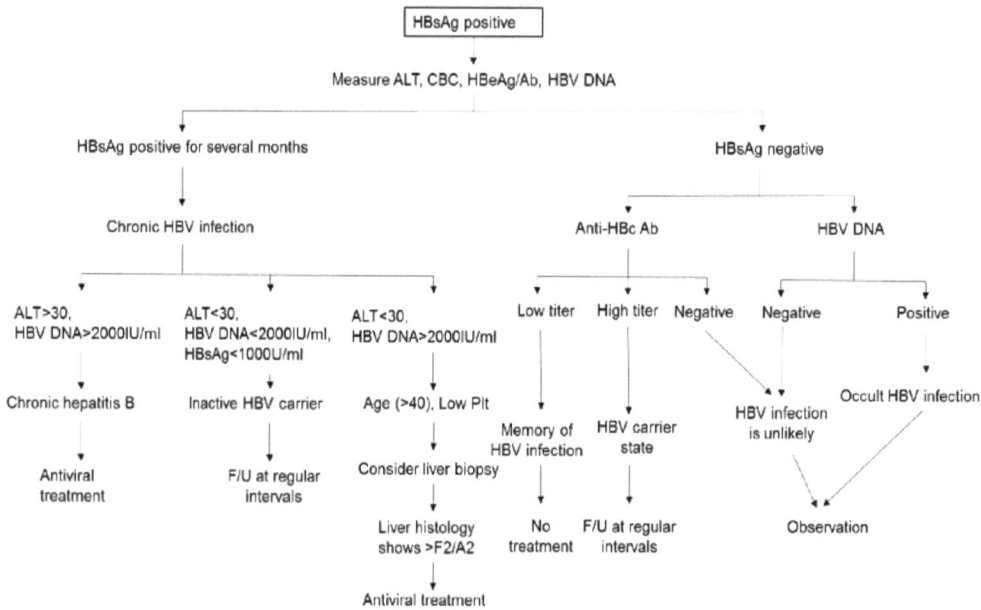

Figure 5: Management of HBsAg-positive patients.

Chronic Hepatitis C

Since not all patients positive for anti-HCV antibody are positive for serum HCV RNA, quantitative PCR should be performed to confirm ongoing HCV infection. A recent study of liver histology in patients positive for anti-HCV antibody but negative for HCV RNA found that most had persistent HCV infection in the liver [19]. Although their natural course of disease is unclear, those patients may have to be followed up for a long time.

In contrast, the sensitivity for anti-HCV antibody is reported to be 92% to 97%, and a negative HCV antibody result does not completely exclude HCV infection. Patients at high risk of HCV infection should also be tested by quantitative PCR test for HCV RNA, even if they are negative for anti-HCV antibody.

Diagnostic Criteria

1. Positive for anti-HCV and HCV RNA in serum

2. HCV positivity for longer than 6 months

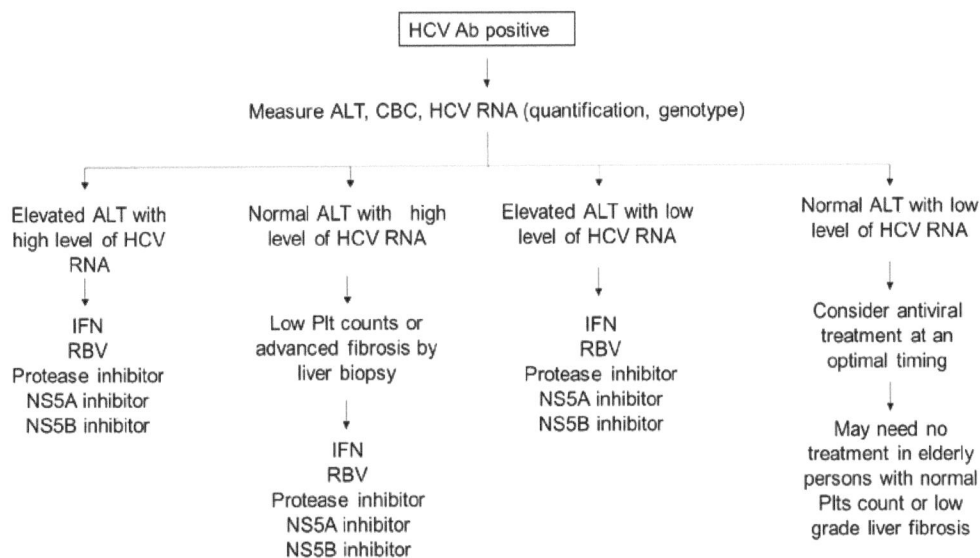

Figure 6: Management of patients positive for anti-HCV Ab.
Abbreviations: CBC, complete blood count; IFN, interferon; RBV, ribavirin

Management

1. Measure complete blood count (platelet) and ALT, and assess chronicity and activity of chronic HCV infection.

2. All patients positive for HCV can be candidates for antiviral treatment.

3. Select treatment depending on HCV viremia and genotype.

4. Several new antiviral drugs have become available with high efficacy.

It has been estimated that 60% to 80% of patients with acute HCV infection develop chronic infection, with most patients chronically infected with HCV having been acutely infected several years earlier. The natural history of chronic HCV infection has been analyzed in various countries and found to vary geographically. HCV infection usually progresses slowly, with 20% to 30% of chronically infected patients developing cirrhosis over 20 to 30 years. An early study from France found that 30% of patients with chronic

HCV infection will not progress to cirrhosis or will require more than 50 years to develop cirrhosis [20]. However, the clinical course may depend on age at time of infection, with individuals infected at >60 years showing rapid progression to cirrhosis and HCC [21]. However, progression from chronic hepatitis to cirrhosis usually occurs slowly and silently, and the development of cirrhosis may be suggested by AST:ALT >1, low platelet counts (less than $10^5/\mu L$) and hypergammaglobulinemia. Although liver biopsy may help diagnose cirrhosis, the bleeding risk of this procedure is high. Thus biopsy is not routinely recommended, especially when laboratory data and/or clinical features strongly suggest the presence of cirrhosis.

Who Should be Treated?

Basically, all individuals with chronic HCV infection can be candidates for antiviral treatment. However, indications for treatment depend on patient age, expected natural history of disease, risks of development of cirrhosis and HCC, serum ALT levels, HCV genotype and viral load (Fig. **6**).

Treatment of patients with chronic hepatitis C has progressed during the last decade, with 40% to 50% of patients with genotype 1b achieving a sustained virological response (SVR), defined as undetectable serum HCV RNA six months after cessation of treatment, using a combination of weekly subcutaneously injected pegylated interferon and daily oral ribavirin.

Even after achieving SVR, patients should be followed up for several years because of the risk of development of HCC. Although this risk is low, it is higher in patients over 65 years of age and in those with advanced liver disease at the time of treatment [22].

Several directly acting antiviral drugs (oral) have been developed recently (Table **1**), with interferon-free combination therapies showing high rates of eradication of HCV genotype 1b [Table **2**, 23-27]. Similarly, over 95% of patients infected with

HCV genotypes 2 and 3 HCV achieve SVR following treatment with sofosbuvir and ribavirin [28]. The introduction of these new combination regimens may make possible the eradication of HCV from all infected patients.

Table 1. Directly acting antiviral agents used to treat HCV.

Antiviral activity	Drugs
NS3 protease inhibitor	Asunaprevir ABT-450 Vedroprevir
NS5A inhibitor	Ledipasvir Daclatasvir ABT-267
NS5B inhibitor	Sofosbuvir (nucleotide) GS-9669 ABT-333 Tegobuvir

Table 2. Interferon-free oral combination therapies for hepatitis C in patients infected with HCV genotype 1b.

Patients	Regimen	Results	Refs.
Treatment-naïve	sofosbuvir+RBV 12W	SVR24 84%	[23]
Prior nonresponder	sofosbuvir+RBV 12W	SVR24 10%	
Treatment-naïve	sofosbuvir+ledipasvir+RBV 12W	SVR12 100%	[24]
	sofosbuvir+GS-9669+RBV 12W	SVR12 92%	
Prior null responder	sofosbuvir+ledipasvir+RBV 12W	SVR12 100%	
(noncirrhotic)	sofosbuvir+GS-9669+RBV 12W	SVR12 100%	
Prior null responder	sofosbuvir+ledipasvir+RBV 12W	SVR12 100%	
(cirrhotic)	sofosbuvir+ledipasvir 12W	SVR12 70%	
Treatment-naïve	daclatasvir+asunaprevir+ BMS-791325 12W or 24W	SVR12 92%	[25]
Treatment-naïve	ABT-450/r+ ABT-267 or	SVR24 83-100%	[26]
Prior null responder	ABT-333 or both		
Treatment-naïve	daclatasvir+sofosbuvir +/- RBV	SVR12 98%	[27]
Prior null responder		SVR12 98%	

Abbreviations: RBV, ribavirin; SVR, sustained virologic response

Autoimmune Hepatitis (AIH)

Diagnostic Criteria

1. Moderate chronic hepatitis with hypergammaglobulinemia (IgG elevation) in young or middle aged women.

2. Positivity for anti-nuclear Ab (ANA) and anti-smooth muscle Ab (ASMA) in type 1 AIH and for anti-liver kidney microsomal-1 (LKM-1) Ab in type 2 AIH.

3. The diagnostic scoring system proposed by the International AIH Study Group is useful (Table **3**) [29].

4. Histologic examination of liver biopsy showing periportal or interface hepatitis with lymphocytic and plasmacytic infiltrates suggests AIH (Fig. **7**).

5. Almost 10% of these patients present with acute hepatitis; their diagnosis may be difficult due to their atypical clinical characteristics [30].

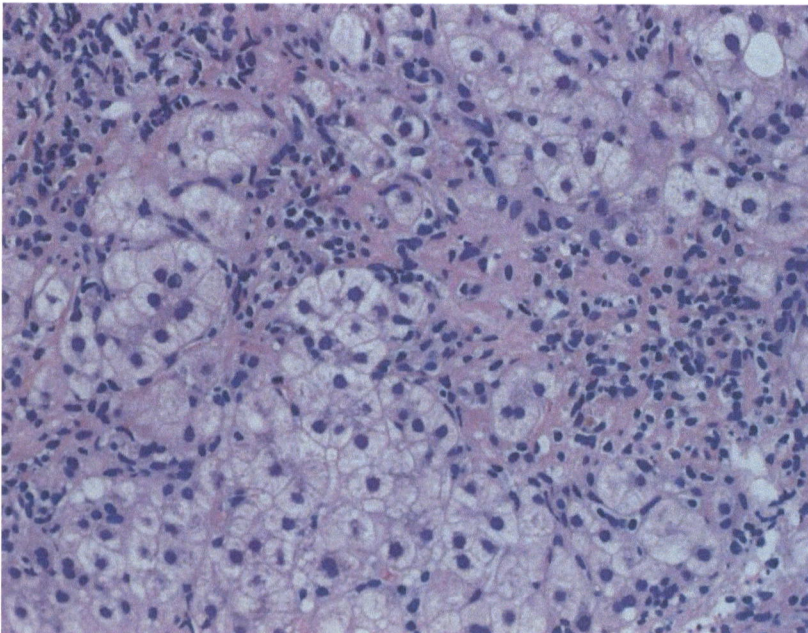

Figure 7: Typical liver histology of a patient with autoimmune hepatitis, showing interface hepatitis and ballooning of hepatocytes with rosette formation.

Table 3. Simplified diagnostic criteria for autoimmune hepatitis [29]

Variable	Cutoff	Points
ANA or SMA	≥1:40	1
ANA or SMA	≥1:40	
or LKM	≥1:40	2*
or SLA	Positive	
IgG	>Upper normal limit	1
	>1.10 times upper normal limit	2
Liver histology (evidence	Compatible with AIH	1
of hepatitis is a necessary	Typical AIH	2
condition)		
Absence of viral hepatitis	Yes	2
		≥6: probable AIH
		≥7: definite AIH

*Addition of points achieved for all autoantibodies (maximum, 2 points)

Management

1.   All patients with high hepatitis activity should be treated with corticosteroids. If patients are resistant to therapy, azathioprine should be added.

2.   Patients who progress to liver cirrhosis and are resistant to immunosuppressive therapy may require liver transplantation.

AIH is a disease found mostly in young and middle aged women, with an estimated prevalence in Western Europe and North America of 50 to 200 patients/million in the general population. As it often shows rapid progression to cirrhosis or liver failure, this disease should always be suspected in patients with moderate to marked elevation of ALT but negative for hepatitis viral infection. Although breaking self-tolerance is thought to cause AIH and several immunological abnormalities have been reported, the key event in its immunopathogenesis is unknown. Early stage patients may show acute hepatitis, with low levels of serum IgG and ANA [30]. These patients are difficult to diagnose with AIH, even after assessment of liver histology. Centrilobular necrosis, a feature of DILI, is often observed during acute clinical presentation of AIH and may reflect an early lesion prior to portal involvement [31].

Symptoms frequently observed in patients with AIH include fatigue (45%), anorexia, jaundice (55%), edema (45%), pruritus (24%), fever (21%), abdominal pain (24%) and arthralgia (18%). Other symptoms may include arthritis, exanthema nodosum, colitis, pleuritis, pericarditis, and sicca syndrome [32].

Analysis of patients with AIH found that 50% present with chronic hepatitis, 34% with cirrhosis, 13% with acute hepatitis and 3% with cholestatic hepatitis. Moreover, a fulminant form of AIH has been described [32].

Three types of AIH have been described. Type 1, or classic type, is associated with ANA, ASMA and anti-asialoglycoprotein receptor antibody; type 2, mostly found in young women and girls, is associated with antibody against LKM-1; and type 3, although not formally recognized and, is associated with anti-soluble liver antigen. Because most patients with AIH have type 1, serum γ-globulin, ANA and ASMA should be first assessed in patients suspected of AIH.

The presence of fatty deposits in the liver does not exclude a diagnosis of AIH, since patients may have AIH with fatty changes. In contrast, serum ANA is present in many patients with NASH [9]. As therapies for NASH and AIH are contrary to each other, assessment of liver histology may be required to differentiate between these two diseases.

Diagnosis of AIH

Serum protein electrophoresis showing hypergammaglobulinemia is useful in screening for AIH. A greater than two-fold polyclonal elevation of immunoglobulins suggests a diagnosis of AIH. If AIH is suspected, patients should be tested for the presence of ANA, ASMA and LKM-1. Since no single test is specific for a diagnosis of AIH, a diagnostic scoring system has been proposed by the International AIH study group [29]. The specificity and sensitivity of this scoring system have been reported satisfactory, enabling this system to be used in daily practice. Although liver histology is not diagnostic, periportal or interface hepatitis with lymphocytic and plasmacytic infiltrates suggests AIH.

Treatment

The prognosis of patients with untreated AIH has been reported poor, with 5- and 10-year overall survival rates of 50% and 10%, respectively. The American Association for the Study of Liver Diseases has recommended immunosuppressive treatment for patients with serum AST or ALT levels greater than 10-times ULN; in patients with AST and ALT greater than five-times ULN and serum γ-globulin level at least 2-times ULN; and/or in patients with histological features of bridging or multilobular necrosis [33]. Progression from chronic hepatitis to cirrhosis is rapid if liver histology shows periportal hepatitis or bridging necrosis. Therefore, all patients with AIH and high inflammatory activity in the liver should start treatment as soon as the diagnosis is established. Corticosteroid is the initial treatment of choice; if patients are resistant to corticosteroid, azathioprine should be added. Almost 90% of patients with AIH respond to treatment. In Japan, UDCA is also used to treat AIH patients with mild activity or during tapering of corticosteroid, and has been shown effective [34].

Primary Biliary Cirrhosis (PBC)

PBC is not a rare disease. Therefore, this disease should be suspected in patients, especially women, showing liver function abnormalities of a cholestatic pattern.

Diagnostic Criteria [36]

1. Most patients are middle-aged women with cholestatic type of liver injury, and anti-mitochondrial Ab (AMA) and its M2 subtype are disease-specific (Fig. **8**).

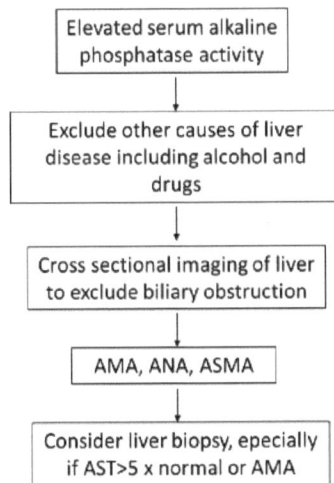

Figure 8: Diagnostic algorithm for primary biliary cirrhosis [35].

2. Liver histology showing chronic nonsupprative destructive cholangitis is characteristic of this disease (Fig. **9**).

Management

1. UDCA is the initial treatment of choice for these patients, especially those with early stage disease [36].

2. Liver transplantation should be considered for patients with end stage PBC, and several clinical trials have attempted to predict the prognosis of these patients [37].

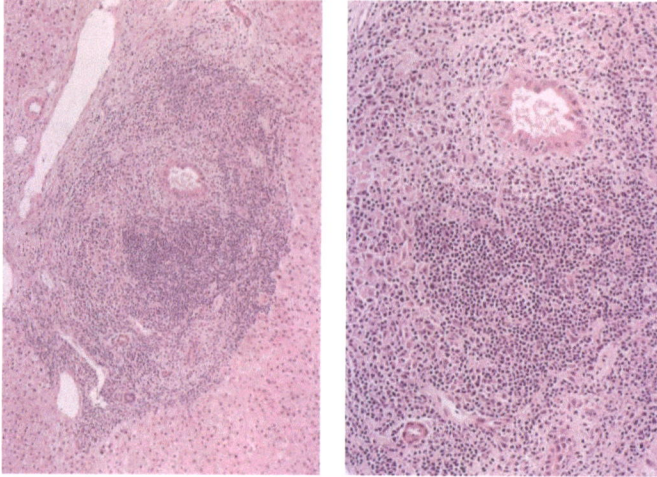

Figure 9: Typical liver histology in a patient with primary biliary cirrhosis, showing a granulomatous lesion with damage to the interlobular bile duct epithelium. Lymphocyte infiltration into the lining of bile duct epithelium and stratification of the epithelium are also characteristic of primary biliary cirrhosis (original magnification, left; x100, right x200).

PBC is an immune-mediated chronic cholestatic liver disease, mostly affecting middle-aged women. In contrast to AIH, PBC is characterized by disease-specific autoantibodies, AMA and its M2 subtype. Although AMA is present in 0.5% of the general population, the natural course of these individuals has not been clarified [38].

Natural History of PBC

Prognosis depends on the presence or absence of liver disease-derived symptoms such as pruritus, and patients with asymptomatic PBC have a better prognosis than those with symptoms. Median survival of asymptomatic patients has been reported to be 10 to 16 years. PBC usually progresses slowly, but some asymptomatic patients do not progress for several years [37].

Diagnosis of PBC

All patients with a cholestatic pattern of abnormal LFTs should be suspected of having PBC, especially if they are middle-aged women. Laboratory findings in patients with PBC include elevated serum ALP and/or γ-GTP; serum aminotransferase may be also elevated, especially at early presentation. Some patients may show little abnormality in LFTs or a mild elevation of γ-GTP alone, but demonstrate bile duct damage surrounded by granulomatous lesions compatible with PBC stage 1. Those patients are thought to be at an early stage of PBC [39]. Therefore, patients with mild abnormalities lacking other etiologies should be screened for PBC. Differential diagnosis should include drug-induced cholestasis, biliary tract malignancy or stone, primary sclerosing cholangitis, alcoholic liver disease, granulomatous formation in the liver, infiltrative liver lesions such as amyloidosis, metastatic liver tumors or hematological malignancies and vanishing bile duct syndrome.

The most specific markers for PBC are serum AMA and M2, and serum IgM and cholesterol concentrations are often elevated. Liver histology is useful for the confirmation of diagnosis and estimation of histological stage. Thus, liver biopsy is recommended when laboratory test results suggest PBC.

Treatments and Prognosis

Ursodeoxycholic acid (UDCA) is the most widely used drug for initial treatment. At a dose of 13-15 mg/kg body weight/day, oral UDCA has been shown to improve LFT results and retard disease progression and may improve patient prognosis [40]. However, its efficacy is limited to patients with Scheuer's stages I and II [36], indicating that diagnosis at an early stage and early start of treatment are important for improving patient prognosis and avoiding liver transplantation. Once these patients develop jaundice, their prognosis can be calculated by several scoring systems, helping select candidates for liver transplantation [37]. Therefore, patient management should aim at not progressing to cirrhosis with jaundice, thus avoiding the need for liver transplantation.

Wilson Disease (WD)

Diagnostic Criteria (Fig. 10)

1. Young patients (<40 years of age) with chronic hepatitis of unknown etiology should be suspected of having WD. However, it should be noted that patients could be at any age.

2. The presence of copper deposition in the cornea (Kayser–Fleischer rings) and/or on brain (MRI) suggests a diagnosis of WD.

3. Low serum ceruloplasmin and excess urinary copper excretion strongly suggest WD [41].

4. A hepatic copper concentration >250 μg/g dry liver is important in the final diagnosis of WD.

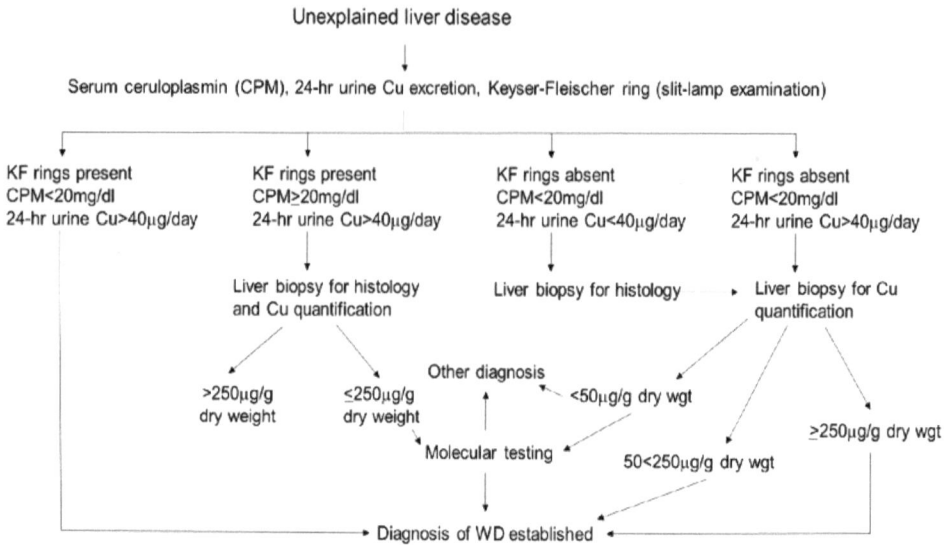

Unexplained liver disease

Serum ceruloplasmin (CPM), 24-hr urine Cu excretion, Keyser-Fleischer ring (slit-lamp examination)

| KF rings present CPM<20mg/dl 24-hr urine Cu>40μg/day | KF rings present CPM≥20mg/dl 24-hr urine Cu>40μg/day | KF rings absent CPM<20mg/dl 24-hr urine Cu<40μg/day | KF rings absent CPM<20mg/dl 24-hr urine Cu>40μg/day |

Liver biopsy for histology and Cu quantification

Liver biopsy for histology

Liver biopsy for Cu quantification

>250μg/g dry weight   ≤250μg/g dry weight

Other diagnosis

<50μg/g dry wgt

Molecular testing

50<250μg/g dry wgt

≥250μg/g dry wgt

Diagnosis of WD established

Figure 10: Diagnostic algorithm for Wilson disease [41].

Management

1. D-penicillamine is the first line drug for the treatment of WD.

2. The patients should be educated to avoid copper-rich foods such as liver, chocolate, nuts, mushrooms, or shellfish.

WD is an autosomal recessive inherited disorder of copper metabolism. Excessive accumulation of copper is observed in virtually all organs, especially in the liver. Clinical spectrums of liver disorders in WD includes mild biochemical abnormalities, chronic active hepatitis, and liver cirrhosis. It is rarely manifested as fulminant hepatitis. Copper accumulation is also detectable in the corneas (Kayser–Fleischer rings) and brains of patients with WD.

Most patients with WD are diagnosed at ages 3 to 40 years. Patients of these ages with unexplained elevation of aminotransferase levels should be suspected of having WD and their serum concentrations of ceruloplasmin measured. A combination of a low serum ceruloplasmin concentration and the presence of Kayser-Fleischer rings is usually sufficient to diagnose WD. If liver biopsy can be performed, hepatic copper content should be measured. A combination of hepatic copper concentration >250μg/g dry liver and low serum ceruloplasmin could establish a final diagnosis of WD [41].

Patients with WD present with various neuropsychiatric symptoms, including dysarthria, dyspraxia, ataxia, tremor-rigidity syndrome and psychoses. Progressive extrapyramidal neurological symptoms are typical features of neurologic WD. Patients usually develop initial neurological symptoms during their mid-teens or twenties and are frequently misdiagnosed with behavioral problems associated with puberty [41].

Treatment

Once WD is diagnosed, patients are advised to avoid foods with high copper contents, such as liver, chocolate, nuts, mushrooms, and shellfish. D-penicillamine is the first line drug for the treatment of WD, and pyridoxine (25 mg/day) should be co-administered. Side effects, including fever, rash, and lymph node swelling, occur in about 20% of these patients within the first months after starting treatment.

Hereditary Hemochromatosis (HHC)

Diagnostic Criteria (Fig. 11)

1. The diagnosis of HHC requires elevated fasting transferrin saturation or ferritin with genetic analysis or measurement of hepatic iron concentration.

2. Elevated serum ferritin alone is not specific for HHE.

Management

1. Phlebotomy has been the conventional treatment to remove excessive iron from the body.

2. Recently, an oral iron chelator, deferasirox, was shown effective in patients with secondary iron overload.

Hereditary hemochromatosis (HHE) is underdiagnosed, because it is thought to be a rare disorder. The genetic abnormality characteristic of HHE (C282 homozygote) has been reported present in 1 of 250 individuals [43]. Some patients with HHE are asymptomatic, whereas others have various symptoms, including arthralgias, diabetes, amenorrhea, congestive heart failure, arrhythmia, increased skin pigmentation, loss of libido, and abdominal pain. Importantly, patients with untreated HHE often develop cirrhosis and may progress to HCC. Therefore, early diagnosis and treatment are mandatory for patient management. Although fasting transferrin saturation and ferritin have been thought to be the standard diagnostic criteria, their sensitivity and specificity are lower in younger patients. Moreover, high serum ferritin concentrations have been observed in patients with NASH, chronic hepatitis C and alcoholic liver disease, hampering a diagnosis of HHE by serum ferritin concentration alone. Therefore patients with fasting transferrin saturation or elevated ferritin should undergo genetic analysis, and their hepatic iron concentration should be measured.

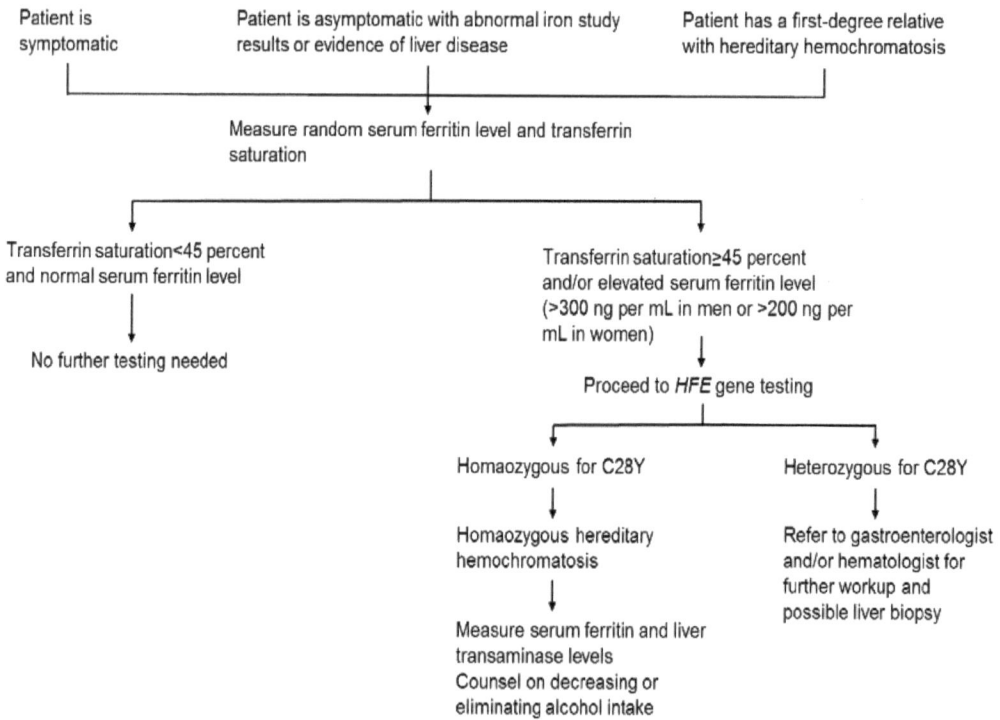

Patient is symptomatic

Patient is asymptomatic with abnormal iron study results or evidence of liver disease

Patient has a first-degree relative with hereditary hemochromatosis

Measure random serum ferritin level and transferrin saturation

Transferrin saturation<45 percent and normal serum ferritin level

No further testing needed

Transferrin saturation≥45 percent and/or elevated serum ferritin level (>300 ng per mL in men or >200 ng per mL in women)

Proceed to *HFE* gene testing

Homaozygous for C28Y

Homozygous hereditary hemochromatosis

Measure serum ferritin and liver transaminase levels
Counsel on decreasing or eliminating alcohol intake

Heterozygous for C28Y

Refer to gastroenterologist and/or hematologist for further workup and possible liver biopsy

Figure 11: Diagnostic algorithm for hereditary hemochromatosis [42].

Treatment

Phlebotomy is the treatment of choice to reduce excess iron deposits, since 500 ml blood contains about 250 mg iron. Phlebotomy should be performed weekly until serum ferritin concentration is less than 20-50ng/ml. Although the oral iron chelator deferasirox was recently shown effective in patients with secondary iron overload, its effects in patients with HHE remain uncertain. Moreover, deferasirox has serious side effects, including renal insufficiency, cytopenias and elevated liver enzymes [44].

Primary Sclerosing Cholangitis (PSC)

PSC is an autoimmune liver disease characterized by segmental bile duct fibrosis and dilatation with dilated normal intervening areas resulting in the characteristic "beads on a string" appearance. Its pathogenesis remains unclear, but may involve immune-mediated destruction of the bile ducts.

Patients are usually diagnosed by endoscopic cholangiography, although magnetic resonance cholangiopancreatography (MRCP) is an alternative method, with an accuracy close to 90%.

In European and North American populations, 70% to 80% of patients with PSC are estimated to have inflammatory bowel disease (IBD), and about 2% to 4% of patients with IBD have PSC [45]. These numbers differ in different countries. However, there is a definite association between PSC and IBD.

In general, only UDCA has been used to treat PSC, but has shown limited efficacy. Recently, IgG4-related sclerosing cholangitis, often associated with autoimmune pancreatitis, has been found to respond very well to corticosteroids. These patients have a good prognosis, in contrast to patients with PSC, who often require liver transplantation. Diffuse cholangiographic abnormalities observed in IgG4-related sclerosing cholangitis may resemble those observed in PSC, but the presence of segmental stenosis may suggest cholangiocarcinoma [46]. Since treatment and prognosis differ in these diseases with similar imaging results, differential diagnosis is important.

DIAGNOSIS AND MANAGEMENT OF LIVER CIRRHOSIS IN THE PRIMARY CARE SETTING

Clinical Diagnosis of Liver Cirrhosis

Cirrhosis is defined as a diffuse process with fibrosis and nodular formation of the liver. Nodular formation without fibrosis is not cirrhosis but is called nodular regenerative hyperplasia. Fibrosis usually occurs following hepatocyte necrosis, through the activation and proliferation of hepatic stellate cells and their production of cytokines, such as TGF-β. Since there are mechanisms for matrix degradation in the liver, the occurrence of fibrosis is determined by the balance between matrix synthesis and degradation.

Etiology of Cirrhosis

1. Hepatitis B and hepatitis C

2. Alcohol overconsumption

3. AIH

4. Metabolic diseases: NAFLD, hemochromatosis, Wilson disease, α1-antitrypsin deficiency

5. Biliary diseases: PBC or PSC

6. Cardiac disease: congestive heart failure

7. Drug-induced disease: methotrexate

8. Cryptogenic

Diagnosis of Cirrhosis

Cirrhosis is diagnosed based on physical examination and the results of laboratory tests and imaging modalities. Patients may complain of fatigue, anorexia, low grade fever, jaundice and/or pruritus (without skin lesions), but only jaundice is relatively specific for cirrhosis, with the other symptoms not contributing to an establishment of diagnosis. Histological examination is the gold standard for the diagnosis of cirrhosis. However, the risk of bleeding is high in patients with cirrhosis, Therefore, if cirrhosis can be diagnosed clinically, liver biopsy may be avoided.

Clinical features suggestive of cirrhosis are abdominal wall vascular collaterals (caput medusa), ascites, asterixis, spider nevi, palmar erythema, gynecomastia, testicular atrophy, splenomegaly, and hepatomegaly at midline. Symptoms include anorexia, fatigue, weakness, and weight loss, but none of them are specific. Other features suggesting cirrhosis include Dupuytren's contracture, fetor hepaticus, nail changes such as Muehrcke's nails; white bands go across the entire nail from side to side, and Terry's nails; white with reddened or dark tips [47].

Imaging methods, such as ultrasound, CT and MRI, are useful in diagnosing cirrhosis. The presence of irregular or nodular surfaces and blunt edge of the liver are indicators of cirrhosis on US, whereas manifestations of portal hypertension and morphological changes in the liver were the predictive signs on MRI and CT [47]. Although MRI and CT were slightly superior to US in predicting cirrhosis

[47], ultrasound can be repeatedly performed at shorter intervals because of its low cost and non-invasiveness [48]. Thus, ultrasound may be suitable as the initial screening method in patients suspected of cirrhosis [48].

Laboratory tests results suggestive of cirrhosis include AST/ALT >1, low serum albumin, prolonged PT, low platelet counts and hypergammaglobulinemia.

Management of Cirrhotic Patients

The treatment of patients with compensated cirrhosis should focus on removing the cause of liver injury, including antiviral agents for patients with viral hepatitis and immunosuppressants for patients with autoimmune liver disease. However, careful observation at regular intervals may be sufficient for patients with no indications for specific treatments and who show low or no inflammation and well preserved liver reserve functions.

Management of cirrhotic patients, especially decompensated patients, is mostly directed toward the treatment of complications.

Complications of Cirrhosis

Major complications of cirrhosis include ascites, spontaneous bacterial peritonitis, hepatic encephalopathy, portal hypertension, variceal bleeding, hepatorenal syndrome and HCC [49]. Pathophysiology and sequel of liver cirrhosis are summarized in Fig. (**12**).

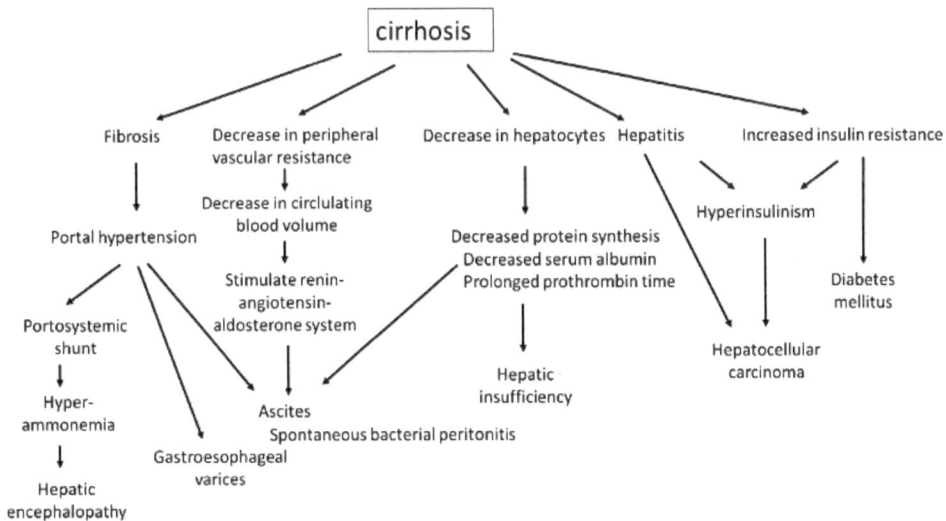

Figure 12: Pathophysiology and sequels of liver cirrhosis.

Ascites and Spontaneous Bacterial Peritonitis;

The pathogenesis of ascites formation in patients with liver diseases is not fully understood, but the renin-angiotensin-aldosterone system is thought to play a significant role. Moreover, hypoalbuminemia and portal hypertension are important causative events leading to ascites formation.

Causes of ascites retention can be estimated by measuring serum-ascites albumin gradient (SAAG), which is calculated by subtracting the albumin concentration in ascites from albumin concentration in serum obtained on the same day. Portal hypertension is indicated if the SAAG is ≥1.1 g/dL, and peritonitis or peritoneal carcinomatosis is suspected if SAAG is <1.1 g/dL. Spontaneous bacterial peritonitis is a common complication and is usually suspected in cirrhotic patients with fever, abdominal pain, ascites retention and >250/μl polymorphonuclear leukocytes in ascites. Ascites culture can be successful only when ascites is transferred to blood culture bottles at the bedside.

Management of Ascites

1. Sodium and fluid restriction and diuretics are essential. Spironolactone is the diuretic of choice, because it can suppress the renin-angiotensin-aldosterone system.

2. Spontaneous bacterial peritonitis can be treated with third generation cephalosporin antibiotics. For prophylaxis, long-term administration of norfloxacin or trimethoprim/sulfamethoxazole may be effective.

3. If ascites is refractory to sodium restriction and oral diuretics, large volume paracentesis may be necessary, with post paracentesis albumin infusion considered if paracentesis is greater than 4 to 5 L.

4. Administration of an oral β-blocker (*e.g.* propranolol, 10-30mg/day), which is effective in reducing portal pressure, may help control ascites retention secondary to portal hypertension. However, this treatment may worsen patient prognosis.

Hepatic Encephalopathy

Hepatic encephalopathy is characterized by changes in consciousness level, behavioral patterns, neurological disturbances, asterixis and/or electroencephalographic abnormalities. Hepatic encephalopathy may be reversible or chronic/progressive depending on its cause.

Pathophysiology; The pathogenesis of hepatic encephalopathy is not well understood. Although elevated plasma ammonia concentrations are important, other factors may be involved, including increased levels of serotonin, endogenous benzodiazepines, alteration of the blood-brain barrier, zinc deficiency, and manganese deposition.

Diagnosis; Overt hepatic encephalopathy is diagnosed by symptoms such as abnormal sleep patterns, lack of awareness, prolonged reaction times, impairments in cognitive and mental function, alterations in behavior and personality, disturbances in attention and coordination, asterixis, and flapping tremors. Electroencephalographic abnormalities may support a diagnosis of hepatic encephalopathy. Patients with encephalopathy experience disturbances in consciousness, which can progress to confusion, stupor, coma and even death. Subclinical hepatic encephalopathy, characterized by an impairment in complex activities such as driving a car, was recently described and can be detected only by specific psychometric tests such as number connection tests.

Precipitants; Elevated blood ammonia may be due to excessive dietary protein, gastrointestinal bleeding, constipation, or infection. Ammonia (NH_3) is converted to ammonium ion (NH_4+) in an acidic milieu. However, only NH_3 can pass from the gut to the blood and move across the blood-brain barrier. This passage may occur more easily in patients with hypokalemia, azotemia, and alkalosis. The presence of a portosystemic shunt, generated by portal hypertension or TIPS, may also elevate blood ammonia. Moreover, an imbalance in amino acids is thought to contribute to the development of hepatic encephalopathy, and low Fischer ratio (branched chain amino acids/phenylalanine+tyrosine, where normal is >3) is often demonstrated in these patients.

Treatment;

1. Lactulose or lactitol, and other laxatives or enemas are effective to reduce the production and absorption of ammonia from the colon. Lactulose and lactitol are the synthetic disaccharides that make the intestinal lumen an acidic environment, leading to the conversion of NH3 to NH4+, reducing the absorption of NH3.

2. Nonabsorbable oral antibiotics may reduce the population of intestinal bacteria.

3. Flumazenil and other benzodiazepine receptor antagonists may be effective.

4. Patients should be intravenously administered solutions containing high concentrations of branched chain amino acids. However, this treatment may not lower blood ammonia levels.

Portal Hypertension and Variceal Hemorrhage [50]

Portal hypertension, defined as portal vein pressure >10 mmHg, is caused by increased outflow resistance or increased portal inflow. Increased outflow resistance may be due to (1) prehepatic causes (*e.g.* portal vein thrombosis), (2) hepatic causes (*e.g.* cirrhosis, liver mass) or (3) posthepatic causes (*e.g.* hepatic vein obstruction, Budd Chiari syndrome). Increased portal inflow results from peripheral vasodilation, hyperdynamic circulation or increased blood flow from an enlarged spleen.

The major complication of portal hypertension is variceal hemorrhage. Approximately 50% of patients with cirrhosis develop varices (5% to 15% per year), with the rate of variceal bleeding being approximately 10% to 30% per year. Three clinical criteria are used to predict the risk of variceal bleeding: (1) variceal size, (2) Child-Pugh class and (3) the presence of red wales (endoscopically identified longitudinal, dilated venules on varices). British Society of Gastroenterology guidelines recommend that patients at high risk of variceal rupture receive prophylactic treatment.

1. Primary prophylaxis of variceal bleeding is aimed at reducing the portal pressure leading to the lowering of variceal pressure. Propranolol at a dosage of 40 to 80 mg twice daily is the drug therapy with evidence. Dosage of propranolol can be determined based on a 25% reduction in pulse rate.

2. If propranolol is not tolerated, isosorbide mononitrate at a dosage of 20 mg twice daily can be used.

If variceal bleeding occurs, it may be controlled by band ligation. If banding procedure is technically difficult, endoscopic sclerotherapy with vasoconstrictors such as vasopressin or insertion of a Sengstaken-Blakemore tube may be useful.

Transjugular intrahepatic portosystemic shunt (TIPS) has been shown to reduce portal hypertension and variceal bleeding more effective than band ligation. However, TIPS may increase the risk of encephalopathy, and it remains unclear whether TIPS improves survival.

Hepatorenal syndrome and HCC are discussed in other chapters.

MESSAGES FROM HEPATOLOGISTS TO GENERAL PHYSICIANS

1. There are five common causes of chronic liver injury: viral hepatitis (B or C), fatty liver disease, alcoholic liver injury, DILI, and autoimmune liver disease (primary biliary cirrhosis, autoimmune hepatitis, and primary sclerosing cholangitis), and tests for these diseases should first be considered.

2. Fatty liver is the most common cause of chronic liver injury, but the presence of fatty deposits does not exclude other accompanying etiologies. The most common pattern of liver injury caused by fatty liver is mild elevation of ALT (> AST) and γ-GTP.

3. Chronic hepatitis B is diagnosed by persistent elevation of ALT and serum HBV DNA. Flare of ALT is usually observed 2 – 4 weeks after elevation of serum HBV DNA and constant low levels of serum HBV DNA with high and fluctuated ALT exclude HBV-related liver injury.

4. High levels of serum anti-HBc are exclusively observed in chronic HBV infection, and some patients with liver cirrhosis B may be positive only for high levels of anti-HBc but negative for both HBsAg and HBV DNA.

5. Serum HBV DNA levels are the most important markers for predicting the possible development of hepatitis and hepatocarcinogenesis. Serum HBV DNA<10^4copies/mL (= 2000 IU/mL) indicates stable hepatitis B with little risk of progression to hepatitis and hepatocarcinogenesis.

6. Chronic hepatitis B often progresses rapidly to liver cirrhosis, which occurs in less than 3 years in most cases. Therefore, prompt and appropriate management of patients with chronic hepatitis B with high activity should be performed by hepatologists.

7. HBV infection persists for a long time, and is essentially a lifelong infection. Therefore, patients positive for anti-HBs or anti-HBc are thought to have HBV in the liver even when HBV DNA is not detectable in serum. Patients with low levels of HBV replication could

show reactivation of the virus after administration of immunosuppressive agents or glucocorticoid. Especially, glucocorticoid can directly stimulate HBV replication *via* interaction with glucocorticoid responsive elements present on the S-region of HBV DNA, and may lead to explosive replication of HBV followed by severe hepatitis.

8. The main treatment for hepatitis B consists of nucleot(s)ide analog administration, and essentially all patients with hepatitis B, from children to the elderly and form chronic hepatitis to decompensated cirrhosis, can be safely treated with these drugs. However, cessation of treatment is difficult in patients with liver cirrhosis.

9. In young patients, pegylated interferon is another treatment of choice.

10. Chronic hepatitis C usually progress slowly and platelet counts are decreased with the progression of fibrosis. Platelet counts below $10^5/\mu L$ are often seen in patients with liver cirrhosis.

11. Treatment of chronic hepatitis C has changed markedly, and interferon-free treatment is now the main strategy. Selection of the treatment method should be done by hepatologists according to the patient's age, activity and chronicity of hepatitis, and the presence of mutations of HCV RNA determining sensitivity of direct-acting antiviral agents.

12. In cases of liver cirrhosis, appropriate management of the complications, such as ascites, hepatic encephalopathy, gastroesophageal varices, and development of HCC, is essential. Ascites retention is caused not only by hypoalbuminemia but also by portal hypertension. Therefore, reducing portal pressure should be considered in addition to salt restriction and diuretics, especially in patients with refractory ascites.

13. Hepatic encephalopathy is usually caused by hyperammonemia, but it should be noted that plasma ammonia is routinely measured as NH_4^+, while NH_3 that is responsible for the pathogenesis of encephalopathy is not measured. Therefore, plasma ammonia level does not correlate well with the degree of encephalopathy. Branched amino acids are used in the management of hepatic encephalopathy, but intravenous

BCAA administration improves encephalopathy not by reducing plasma ammonia levels, but mainly by correcting amino acid imbalance in the plasma and brain. The essential treatment for reduction of plasma ammonia is administration of lactulose or lactitol. Recent studies demonstrated the efficacy of probiotics for prevention and amelioration of hepatic encephalopathy.

14. Suppression and early detection of HCC development are important for the management of patients with liver cirrhosis, and several antiviral drugs that are administered even in cirrhotic patients with hepatitis B and C can reduce the development of HCC in these patients.

ACKNOWLEDGEMENTS

We are very thankful to Ms. Asma Ahmed, manager publications, Bentham Science Publishers, for her patience and long-term assistance.

CONFLICT OF INTEREST

The author confirms that he has no conflict of interest to declare for this publication.

REFERENCES

[1]   Lazo M, Selvin E, Clark JM. Brief communication: clinical implications of short-term variability in liver function test results. Ann Intern Med 2008;148:348-352.
[2]   Penna A, Artini M, Cavalli A, Levrero M, Bertoletti A, Pilli M, Chisari FV, Rehermann B, Del Prete G, Fiaccadori F, Ferrari C. Long-lasting memory T cell responses following self-limited acute hepatitis B. J Clin Invest 1996;98:1185-1194.
[3]   Powell LW, George DK, McDonnell SM, Kowdley KV. Diagnosis of hemochromatosis. Ann Intern Med 1998;129:925-931.
[4]   Maddrey WC. Clinicopathological patterns of drug-induced liver disease. In Drug-induced liver disease. Kaplowitz N and DeLeve LD Eds. Pp227-242. Marcel DEKKER, Inc., 2003.
[5]   Björnsson E. The natural history of drug-induced liver injury. Semin Liver Dis 2009;29:357-363.
[6]   Danan G, Benichou C. Causality assessment of adverse reactions to drugs--I. A novel method based on the conclusions of international consensus meetings: application to drug-induced liver injuries. J Clin Epidemiol 1993;46:1323-1330.
[7]   Janus PO, Younossi ZM. Epidemiology and Natural History of NAFLD and NASH. Clin Liver Dis 2007;11:1–16.
[8]   Bayard M, Holt J, Boroughs E. Nonalcoholic fatty liver disease. Am Fam Physician 2006;73:1961-1968.
[9]   Adams LA, Lindor KD, Angulo P. The prevalence of autoantibodies and autoimmune hepatitis in patients with nonalcoholic fatty liver disease. Am J Gastroenterol 2004;99:1316-1320.
[10]   Angulo P, Hui JM, Marchesini G, Bugianesi E, George J, Farrell GC, Enders F, Saksena S, Burt AD, Bida JP, Lindor K, Sanderson SO, Lenzi M, Adams LA, Kench J, Therneau TM, Day CP. The NAFLD fibrosis score: a noninvasive system that identifies liver fibrosis in patients with NAFLD. Hepatology 2007;45:846-854.

[11]   Tanwar S, Trembling PM, Guha IN, Parkes J, Kaye P, Burt AD, Ryder SD, Aithal GP, Day CP, Rosenberg WM. Validation of terminal peptide of procollagen III for the detection and assessment of nonalcoholic steatohepatitis in patients with nonalcoholic fatty liver disease. Hepatology 2013;57:103-111.

[12]   Cichoż-Lach H, Celiński K, Prozorow-Król B, Swatek J, Słomka M, Lach T. The BARD score and the NAFLD fibrosis score in the assessment of advanced liver fibrosis in nonalcoholic fatty liver disease. Med Sci Monit 2012;18:CR735-40.

[13]   Lee TH, Han SH, Yang JD, Kim D, Ahmed M. Prediction of advanced fibrosis in nonalcoholic fatty liver disease: An enhanced model of BARD score. Gut Liver 2013;7:323-338.

[14]   Hashimoto E, Yatsuji S, Tobari M, Taniai M, Torii N, Tokushige K, Shiratori K. Hepatocellular carcinoma in patients with nonalcoholic steatohepatitis. J Gastroenterol 2009;44 Suppl 19:89-95.

[15]   Katsurada A, Marusawa H, Uemoto S, Kaburagi A, Tanaka K, Chiba T. Circulating antibody to hepatitis B core antigen does NOT always reflect the latent hepatitis B virus infection in the liver tissue. Hepatol Res 2003;25:105-114.

[16]   Ikeda K, Kobayashi M, Someya T, Saitoh S, Hosaka T, Akuta N, Suzuki F, Suzuki Y, Arase Y, Kumada H. Occult hepatitis B virus infection increases hepatocellular carcinogenesis by eight times in patients with non-B, non-C liver cirrhosis: a cohort study. J Viral Hepat 2009;16:437-443.

[17]   Tseng TC, Liu CJ, Yang HC, Su TH, Wang CC, Chen CL, Hsu CA, Kuo SF, Liu CH, Chen PJ, Chen DS, Kao JH. Serum hepatitis B surface antigen levels help predict disease progression in patients with low hepatitis B virus loads. Hepatology 2013;57:441-450.

[18]   Kumada T, Toyoda H, Tada T, Kiriyama S, Tanikawa M, Hisanaga Y, Kanamori A, Niinomi T, Yasuda S, Andou Y, Yamamoto K, Tanaka J. Effect of nucleos(t)ide analogue therapy on hepatocarcinogenesis in chronic hepatitis B patients: a propensity score analysis. J Hepatol 2013;58:427-433.

[19]   Hoare M, Gelson WT, Rushbrook SM, Curran MD, Woodall T, Coleman N, Davies SE, Alexander GJ. Histological changes in HCV antibody-positive, HCV RNA-negative subjects suggest persistent virus infection. Hepatology 2008;48:1737-1745.

[20]   Poynard T, Ratziu V, Benhamou Y, Opolon P, Cacoub P, Bedossa P. Natural history of HCV infection. Baillieres Best Pract Res Clin Gastroenterol 2000;14:211-228.

[21]   Hamada H, Yatsuhashi H, Yano K, Daikoku M, Arisawa K, Inoue O, Koga M, Nakata K, Eguchi K, Yano M. Impact of aging on the development of hepatocellular carcinoma in patients with posttransfusion chronic hepatitis C. Cancer 2002;95:331-339.

[22]   Tokita H, Fukui H, Tanaka A, Kamitsukasa H, Yagura M, Harada H, Okamoto H. Risk factors for the development of hepatocellular carcinoma among patients with chronic hepatitis C who achieved a sustained virological response to interferon therapy. J Gastroenterol Hepatol 2005;20:752-758.

[23]   Gane EJ, Stedman CA, Hyland RH, Ding X, Svarovskaia E, Symonds WT, Hindes RG, Berrey MM. Nucleotide polymerase inhibitor sofosbuvir plus ribavirin for hepatitis C. N Engl J Med 2013;368:34-44.

[24]   Gane EJ, Stedman CA, Hyland RH, Ding X, Svarovskaia E, Subramanian GM, Symonds WT, McHutchison JG, Pang PS. Efficacy of nucleotide polymerase inhibitor sofosbuvir plus the NS5A inhibitor ledipasvir or the NS5B non-nucleoside inhibitor GS-9669 against HCV genotype 1 infection. Gastroenterology 2014;146:736-743.

[25]   Everson GT, Sims KD, Rodriguez-Torres M, Hézode C, Lawitz E, Bourlière M, Loustaud-Ratti V, Rustgi V, Schwartz H, Tatum H, Marcellin P, Pol S, Thuluvath PJ, Eley T, Wang X, Huang SP, McPhee F, Wind-Rotolo M, Chung E, Pasquinelli C, Grasela DM, Gardiner DF. Efficacy of an interferon- and ribavirin-free regimen of daclatasvir, asunaprevir, and BMS-791325 in treatment-naive patients with HCV genotype 1 infection. Gastroenterology 2014;146:420-429.

[26]   Kowdley KV, Lawitz E, Poordad F, Cohen DE, Nelson DR, Zeuzem S, Everson GT, Kwo P, Foster GR, Sulkowski MS, Xie W, Pilot-Matias T, Liossis G, Larsen L, Khatri A, Podsadecki T, Bernstein B. Phase 2b trial of interferon-free therapy for hepatitis C virus genotype 1. N Engl J Med 2014;370:222-232.

[27]   Sulkowski MS, Gardiner DF, Rodriguez-Torres M, Reddy KR, Hassanein T, Jacobson I, Lawitz E, Lok AS, Hinestrosa F, Thuluvath PJ, Schwartz H, Nelson DR, Everson GT, Eley T, Wind-Rotolo M, Huang SP, Gao M, Hernandez D, McPhee F, Sherman D, Hindes R, Symonds W, Pasquinelli C,

Grasela DM; AI444040 Study Group. Daclatasvir plus sofosbuvir for previously treated or untreated chronic HCV infection. N Engl J Med 2014;370:211-221.

[28]   Zeuzem S1, Dusheiko GM, Salupere R, Mangia A, Flisiak R, Hyland RH, Illeperuma A, Svarovskaia E, Brainard DM, Symonds WT, Subramanian GM, McHutchison JG, Weiland O, Reesink HW, Ferenci P, Hézode C, Esteban R; VALENCE Investigators. Sofosbuvir and ribavirin in HCV genotypes 2 and 3. N Engl J Med 2014;370:1993-2001.

[29]   Hennes EM, Zeniya M, Czaja AJ, Parés A, Dalekos GN, Krawitt EL, Bittencourt PL, Porta G, Boberg KM, Hofer H, Bianchi FB, Shibata M, Schramm C, Eisenmann de Torres B, Galle PR, McFarlane I, Dienes HP, Lohse AW; International Autoimmune Hepatitis Group. Simplified criteria for the diagnosis of autoimmune hepatitis. Hepatology 2008;48:169-176.

[30]   Abe M, Hiasa Y, Masumoto T, Kumagi T, Akbar SM, Ninomiya T, Matsui H, Michitaka K, Horiike N, Onji M. Clinical characteristics of autoimmune hepatitis with histological features of acute hepatitis. Hepatol Res 2001;21:213-219.

[31]   Hofer H, Oesterreicher C, Wrba F, Ferenci P, Penner E. Centrilobular necrosis in autoimmune hepatitis: a histological feature associated with acute clinical presentation. J Clin Pathol 2006;59:246-249.

[32]   Choudhuri G, Somani SK, Baba CS, Alexander G. Autoimmune hepatitis in India: profile of an uncommon disease. BMC Gastroenterol 2005;5:27.

[33]   Manns MP, Czaja AJ, Gorham JD, Krawitt EL, Mieli-Vergani G, Vergani D, Vierling JM; American Association for the Study of Liver Diseases. Diagnosis and management of autoimmune hepatitis. Hepatology 2010;51:2193-2213.

[34]   Miyake Y, Iwasaki Y, Kobashi H, Yasunaka T, Ikeda F, Takaki A, Okamoto R, Takaguchi K, Ikeda H, Makino Y, Ando M, Sakaguchi K, Yamamoto K. Efficacy of ursodeoxycholic acid for Japanese patients with autoimmune hepatitis. Hepatol Int 2009;3:556-562.

[35]   Lindor KD, Gershwin ME, Poupon R, Kaplan M, Bergasa NV, Heathcote EJ; American Association for Study of Liver Disease. Primary biliary cirrhosis. Hepatology 2009;50:291-308.

[36]   Corpechot C, Carrat F, Bahr A, Chrétien Y, Poupon RE, Poupon R. The effect of ursodeoxycholic acid therapy on the natural course of primary biliary cirrhosis. Gastroenterology 2005;128:297-303.

[37]   Parés A, Rodés J. Natural history of primary biliary cirrhosis. Clin Liver Dis 2003;7:779-794.

[38]   Mattalia A, Quaranta S, Leung PS, Bauducci M, Van de Water J, Calvo PL, Danielle F, Rizzetto M, Ansari A, Coppel RL, Rosina F, Gershwin ME. Characterization of antimitochondrial antibodies in health adults. Hepatology 1998;27:656-661.

[39]   Metcalf JV, Mitchison HC, Palmer JM, Jones DE, Bassendine MF, James OF. Natural history of early primary biliary cirrhosis. Lancet 1996;348(9039):1399-1402.

[40]   Jackson H, Solaymani-Dodaran M, Card TR, Aithal GP, Logan R, West J. Influence of ursodeoxycholic acid on the mortality and malignancy associated with primary biliary cirrhosis: a population-based cohort study. Hepatology 2007;46:1131-1137.

[41]   Roberts EA, Schilsky ML; American Association for Study of Liver Diseases (AASLD). Diagnosis and treatment of Wilson disease: an update. Hepatology 2008;47:2089-2111.

[42]   Crownover BK1, Covey CJ. Hereditary hemochromatosis. Am Fam Physician 2013;87:183-190.

[43]   Bacon BR. Genetic hemochromatosis and iron overload. In Practical management of liver diseases. Younossi ZM Eds. Pp117-130. Cambridge University Press, 2008.

[44]   Gattermann N. The treatment of secondary hemochromatosis. Dtsch Arztebl Int 2009;106:499-450.

[45]   Talwalkar JA, Lindor KD. Autoimmune Liver Disease. In Practical Gastroenterology and Hepatology; Liver and Biliary Disease. Talley NJ, Lindor KD, Vargas HE Eds. Pp250-260. WILEY-BLACKWELL, 2010.

[46]   Nakazawa T, Naitoh I, Hayashi K, Miyabe K, Simizu S, Joh T. Diagnosis of IgG4-related sclerosing cholangitis. World J Gastroenterol 2013;19:7661-7670.

[47]   Heidelbaugh JJ, Bruderly M. Cirrhosis and chronic liver failure: part I. Diagnosis and evaluation. Am Fam Physician 2006;74:756-762.

[48]   Kudo M, Zheng RQ, Kim SR, Okabe Y, Osaki Y, Iijima H, Itani T, Kasugai H, Kanematsu M, Ito K, Usuki N, Shimamatsu K, Kage M, Kojiro M. Diagnostic accuracy of imaging for liver cirrhosis compared to histologically proven liver cirrhosis. A multicenter collaborative study. Intervirology 2008;51 Suppl 1:17-26.

[49]   Heidelbaugh JJ, Sherbondy M. Cirrhosis and chronic liver failure: part II. Complications and treatment. Am Fam Physician 2006;74:767-776.

[50]   Bosch J1, García-Pagán JC. Complications of cirrhosis. I. Portal hypertension. J Hepatol 2000;32(1 Suppl):141-156.

CHAPTER 5

Diagnostic Strategies and Treatment of Liver Tumors

Yoshiharu Tokimitsu[1],* and Yukihiro Shimizu[2]

[1]Department of Internal Medicine, Toyama Red Cross Hospital, Japan and [2]Gastroenterology Center, Nanto Municipal Hospital, Toyama, Japan

Abstract: Because liver tumors are usually asymptomatic, they are frequently observed incidentally on imaging tests performed for other purposes. The most common types of liver tumors are cysts and hemangiomas, which do not require any treatment unless they are accompanied by infection, hemorrhage, or rupture. In contrast, primary liver cancer and metastatic liver tumors are usually found in patients at high risk during regular checkups or close examination. Other benign masses found in the liver often need CT, MRI, or even liver biopsy for a final diagnosis. Radiofrequency ablation has been shown effective in the treatment of hepatocellular carcinomas and liver metastases from colorectal cancer, with liver resection also effective for those tumors.

Keywords: Adenoma, cholangiocarcinoma, computed tomography, cysts, focal nodular hyperplasia, hemangioma, hepatocellular carcinoma, liver tumor, magnetic resonance imaging, metastatic liver tumor, radiofrequency ablation, tumor marker, ultrasonography.

KEY POINTS

1. Patients usually do not have any specific complaints.

2. Patients at high risk of developing liver cancer require regular checkups.

3. Liver masses are often found incidentally by ultrasonography, but ultrasonography alone is usually insufficient for a final diagnosis.

4. Liver cysts and hemangiomas are the most common liver tumors found on ultrasonography, but hemangiomas are sometimes difficult to differentiate from well-differentiated hepatocellular carcinoma.

*Corresponding author Yoshiharu Tokimitsu: Gastroenterology Unit, Toyama Red Cross Hospital, Toayama, Japan; E-mail: ytokimitsu@gmail.com

5.   Liver solid masses >1cm in diameter should be further examined by contrast-medium enhanced CT or MRI.

INTRODUCTION

Patients with liver tumors are frequently encountered in primary care. As most liver tumors are asymptomatic, they are usually discovered incidentally during ultrasonography (US) or computed tomography (CT) scans performed for other purposes. Liver tumors rarely cause marked swelling of the liver unless they are present in significant numbers or are large in size. Thus, palpation is usually unable to detect their presence. Although biliary tract enzymes and transaminases may be elevated in patients with multiple lesions or large tumors, most patients with liver tumors do not show abnormal results on liver function tests. Primary care providers must know how to diagnose small liver tumors and determine whether or not these lesions require immediate treatment (Table **1**).

Many clinical practice guidelines have been formulated for hepatocellular carcinoma (HCC), including the guidelines of the American Association for the Study of Liver Diseases (AASLD) [1] and the European Association for the Study of the Liver/the European Organization for Research and Treatment of Cancer (EASL-EORTC) [2]. Physicians caring for patients at high risk for HCC must provide high-quality screening, properly manage the detected lesions, and provide therapy most appropriate for the stage of disease [1].

DIAGNOSTIC STRATEGY

If a liver tumor is detected during abdominal US or CT, what are the next steps? This section will describe a strategy for the differential diagnosis of liver tumors.

General Considerations

US is a non-invasive and economical imaging method, allowing repeat scans at short intervals. Their sensitivity in detecting lesions, however, depends on the skill and knowledge of the person performing the examination. US also has several disadvantages. As ultrasound waves are strongly reflected from the surface of air within the body, US cannot produce detailed images of the intestines, as these contain large amounts of air, or of the organs lying behind the intestines. Fatty tissue also attenuates ultrasound waves, making US more difficult in obese patients. Gallstones, cholecystitis, obstructive jaundice, pancreatitis, pleural effusion, and peritoneal ascites may all be easily diagnosed by abdominal

US. Diagnosis of liver tumors requires ascertaining their characteristics, including tumor size, shape, echogenicity, echo pattern, marginal properties, and relationships to adjacent blood vessels. Both the qualitative properties of the liver tumors themselves and the patient's clinical background are important for the differential diagnosis of liver tumors. In particular, patients with chronic liver disease are at higher risk for HCC, and the detection of a liver tumor in a febrile patient may suggest a liver abscess. A history of oral contraceptive use suggests the possibility of adenoma. The simultaneous detection of a liver and an extrahepatic tumor suggests the possibility that the liver tumor is metastatic from the primary extrahepatic tumor.

Table 1. Solid liver tumors.

	Benign	Malignant
Hepatocyte origin	Hepatocellular adenoma [§ +]	Hepatocellular carcinoma*
	Focal nodular hyperplasia	Hepatoblastoma*
	Nodular regenerative hyperplasia	
	Adenomatous hyperplaisa[++]	
	Partial nodular transformation	
Cholangiocellular orgin	Bile duct adenoma	Cholangiocarcinoma*
	Biliary microhemartoma	
	Biliary cystadenoma[+]	
	Biliary papillomatosis[+]	
Others	Hemangioma[§]	Epitheloid hemangioendothelioma*
	Mesenchymal hamartoma	Angiosarcoma*
	Inflammatory pseudotumor	Primary hepatic lymphoma*
	Lipoma, Angiomyolipoma	
	Infatile hemangioendothelioma [§]	
	Lymphangiomatosis, Leiomyoma	
	Fibroma, Myxoma	

* Treatment including resection, chemotherapy or radiation should be required.

[+] Malignant transformation should be considered.

++ No specific therapy is needed..

[§] Treatment including resection may be required in symptomatic cases.

Cysts and hemangiomas are the most often encountered mass lesions in the liver, and the former can be diagnosed accurately by US alone. Hemangiomas characteristically appear hyperechoic (Fig. **1**), but their images may vary greatly among patients [3]. Well-differentiated HCC and hemangioma appear extremely similar on US images and are frequently difficult to distinguish. A tumor detected in a patient with severe chronic liver disease, particularly a large tumor, is more likely to be HCC than hemangioma. Cysts, hemangiomas, and metastatic liver tumors are more common than benign liver tumors such as adenoma and focal nodular hyperplasia (Fig. **2**). In the United States, colorectal cancer is the most common cause of metastatic liver tumors (Fig. **3**). If a liver tumor cannot be diagnosed by US alone, then CT (Fig. **4**) or magnetic resonance imaging (MRI) should be performed. If imaging alone is not diagnostic, a tumor biopsy should be performed for histological diagnosis (Fig. **5**). However, as biopsy procedures carry several risks, including hemorrhage and dissemination, they should only be performed in selected patients. In general, solid liver masses less than 1 cm in diameter, found in patients with chronic liver disease, should be followed-up at regular intervals, whereas larger tumors above 1 cm in diameter, usually require additional examination, by dynamic contrast enhanced CT or MRI. A suggested strategy for a patient with a liver mass found during ultrasound screening is shown in Fig. (**5**) [4].

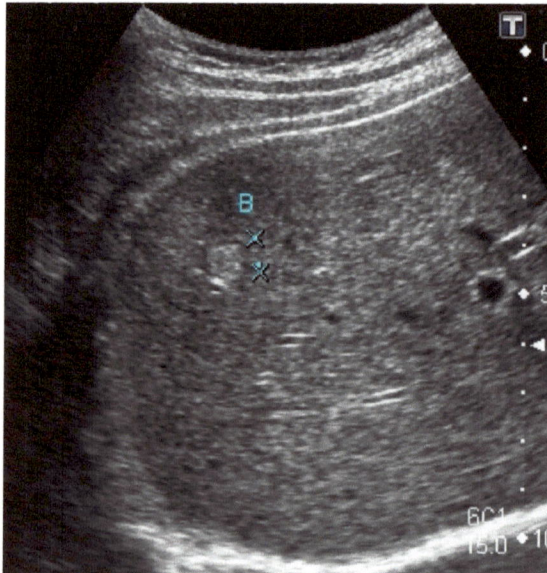

Figure 1: US imaging of a hemangioma. Hemangiomas characteristically appear as homogeneously hyperechoic lesions with clearly demarcated margins. Small hemangiomas (<30 mm) are usually hyperechoic.

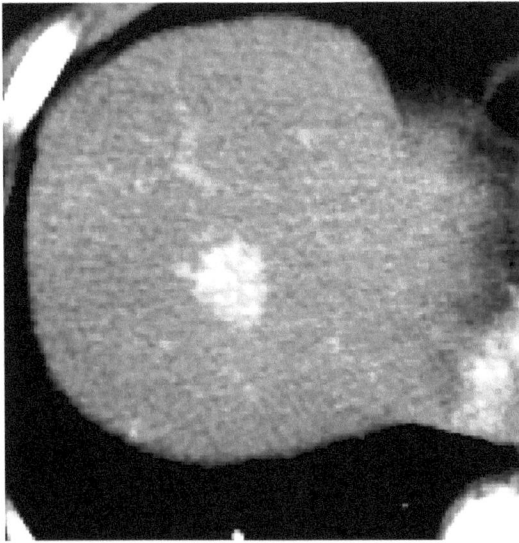

Figure 2: Dynamic CT imaging of a focal nodular hyperplasia (FNH). FNHs appear as hypervascular tumors without capsule, and may be difficult to differentiate from hepatocellular carcinoma. A central fibrous scar, appearing as a central hypodense area, is observed in 43.5% of FNHs during the early vascular phase [5].

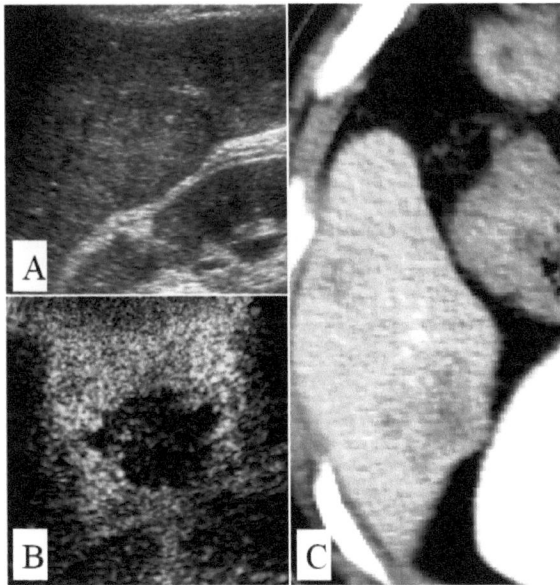

Figure 3: US and CT images of liver metastases from colorectal cancer. **A:** On US, these metastatic tumors are often hyperechoic. **B:** Contrast-enhanced ultrasound (CEUS) is also extremely useful for diagnosis. Malignant tumors appear hypoechoic compared with their surroundings during the Kupffer phase. **C:** On contrast-enhanced CT, the interiors of metastatic liver tumors are often hypovascular.

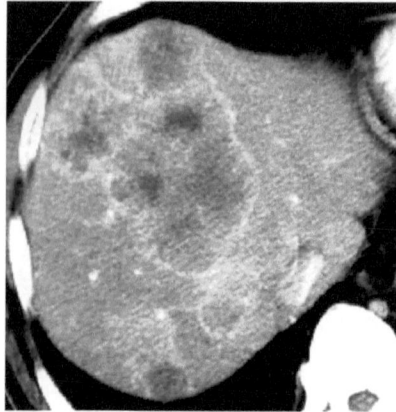

Figure 4: Contrast-enhanced imaging of liver metastases from colorectal cancer. In most cases, multiple nodules are observed in the liver. The margins of metastatic liver tumors are slightly enhanced, but their interiors are hypovascular.

Diagnostic Considerations for Liver Tumors

Liver Cysts

Most liver cysts are discovered by chance during imaging scans, with the majority being asymptomatic. Ultrasound scanning is the simplest and most effective method of detecting liver cysts, which appear as anechoic areas with posterior echo enhancement. Very small cysts, however, may be difficult to diagnose by US scan alone; CT scans are more sensitive than US in detecting small cysts.

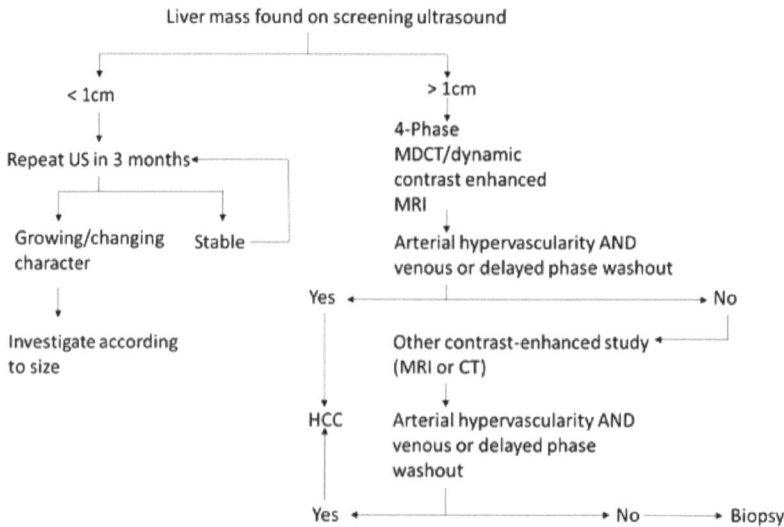

Figure 5: Diagnostic strategy for liver masses found during ultrasound screening [4].

Almost all cysts are asymptomatic and do not cause any abnormal liver function test results. However, large cysts and those present in very large numbers may cause abdominal distension or other symptoms, as well as abnormal liver function, particularly elevated gamma-glutamyltransferase (γ-GTP) and alkaline phosphatase (ALP). Large (>4 cm) cysts may be accompanied by intracystic hemorrhage and/or sudden abdominal pain. Simple cysts appear hypointense on CT. The differential diagnosis for simple cysts includes cystic metastatic tumors such as ovarian cancer, cystadenocarcinoma, cystadenoma, liver abscess, and necrotic malignant tumor. Necrosis frequently appears as a cystic lesion within liver metastases from squamous cell carcinoma, neuroendocrine tumor, and sarcoma. In most cases, US scanning is sufficient for the diagnosis of simple cyst, but CT or MRI may be required for the final diagnosis of cysts complicated by hemorrhage or infection.

Hemangioma

Cavernous hemangioma is the most frequent type of benign liver tumor, with a prevalence estimated at 0.4% to 20%. Hemangiomas are usually asymptomatic, and are detected incidentally in most patients. Hemangiomas appearing as homogeneous, hyperechoic lesions with clearly demarcated margins can be diagnosed by US alone. However, complications such as thrombi, fibrosis, hemorrhage, and calcification result in a range of modes, from isoechoic to hypoechoic, making it difficult to diagnose hemangiomas with complications by US alone. This variation in internal echogenicity is a phenomenon unique to hemangiomas. Hemangiomas ≤30 mm in size do not require any particular monitoring, and those in adults ≤50 mm in diameter have been reported not to increase in size [6].

Hyperechoic lesions in cirrhotic livers may be hemangiomas or well-differentiated HCCs. Contrast-enhanced CT or MRI is therefore required for the diagnosis of hemangioma in patients at high risk of HCC or metastatic liver cancer. Biopsy may be attempted for diagnostic purposes, but its usefulness is limited if sufficient tissue cannot be obtained.

Malignant Liver Tumors

Malignant liver tumors include HCC, cholangiocarcinoma and metastatic liver tumor. A malignant liver tumor is often detected by chance or inevitably during the diagnostic process. Space-occupying lesions ≤5 mm in size are not often recognized as tumors. Patients at high risk of cancer should be assessed by CT scanning and tumor marker tests, in addition to US. Lesions that are not identified on US scans may be detected on CT.

Patients at risk of HCC are recommended to undergo US scans at three- to six-month intervals. Malignant liver tumors ≤20 mm in size rarely exhibit a normal isoechoic pattern. Of HCCs ≤10 mm in size, 92.3% of lesions were found to be hypoechoic and 7.6% hyperechoic, whereas, of those lesions 10–20 mm in size, 59.5% have been reported hypoechoic and 5.4% hyperechoic [7]. HCC lesions ≥20 mm in size often exhibit signs specific for HCC, including a mosaic pattern, posterior echo enhancement, and lateral shadow patterns. Assessment of all nodules ≤30 mm in diameter showed that 91% exhibited a mosaic pattern and that 92% of hypoechoic lesions were HCC. Clearly demarcated margins and a mosaic pattern in lesions ≥30 mm in size each had a sensitivity ≥80% for HCC [8]. In contrast, metastatic liver tumors, especially those originating from the gastrointestinal tract, are frequently hyperechoic, with a bull's-eye like pattern characteristic of metastatic liver tumors.

Contrast-enhanced ultrasound (CEUS) is also extremely useful for the diagnosis of HCC (Fig. **6**). Microbubbles clearly demonstrate the presence of tumors in the liver. During the early vascular phase, most HCCs are hyperechoic, reflecting tumor neovascularization with abundant blood circulation. Microbubbles are subsequently phagocytosed by Kupffer cells. As fewer Kupffer cells are present in malignant tumors than in the surrounding liver, these tumors appear hypoechoic compared with surrounding non-malignant tissue during the Kupffer phase.

Attention should also be paid to the tissue surrounding the tumor. Partial dilatation of the intrahepatic bile ducts suggests that the tumor may be located downstream. Small cholangiocarcinomas may exist in such area, which are usually irregular with poorly demarcated margins and variations in internal echo intensity. The progression of intrahepatic cholangiocarcinoma into its surroundings may be diagnosed by careful observation, although, in some patients, the only indication may be thickening of the bile duct wall. Vascular invasion occurs not only in HCC but also in cholangiocarcinoma. Portal vein infiltration is seen in approximately 50% of patients with cholangiocarcinoma. Color Doppler should be used to assess blood flow in the vessels.

If US results suggest a metastatic liver tumor, HCC, or cholangiocarcinoma, the patient should be referred to a specialist. Dynamic CT, contrast-enhanced MRI, and/or CEUS are required for a more accurate diagnosis. These imaging modalities can be used to assess blood flow within the tumor and possible portal vein tumor thrombus. These imaging tests are essential for the differential diagnosis, not only of malignant tumors, but of benign tumors such as hemangioma and focal nodular hyperplasia.

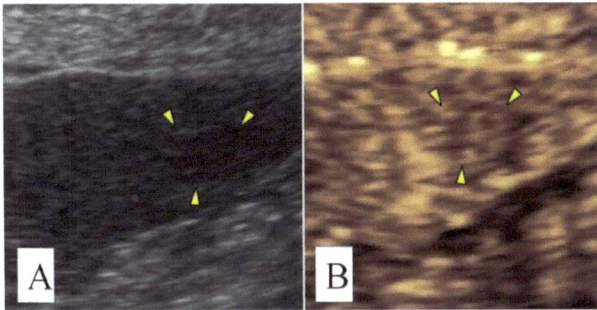

Figure 6: US imagings of small HCCs. **A:** On US scanning, tumors are hypoechoic. **B:** On CEUS using Sonazoid^R, microbubbles are phagocytosed by Kupffer cells. As fewer Kupffer cells are present in HCC than in nontumor liver tissue, HCCs appear hypoechoic when compared with surrounding non-malignant tissue during the Kupffer phase.

SYMPTOMS ASSOCIATED WITH LIVER TUMORS

Patients with liver tumors tend to exhibit a range of nonspecific symptoms, although many patients are asymptomatic. As many patients with large tumors, including those seriously affected, do not always report symptoms of any urgency, careful attention is required not to overlook liver tumors.

Pain

Pain is one of the symptoms frequently encountered in primary care. Pain spontaneously appearing in the abdominal region may indicate a liver tumor at the same location. Bile duct occlusion by a tumor may also cause pain. HCC rupture may be accompanied by severe abdominal pain, with many of these patients developing shock. Pain in the right upper abdomen may occur in patients with a liver abscess, accompanied by percussion tenderness in the same area.

General Malaise

General malaise is a common symptom in patients with malignant tumors. Since general malaise accompanies many different conditions, the tumor cannot be diagnosed by the presence of malaise alone. Rather, a disease must be based on a detailed medical history and physical signs. Patients unable to get up due to extreme fatigue may have experienced severe liver damage or general debility by malignancy.

Weight Loss or Gain

The discovery of a liver tumor in a patient who has lost or gained weight should lead to a suspicion of malignant tumor or cirrhosis of the liver. Reduced food intake or poor nutritional status over several months is associated with weight loss. A highly distended abdomen, often caused by ascites due to a liver disease or malignant tumor, may also be evident. A hard abdomen on palpation may indicate a very advanced malignant tumor or malignant ascites. Patients who experience rapid weight gain without obesity may be due to ascites or edema. Pleural effusion may accumulate, with pleural effusion accumulating in 85% of patients with cirrhosis of the liver only on the right-hand side. Most patients with large amounts of pleural effusion complain of dyspnea.

Fever

Fever may be caused by a malignant tumor. If a fever is accompanied by chills, infection should first be suspected. Liver abscess and infection with *Echinococcus multilocularis* or *E. granulosus* should be distinguished from a liver tumor. Liver tumors may also cause secondary infection. Bacterial infection in bile ducts obstructed by cholangiocarcinoma may easily cause bacteremia.

Jaundice

Jaundice occurs in a variety of diseases. Jaundice is not only due to a decreased capacity to metabolize bilirubin in patients with acute hepatitis or liver failure, but may be caused by bile duct occlusion in many diseases. Jaundice is often observed in patients with cholangiocarcinoma because tumor growth into the bile duct can cause obstruction of the bile duct. Jaundice may also be seen in patients with HCC, albeit rarely; in these patients, obstructive jaundice may result from hemorrhage into the bile duct or liver failure due to tumor progression or portal vein tumor thrombus.

Abdominal Distension

Abdominal distension may be due to intestinal gas or the accumulation of ascites. If ascites has accumulated, an ascites puncture test should be performed as soon as possible to examine the nature of the ascites. Examination of ascites enables the diagnosis of peritonitis carcinomatosa, intraperitoneal hemorrhage, or bacterial infection. Ascites puncture should be performed under ultrasound guidance to avoid abdominal organ damage during the procedure. Patients with ascites containing an extremely high red blood cell count should be suspected of HCC rupture; if rupture has occurred, emergency treatment such as radiological intervention should be arranged.

Gastrointestinal Hemorrhage

In most cases of hemorrhage from gastrointestinal lesions such as stomach or colorectal cancer, the volume of hemorrhage is relatively small. Patients who repeatedly vomit large quantities of fresh blood are likely to have experienced rupture of esophageal varices secondary to cirrhosis of the liver. If the portal vein is infiltrated by HCC, esophageal varices may grow rapidly secondary to acute exacerbation of portal hypertension, causing a sudden hemorrhage. Following an initial emergency procedure for gastrointestinal hemorrhage, the patient may require transfer to a suitable facility such as a gastroenterology center. As they grow, HCC, cholangiocarcinoma, and pancreatic cancer may infiltrate the adjacent gastrointestinal tract and may cause hemorrhage.

Dyspnea

The accumulation of pleural effusion as a result of liver disease may cause dyspnea. Dyspnea, however, may also be caused by pleural effusion due to pneumonia or lung cancer. Heart failure and chronic obstructive pulmonary disease should be eliminated as possible causes of dyspnea. A chest X-ray of the patient should always be obtained and used to check for the possible site of a primary liver tumor or metastasis from lung cancer, as well as to determine the degree of retention of pleural effusion.

BIOCHEMICAL TESTS

Although routine blood biochemistry tests provide limited information in the diagnosis of liver tumors, hepatobiliary enzymes may be mildly elevated.

Infection

Liver abscesses often occur in immunocompromised patients, for example transplant recipients, elderly individuals, and patients with diabetes. Abscesses, however, may also occur in patients without any particular underlying causes. A liver abscess initially presents as abdominal pain and fever, an increased white blood cell count with a shift to the left, elevated ALP, and markedly elevated C-reactive protein (CRP). If the abscess is pyogenic, bacteria may be detected in blood cultures.

Amoebic liver abscesses caused by *Entamoeba histolytica* have a viscous reddish-brown appearance. These patients have an increased white blood cell count and elevated ALP, aspartate aminotransferase (AST), alanine aminotransferase (ALT), and bilirubin concentrations. If the condition becomes chronic, anemia may appear. Patients will be positive for serum anti-amoeba antibodies. In patients infected with human immunodeficiency virus (HIV), malignant lymphoma may present as a liver tumor with elevated levels of AST, ALT, ALP, and bilirubin.

Benign Liver Tumors

Blood test results will likely be normal in patients with benign liver tumors. For example, in patients with benign liver tumors such as hemangiomas and cysts, ALP and γ-GTP are elevated only if the tumor is extremely large or if there are multiple lesions. Tumor markers should be negative. Patients with tumors diagnosed as benign usually do not require treatment, except for those with hepatic adenoma. If the tumor grows rapidly in size or symptoms such as severe pain appear, surgical removal should be considered.

HCC

Clinical characteristics, including patient history, symptoms and underlying liver disease, are important for accurate diagnosis in patients with liver tumors. Chronic viral hepatitis and cirrhosis have been associated with high risks of HCC (Table **2**), as have chemical agents such as aflatoxin and thorotrast. Patients in these circumstances should undergo careful screening for HCC at regular intervals.

Table 2. Patients whom surveillance for HCC is recommended

Hepatitis B carriers
Asian males ≥ 40 years
Asian females ≥ 50 years
All cirrhotic hepatitis B carriers
Family history of HCC
Africans over age 20
For non-cirrhotic hepatitis B carriers not listed above the risk of HCC varies
    depending on the severity of the underlying liver disease, and current and
    past hepatic inflammatory activity. Patients with high HBV-DNA
    concentrations and those with ongoing hepatic inflammatory activity remain at
    risk for HCC.

Non-hepatitis B cirrhosis
Hepatitis C
Alcoholic cirrhosis
Genetic hemochromatosis
Primary biliary cirrhosis
Although the following groups have an increased risk of HCC, no
    recommendations for or against surveillance can be made because a lack of
    data precludes an assessment of whether surveillance would be beneficial.
Alpha1-antitrypsin deficiency
Nonalcoholic steatohepatitis
Autoimmune hepatitis

Since hepatitis virus infection is associated with hepatocarcinogenesis, patients with HCC should be screened for hepatitis B surface (HBs) antigens and anti-hepatitis C virus (HCV) antibodies. Patients negative for both but positive for anti-hepatitis B core (HBc) antibody have a previous history of hepatitis B virus (HBV) infection. High serum HBV DNA and HBsAg or incorporation of HBV DNA into the host genomes of liver cells is associated with a higher risk for HCC, although most clinics are not equipped to perform tests for HBV DNA integration. Blood biochemistry test results in HCC patients are almost identical to those of patients with cirrhosis of the liver. The inability to diagnose patients by these results alone makes tumor markers useful for diagnosis. For example, alpha-fetoprotein (AFP) concentration has been found to correlate with tumor size and patient prognosis. However, the ratio of AFP-L3 to total AFP and the concentration of des-γ-carboxy prothrombin (DCP) are more specific for HCC than total AFP levels.

Cholangiocarcinoma

Bilirubin is frequently elevated in patients with cholangiocarcinoma. Blood biochemistry test results do not exhibit any specific signs. Unlike in HCC, AFP and DCP concentrations are not elevated, although carcinoembryonic antigen (CEA) and carbohydrate antigen (CA)19-9 concentrations are often increased.

Metastatic Liver Tumor

Identification of the primary tumor may be difficult in patients with poorly-differentiated or highly abundant metastatic foci. Pathological examination of these liver tumors may identify the primary lesion, however, as metastatic liver tumors frequently have the same properties as the primary tumors. Increases in ALP and lactate dehydrogenase (LDH) concentrations are indicators of the growth of liver metastases, despite their non-specificity for primary sites. The tumor markers CEA and CA19-9 are frequently elevated, especially in patients with liver tumors originating from the gastrointestinal tract. In general, tumor markers remain within their normal ranges in patients with tumors located at the primary site with little infiltration into vessels or surrounding tissues. Tumor marker concentrations usually become significantly higher when metastatic foci have grown and occupy a large volume.

DIAGNOSTIC IMAGING FOR LIVER TUMORS

This section describes the use of diagnostic imaging in diagnosing liver tumors in clinical practice.

Plain X-ray examination: Although X-ray images contain less information than those produced by the latest imaging tests, chest X-rays can indicate the presence of a liver tumor. If the diaphragm is elevated, a large liver tumor may be suspected. Abnormal calcifications may also be useful in patient diagnosis. Kidney stones, gallstones, and calcifications of the prostate are often observed, although calcifications in the upper abdomen may be associated with liver tumors.

Liver Abscesses

The multiple forms of liver abscesses complicate patient diagnosis. Monolocular abscesses may be identified as nodules, and multilocular abscesses may form multiple nodules. Treatment of patients with multiple liver abscesses is difficult. On US scans, newly formed liver abscesses may show a hyperechoic internal echo pattern, whereas necrotic areas are hypoechoic regions (Fig. 7. **A**). If gases are produced by bacteria in an abscess, the interior of the abscess exhibits intense hyperechoicity. On plain CT, it appears as a hypointense region. The interior of a liver abscess is not enhanced on contrast-enhanced CT, while the area around the septa is enhanced with an irregular ring-like appearance (Fig. 7. **B**). Typically, the ring-shaped region of enhancement gradually thickens from the arterial to the portal phase. During the early arterial phase, a hypointense region indicating edema is visible around the liver abscess. The possible routes of bacterial infection are *via* the arteries, portal vein, and biliary tract. Liver abscesses >5cm in diameter and those resistant to intravenous antibiotics should be drained. Patients with liver abscesses should be treated with antibiotics for 4 to 6 weeks.

Benign Liver Tumors

Although liver cysts are often found on screening US, their etiology is unknown. On US scans, the interior is anechoic, with the echo enhanced behind the lesion (Fig. **8**). However, these findings are not necessarily observed in small cysts. Infected or hemorrhagic cysts show some echogenicity, making it difficult to differentiate these complicated cysts from other nodular diseases. On CT, liver cysts can be recognized as hypointense regions and show absolutely no contrast enhancement, making it difficult to differentiate between simple liver cysts and primary or metastatic cystic liver tumors. Attention must be paid to the possible nodular hyperplasia of the cyst wall, suggesting cystadenocarcinoma or cystadenoma.

Hemangioma is a benign liver tumor often found on screening US. Patients with hemorrhage from the rupture of large hemangiomas or complicated with disseminated intravascular coagulation (DIC) have been described. Hyperechoic hemangiomas may show clearly demarcated margins on US, but this finding is not specific for hemangiomas (Fig. **9**).

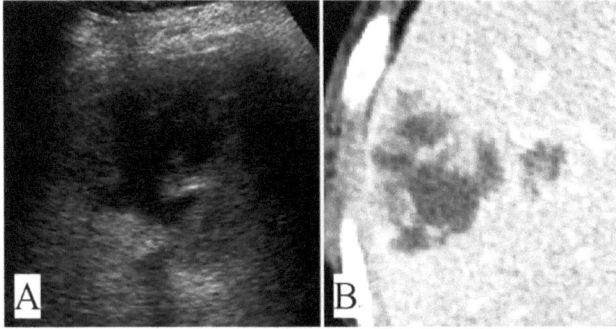

Figure 7: US (**A**) and contrast-enhanced CT (**B**) images of multilocular liver abscesses. **A:** Nodule necrosis appearing as hypoechoic regions. **B:** The interior of liver abscess is not enhanced on contrast-enhanced CT, while the area around the septa is enhanced with a ring-like appearance.

Change in the mode of echogenicity, a phenomenon called the "wax and wane sign," is a finding specific for hemangioma. Larger hemangiomas may include hypoechoic regions. Dynamic CT is useful in the diagnosis of hemangioma, whereas plain CT is not (Fig. **10**). Typically, hemangiomas appear hypointense on plain CT, whereas the area around the tumor is contrast-enhanced during in the early arterial phase of dynamic CT. Hyperintense regions gradually expand to the interior of hemangiomas from the portal to the venous phase. Dynamic CT, dynamic MRI, and CEUS are all reliable diagnostic methods [9]. Hemangiomas appear hyperintense on T2WI MRI (Fig. **11**), whereas 70% exhibit contrast enhancement, extending internally from the margins, on gadolinium-enhanced MRI [10].

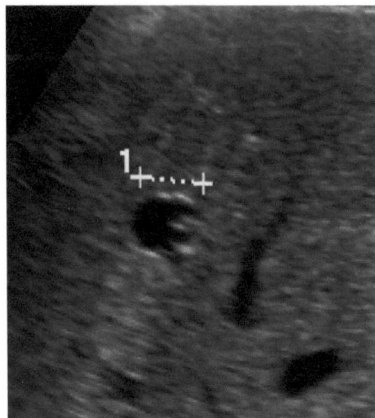

Figure 8: US image of a liver cyst. The interior of the cyst is anechoic, with the echo being enhanced behind the lesion.

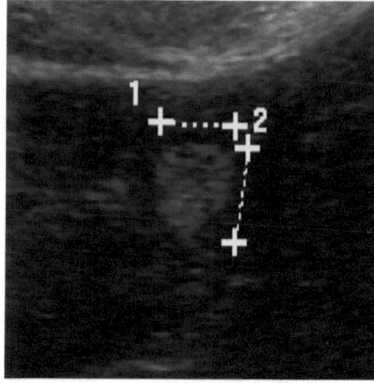

Figure 9: US image of a hemangioma. Hemangiomas appear homogeneously hyperechoic, but their findings may vary greatly among patients. Echogenicity may change during the observation.

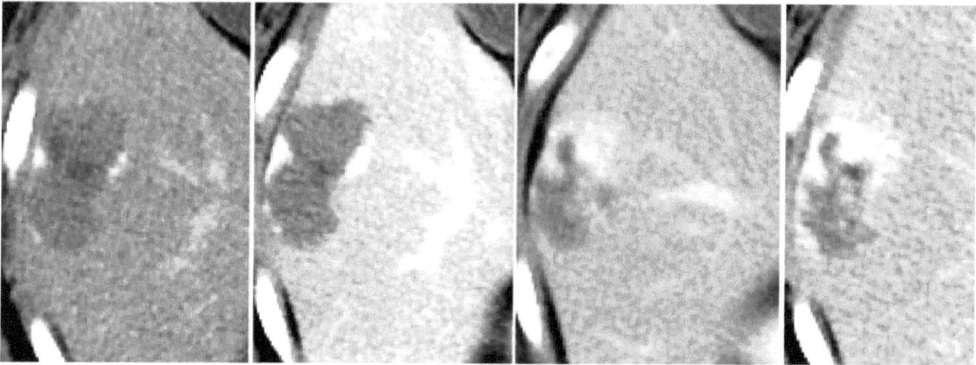

Figure 10: Dynamic CT images of a cavernous hemangioma. This tumor appears hypointense on plain CT, whereas the area around the tumor shows contrast enhancement during the early arterial phase of dynamic CT. A hyperintense region gradually extends inside the mass from the portal phase to the venous phase.

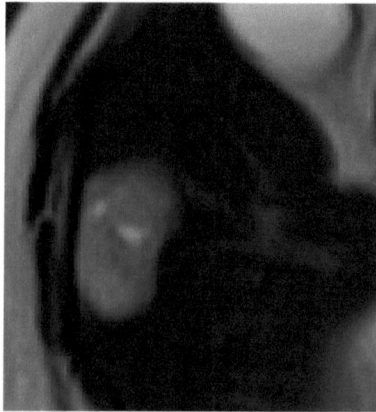

Figure 11: MRI image of a cavernous hemangioma showing a hyperintense mass on T2WI.

Malignant Liver Tumors

HCC

On dynamic CT, HCCs are typically stained intensely during the arterial phase, with washout occurring from the portal phase to the equilibrium phase. Well-differentiated HCCs often appear as isointense nodules in the arterial phase (Fig. **12. A**). Nodules that show weak washout in the portal phase may be well-differentiated HCCs (Fig. **12. B**). HCC is often undetected by fluorodeoxyglucose-positron emission tomography (FDG-PET), because FDG is dephosphorylated and transported outside the cells by glucose transporters expressed on HCC.

Superparamagnetic iron oxide (SPIO) particles are taken up into Kupffer cells in healthy liver tissue. The principal effect of the SPIO particles is on T2* relaxation and the tissue signal is markedly decreased by uptake of the particles in T2/T2*-weighted sequences. Healthy liver tissue thus appears hypointense on SPIO-MRI. On the contrary, cancer tissues, which contains few Kupffer cells, appears comparatively hyperintense. Since pathological studies of small nodules in the liver found that Kupffer cell counts are slightly lower in well-differentiated HCCs than in adjacent healthy areas of the liver, intensity of SPIO-MRI of well-differentiated HCCs may mildly increase as compared with the surrounding tissue. SPIO-MRI can be also used for diagnosis if contrast enhanced CT cannot distinguish between a tumor and an arterioportal (AP) shunt, with hyperintense nodules on SPIO-MRI being a malignant tumor, not an AP shunt.

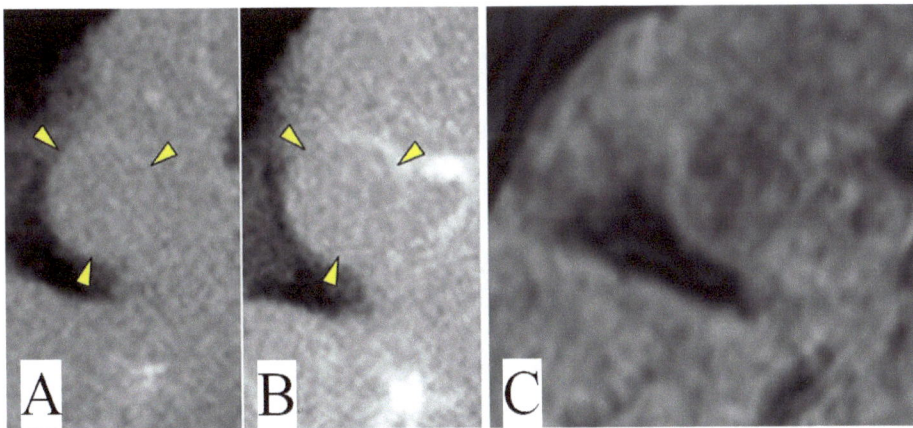

Figure 12: Contrast-enhanced CT and MRI images of well-differentiated HCC. **A:** Dynamic CT, showing a well-differentiated HCC appearing as an isointense nodule s during the arterial phase. **B:** Nodule showing weak washout in the portal phase. **C:** Gd-EOB-DTPA-MRI showing a defect in the hepatobiliary phase without arterial phase staining, making it extremely useful in the detection of well-differentiated HCCs.

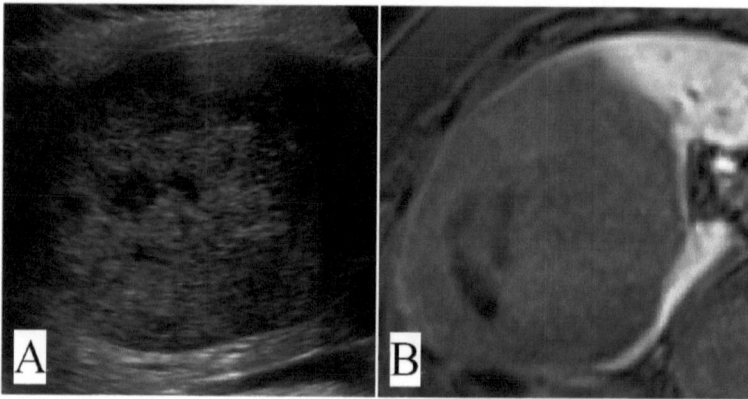

Figure 13: US and contrast-enhanced MRI images of a huge HCC. **A:** US imaging showing a mosaic pattern. **B:** Gd-EOB-DTPA-MRI showing a defect in the hepatobiliary phase.

On CEUS, well-differentiated HCCs can be detected as isoechoic or slightly hypoechoic lesions during the Kupffer phase [11]. In contrast, Kupffer cell counts are similar in dysplastic nodules, representing precancerous lesions, and their surrounding tissue, making CEUS useful for the differential diagnosis of dysplastic nodules and well- differentiated HCC.

Recently, gadolinium-ethoxybenzyl-diethylenetriamine pentaacetic acid (Gd-EOB-DTPA) -enhanced MRI has been mainly used for the differential diagnosis of liver tumors and has been shown to be useful for the detection of malignant tumors (Fig. **12. C**), which are often characterized by a defect in the hepatobiliary phase (Fig. **13**). Gd-EOB-DTPA-MRI is capable of detecting not only moderately- or poorly-differentiated HCC but also well-differentiated HCC.

Cholangiocarcinoma

Almost all mass-forming cholangiocarcinomas are hypovascular tumors (Fig. **14**), although hypervascular nodules may be present. Especially, small, well-differentiated cholangiocarcinomas often show hypervascular nodules. Diagnostic imaging alone is insufficient for differentiating between well-differentiated cholangiocarcinoma and HCC nodules. Multiple tumor markers should be assayed and the presence/absence of underlying chronic liver disease should be utilized in diagnosis.

Metastatic Liver Tumors

On contrast-enhanced CT, the margins of metastatic liver tumors are slightly enhanced, but their interiors are usually hypovascular (Fig. **15**). This enhancement of tumor margins is used to differentiate these tumors from well-differentiated HCCs, which are also often detected as hypointense nodules. Many patients with metastatic liver tumors present with multiple nodules within the liver. During the Kupffer phase on both SPIO-MRI and CEUS, metastatic liver tumors exhibit more intense contrast than early HCCs, because Kupffer cell counts are lower in metastatic liver tumors than in early phase HCC and healthy liver tissue. FDG-PET is useful for the diagnosis of metastatic liver tumors.

Contrast-enhanced CT, showing that the interiors of the tumors are usually hypovascular.

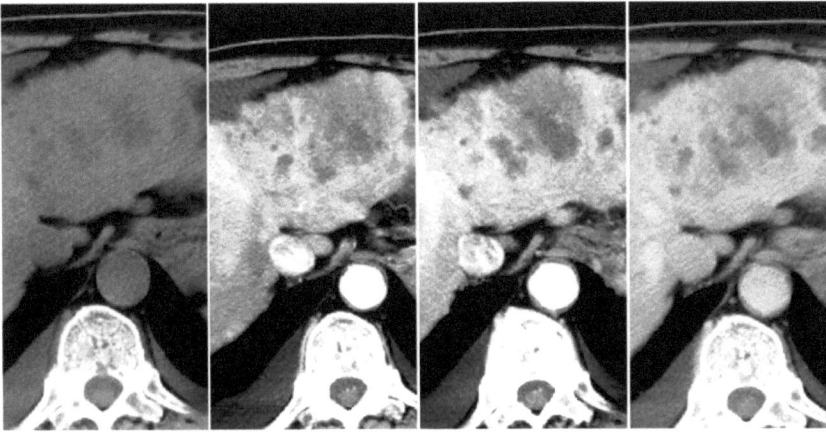

Figure 14: Contrast-enhanced CT images of a mass-forming cholangiocarcinoma. The tumor appears hypovascular, with its margins often slightly enhanced.

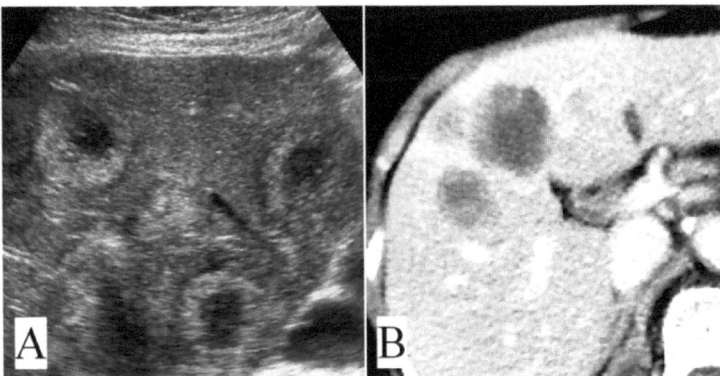

Figure 15: US and contrast-enhanced CT images of liver metastases from gastric cancer. **A:** US scanning showing multiple nodules within the liver, with tumors appearing as hyperechoic regions and necrosis of nodules as hypoechoic regions. **B:** Multiple hypodense nodules with ring-like enhancement.

Clinical and imaging characteristics of liver tumors are summarized in Table **3** [12].

Table 3(1). Typical features of liver focal lesions.

	Simple cyst	Hemangioma	Abscess (pyogenic)
Clinical	Extremely common More common in women	Common Can grow slowly	Causes right upper quadrant pain and tenderness, fever, and leukocytosis
Imaging *General*	Sharply denmarcated thin wall May occasionally have thin septataion	Calcification rare Larger lesions may have lobular border or central scar	Abscess of biliary origin are frequently multiple and scattered; abscess of portal origin are often solitary
US	Anechoic Posterior acoustic enhancement	Well-defined homogeneously hyperechoic when small Sometimes have less echogenic center and uniform echogenic border	Early abscesses are often hyperechoic, whereas mature abscesses may demonstrate decreased echogenicity
CT	Uniform low attenuation (<10HU)	Progressively enhancing from periphery to center	Generally hypoattenuating; a low-attenuation region surrounding the wall may be present. Representing periabscess edema or inflammation
MRI	Low SI on T1WI Very high SI on T2WI	Hypointense on T1WI Hyperintense on T2WI	Usually low SI on T1WI and high SI on T2WI Perilesional edema mey be present as a rim of high SI parenchyma surrounding the abscess wall on T2WI

Table 3(2). Typical features of liver focal lesions.

	Adenoma	FNH	Abscess (amebic)
Clinical	Much common in women Associated with oral contraceptives or anabolic steroid use or glycogen storage disease Frequently hemorrhage Malignant transformation rare	More common in women Common incidental, asymptomatic lesion	Caused by entamoeba histolyca Found in developing tropical areas of the world Cause of right upper quadrant pain and diarrhea Serology is positive in 90%
Imaging *General*	Intralesional hemorrhage or steatosis common Psudocapsule common	Nearly isoechoic to liver Low attenuation central scar	Well-defined, round or oval, unilocular or multilocular Look for evidence of colitis
US	Variable echogenicity Echogenic foci related to fat or calccification	Nearly isodense on unenhanced CT images Low attenuation central scar	Hypoechoic with homogeneously distributed low-level echoes and distal acoustic enhancement
CT	Variable attenuation depending on presence of fat, hemorrhage, or calcification	Nearly isointense to liver on T1WI and T2WI High SI central scar on T2WI (low SI on T1WI) Low attenuation central scar	Abscess cavity is usually hypoattenuating with a well-defined, continuous wall; some mural irregularity may be present
MRI	High SI areas on T1WI caused by hemorrhage or fat Heterogeneous but generally increased SI on T2WI	Brisk arterial-phase enhancement Radiating septa on early-phase contrast-enhanced phases Nearly isodense /isointense on subsequent phases Enhancement of central scar on equilibrium-phase images Significant uptake of SPIO	Abscess cavity is lower SI than hepatic parenchyma on T1WI and hyperintense on T2WI

Table 3(3). Typical features of liver focal lesions.

	Metastasis
Clinical	Most common primary sites include colon, stomach pancreas, lung, melanoma and gallbladder
Imaging General	Cystic metastasis; cystadenocarcimnoma of ovary and pancreas, mucinous adenocarcinoma of colon, sarcoma, squamaous cell carcinoma
US	Hypoechoic halo on US Hyperechoic; gastrointestinal primaries, neuroendocrine tumors, renal cell carcinoma Hypoechoic; breast cancer, lung cancer, lymphoma, esophageal, gastric and pancreatic cancer
CT	Usually isodense or hypodense to liver on enhanced CT Calcified metastasis; colon cancer, osteogenic sarcoma, chondrosarcoma, malignant teratoma, neuroblastoma
MRI	Usually isodense or hypodense to liver on T1WI Hemorrhagic metastasis; metastatic melanoma, and fat-containing (liposarcoma or malignant teratoma) may be hyperintence to liver on T1WI. Usually hyperintense to liver on T2WI
Contrast enhancement	Typical hypervascular liver metastasis; neuroendocrine tumors, renal cell carcinoma, thyroid cancer, breast cancer, pheochromocytoma, Typical hypovascular liver metastasis; colon cancer, lung cancer, prostate cancer, stomach cancer, transitional cell carcinoma, pancreatic cancer, lymphoma

Table 3(4). Typical features of liver focal lesions.

	HCC
Clinical	Common risk factors; cirrhosis, viral hepatitis, hemochromatosis AFP levels often, but not always, elevated
Imaging General	Nodule-within-nodule appearnce suggests HCC Intralesional steatosis or foci of fat ,ay be present Venous invasion by tumor common (portal vein>hepatic vein)
US	Variable echogenicity, almost half of small HCCs are hyperechoic due to fat deposition Hypoechoic halo may be seen Large lesions tend to be of heterogeneous echogenicity Hypervascular and hjgh-velocity flow with Doppler
CT	Small lesions often not visible in cirrhotic liver on unenhanced CT Low-attenuation regions because of fat or necrosis
MRI	Isointense or hypointense on T1WI Isointense or hyperintense on T2W1
Contrast enhancement	Early mosaic enhancement Washout on portal phase Enhancing capsule on equiliblium phase Arterioportal shunting

Table 3(5). Typical features of liver focal lesions.

	Cholangiocarcinoma
Clinical	Risk factors; primary sclerosing cholangitis, choledochal cyst, biliary lithiasis, congenital hepatic fibrosis, and Clonorchis sinensis
Imaging General	Satellite nodules common Can grow into or along bile ducts Can be associated with capsular retraction Dilated bile ducts variably present Calcifications uncommon but can be present
US	Variable echogenicity, more often than hypoechoic
CT	Well-defined Lobular margins
MRI	Hypointense to liver on T1WI Mildly hyperintense to liver on T2W1 Central portion of tumor often hypointense on T2WI because of fibrosis
Contrast enhancement	Early rim enhancement common Progressive and persistent enhancement on subsequent phases of enhancement Peripheral washout on delayed images

Table 3(6). Typical features of liver focal lesions.

	Fibrolammelar hepatocellular carcinoma	Epithelioid hemangioendothelioma
Clinical	More common in young adults AFP levels usually normal Cirrhosis usually absent Better prognosis than conventional HCC	Rare Most common in middle-aged women Variable prognosis
Imaging General	Usually large, lobulated mass Central scar common	Lesions often peripheral, extending to capsule Often multifocal Lesions become confluent as they enlarge Occasionally have calcifications Can metastasize
US	Variable echogenicity Echogenic central scar	Typically hypoechoic Peripheral hypoechoic rim may be present
CT	Well-defined mass with radiating septa Central scar may be hypodense or calcified	Decreased attenuation on unenhanced CT
MRI	Hypointense to liver on T1WI Hyperintense to liver on T2W1 Central scar is hypointense to liver and lesion on T1WI and T2WI Hypointense radiating septa	Lower SI than liver on T1WI Higher SI than liver on T2WI
Contrast enhancement	Heterologous enhancement Scar does not enhance or enhance very late	Target pattern of enhancement: nonenhancing center, enhancing inner rim, poorly enhancing outer rim

TREATMENT OF LIVER TUMORS

Patients with cholangitis and liver abscess should be started immediately on treatment with antibiotics. The causative bacteria and their sensitivity to antibiotics should be determined for proper selection of antibiotics.

Most benign liver tumors require only regular follow-up. However, if the nodular size increases, similar to a malignant tumor, further detailed investigation is required. Patients diagnosed with benign tumors do not require treatment as long as the tumors remain asymptomatic. Surgical resection should be considered for patients who experience abdominal pain and liver dysfunction due to an extremely large benign liver tumor. Laparoscopic fenestration surgery was recently shown to yield good long-term results in patients with symptomatic liver cysts, as well as to be both safe and effective [13]. Surgery should be considered for patients with malignant liver tumors, taking into account the tumor numbers and sizes, as well as underlying liver function. Radiofrequency ablation (RFA) may be used to treat HCC or metastatic liver tumors. Liver transplantation may be indicated in some patients with HCC. Patients in the middle stages of HCC may be treated with hepatic artery chemoembolization or chemotherapy. Improved techniques for hepatic artery chemoembolization and the development of effective molecularly targeted drugs have improved patient prognosis. Moreover, heavy ion radiotherapy and proton-beam radiotherapy have shown good therapeutic outcomes and are now a focus of attention [14].

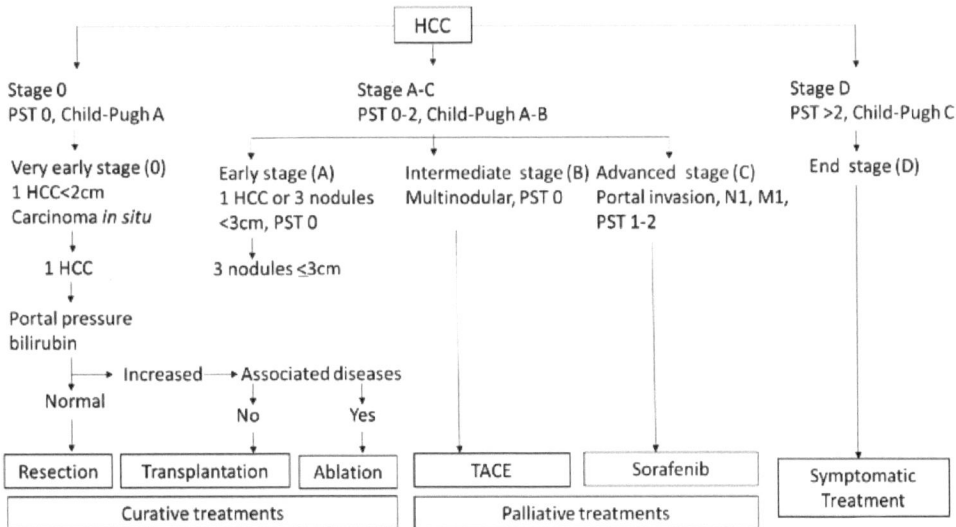

Figure 16: Standard therapeutic strategy proposed by the Barcelona group [15]. Abbreviations: PST, performance status; TACE, transcatheter arterial chemoembolization

The standard therapeutic strategy for HCC proposed by the Barcelona group is shown in Fig. (**16**) [15]. Patients with malignant liver tumors must be treated in medical institutions with sufficient experience in this area.

MESSAGES FROM HEPATOLOGISTS TO GENERAL PHYSICIANS

1. Liver cysts and hemangiomas are the most common liver masses found on routine ultrasound examination, and they do not require any treatment unless they are symptomatic or complicated by infections or abnormalities in liver function tests.

2. For the diagnosis of liver tumors, it is important to identify hepatitis virus B or C infection and the presence of liver cirrhosis, because HCC is only rarely found in patients without hepatitis virus infection or advanced liver diseases.

3. Focal nodular hyperplasia (FNH) and hepatic adenoma are the most common benign liver tumors; the former does not need treatment, whereas the latter often requires liver resection because it is sometimes complicated by hemorrhage or the development of HCC. They are sometimes difficult to differentiate, but normal enhancement of the tumor on MRI with Gd-EOB-DTPA and US with Sonazoid can be taken to indicate FNH.

4. The final diagnosis of a liver mass is done by CT, MRI, or US with contrast medium enhancement. Contrast-enhanced MRI with Gd-EOB-DTPA is used to examine hepatocyte function and contrast-enhanced US with Sonazoid (perfluorobutane microbubbles) is performed to examine the presence of Kupffer cells. The combination of imaging examinations is therefore helpful for the final diagnosis by providing different information on the character of the tumor.

5. Liver solid masses less than 1 cm in diameter found on US can be carefully followed up, and the recommended interval is 3 months. Contrast-enhanced CT or MRI must be performed if the liver mass is over 1 cm in diameter.

6. Compared with HCC, cholangiocarcinomas usually show vague demarcation on US or CT imaging, and localized dilatation of intrahepatic bile ducts often suggests the presence of these lesions.

7. In patients with metastatic liver tumors and cholangiocarcinomas but not HCC, elevation of serum biliary enzyme levels is usually predominant to that of transaminases.

8. The prognosis of patients with solitary liver tumors less than 2 cm in diameter is not different after treatment by radiofrequency ablation (RFA) or surgical resection. On the other hand, liver tumor over 3cm in diameter should be considered for surgical resection, or treated with a combination with transcatheter arterial chemoembolization and RFA.

ACKNOWLEDGEMENTS

We are very thankful to Ms. Asma Ahmed, manager publications, Bentham Science Publishers, for her patience and long-term assistance.

CONFLICT OF INTEREST

The author confirms that he has no conflict of interest to declare for this publication.

REFERENCES

[1]   Bruix J, Sherman M. Management of hepatocellular carcinoma: An update. Hepatology 2011;53:1020-1022.
[2]   European Association for the Study of the Liver; European Organisation for Research and Treatment of Cancer. EASL-EORTC clinical practice guidelines: management of hepatocellular carcinoma. J Hepatol 2012;56:908-943.
[3]   Ricci OE, *et al.* Diagnostic approach to hepatic hemangiomas detected by ultrasound. Hepatogastroenterology 1985;32:53-56.
[4]   Sherman M. Masses in the liver. In Hepatology-Diagnosis and Clinical Management. Heathcote EJ Ed. Pp93-111. Wiley-Blackwell, 2012.
[5]   Mathieu D, *et al.* Hepatic adenomas and focal nodular hyperplasia, dynamic CT study. Radiology 1986;160:53-58.
[6]   Mungovan JA, *et al.* Hepatic cavernous hemagiomas:lack of enlargement over time. Radiology 1994;191:111-113.
[7]   Ebara M, *et al.* Strategy for early diagnosis of hepatocellular carcinoma (HCC). Ann Acad Med Singapore 1989;18:83-89.
[8]   Yoshida T, *et al.* Ultrasonographic differentiation of hepatocellular carcinoma from metastatic liver cancer. J Clin Ultrasound 1987;15:431-437.
[9]   Brancatelli G, *et al.* Hemangioma in the cirrhotic liver: diagnosis and natural history. Radiology 2001;219:69-74.
[10]   Kato H, *et al.* Atypically enhancing hepatic cavernous hemangiomas: high-spatial-resolution gadolinium-enhanced triphasic dynamic gradient-recalled-echo imaging findings. Eur Radiol 2001;11:2510-2515.
[11]   Korenaga K, *et al.* Usefulness of sonazoid contrast-enhanced ultrasonography for hepatocellular carcinoma: comparison with pathological diagnosis and superparamagnetic iron magnetic resonance images. J Gastroenterol 2009;44:733-741.

[12]   Leyendecker JR, Chapter 12 Liver, Dalrymple NC, Leyendecker JR, Oliphant M (Edt), Problem solving in abdominal imageing, 2009, Mosby Elesevier :275-339.

[13]   Ardito F, *et al*. Long-term outcome after laparoscopic fenestration of simple liver cysts. Surg Endosc 2013;27:4670-4674.

[14]   Abei M, *et al*. A phase I study on combined therapy with proton-beam radiotherapy and *in situ* tumor vaccination for locally advanced recurrent hepatocellular carcinoma. Radiat Oncol 2013;8:239-248.

[15]   Bruix J, Llovet JM. Prognostic prediction and treatment strategy in hepatocellular carcinoma. Hepatology 2002;35:519-524.

CHAPTER 6

Liver Function Abnormalities in Systemic Disease

Yukihiro Shimizu*

Gastroenterology Center, Nanto Municipal Hospital, Japan

Abstract: There are many possible causes of abnormal liver function test results, including viral hepatitis, alcohol consumption, nonalcoholic fatty liver disease, autoimmune liver diseases, hereditary diseases, hepatobiliary malignancies or infection, gallstones, and drug-induced liver injury. Moreover, the liver may be involved in systemic diseases that mainly affect other organs. Therefore, in patients without etiology of liver injury based on screening serology and diagnostic imaging analysis, abnormal liver function test results may be due to systemic disease. In most of these patients, systemic disease should be the primary focus of treatment. However, some patients with systemic disease and severe liver injury or fulminant hepatic failure require intensive treatment of the liver.

Keywords: Adrenal gland disease, amyloidosis, connective tissue disease, diabetes mellitus, granuloma, heart failure, metastatic liver tumor, postoperative liver injury, sepsis, shock liver, systemic infection, thyroid disease, total parental nutrition.

KEY POINTS

1. If patients with liver function abnormalities show systemic symptoms or have concomitant systemic disease, abnormal liver function test results may be due to the systemic disease.

2. Treatment of the underlying systemic disease is sufficient to improve liver function test results, but it should be noted that these patients may develop liver failure.

INTRODUCTION

There are several common causes of abnormal liver function test results, including viral hepatitis, alcohol consumption, drug-induced liver injury, nonalcoholic fatty liver disease, autoimmune liver disease, and hereditary disease

"Part of this chapter has been previously published in World J Gastroenterol. 2008 Jul 14; 14(26): 4111–4119. DOI: 10.3748/wjg.14.4111".

***Corresponding author Yukihiro Shimizu:** Gastroenterology Center, Nanto Municipal Hospital, Toyama, Japan; E-mail: rsf14240@nifty.com

involving the liver. Therefore, patients with abnormal liver function test (LFT) results are first assessed for these diseases. However, it is also possible that an underlying systemic disease is responsible for the liver function abnormalities [1]. Several symptoms provide important information to identify the possible cause of liver function abnormalities.

INFECTION

The presence of fever suggests infection, malignant disease, or connective tissue disease. Infection may be systemic or localized in the hepatobiliary system, such as liver abscess or cholangitis. Systemic infection, both viral and bacterial, often causes abnormal LFT results.

Systemic viral infections affecting the liver include Epstein–Barr virus, cytomegalovirus, herpes simplex virus, parvovirus B19, coxsackie virus B2, and human herpesvirus-6, most of which have been reported to cause acute hepatic failure. In younger patients, Epstein–Barr virus and cytomegalovirus infection should always be considered especially in patients showing mononucleosis on blood tests.

Bacterial infection often causes abnormal LFT results, especially in patients with bacteremia or sepsis. Sepsis with either gram-positive (*Staphylococcus aureus*) or gram-negative (*Escherichia coli* and *Klebsiella* spp.) bacteria [2, 3] has been shown to cause cholestasis through inhibition of canalicular excretion of conjugated bilirubin by proinflammatory cytokines [4]. Laboratory findings of sepsis include mild elevation of alkaline phosphatase (ALP), mostly $1 - 3$ times the upper limit of normal (ULN), and modest elevation of alanine aminotransferase (ALT). Jaundice is often seen and the bilirubin levels typically range from 5 to 10 mg/dL [5]. Serum levels of ALP and bilirubin may be discordant, with deeply jaundiced patients often having normal serum ALP levels, while anicteric patients may show marked elevation of ALP or γ-GTP levels [6-8]. Although differential diagnosis of sepsis-induced cholestasis includes cholangitis, cholestasis without any abnormalities in the biliary tree or gallbladder by ultrasonography or computed tomography (CT) usually suggests the former diagnosis. Another differential diagnosis should be made with antibiotic-induced liver injury, if the patient has been treated with antibiotics. The temporal relationship between the course of infection or drug use and the manifestation of abnormal LFT results is important in determining the possible cause of the liver abnormality.

Several other infections can also cause liver injury, including pneumonia due to *Legionella pneumophila, Mycoplasma pneumoniae*, or *Streptococcus pneumoniae*, or infection with *Clostridium perfringens, Salmonella typhi, Campylobacter, Chlamydia, Neisseria, Mycobacteria*, or HIV, Lyme disease, Q fever, and syphilis. The mechanism of liver injury by these pathogens may involve direct invasion of the liver *via* gumma (in the case of syphilis) or granuloma formation. Although some patients show jaundice, severe liver injury is rare and can subside with improvement of infection.

MALIGNANT DISEASE OR METASTATIC LIVER TUMOR

Many malignant diseases invade the liver and cause abnormal LFT results. Metastatic liver tumors are frequently found from the large intestine, lung, breast, kidney, stomach, pancreas, sarcoma, and malignant melanoma. In addition, direct extension of primary malignant tumors of the gallbladder, extrahepatic bile duct, stomach, and pancreas sometimes occurs. Patients often show hepatomegaly with increased consistency and the laboratory data demonstrate predominant elevation of γ-GTP and ALP without any abnormalities in the biliary tree or gallbladder. Although the characteristics of the tumor on ultrasound, contrast-enhanced CT, and magnetic resonance imaging (MRI) may suggest the nature of the primary lesion, percutaneous tumor biopsy with immunohistochemical staining is helpful for identification of the primary lesion.

Liver involvement of malignant disease is often seen in patients with hematological malignancy, such as Hodgkin's disease, non-Hodgkin lymphoma, chronic lymphoid leukemia, chronic myeloid leukemia, acute leukemia, hairy cell leukemia, and multiple myeloma. Hepatomegaly and elevation of γ-GTP, ALP or transaminases are often observed in such cases.

CONNECTIVE TISSUE DISEASE

Patients with fever, arthralgia, or skin lesions may have connective tissue disease. Most connective tissue diseases, including juvenile rheumatoid arthritis, Felty syndrome, rheumatoid arthritis, polymyalgia rheumatica, Sjögren's syndrome, scleroderma, systemic lupus erythematosus, and adult Still's disease, are known to cause abnormal LFT results, especially elevation of ALP and transaminase levels. The mechanisms of liver injury in these diseases are variable. Lupus-related abnormal LFT results and chronic hepatitis are often confused with autoimmune hepatitis. Elevated serum ALT has been reported in 20% of patients with systemic lupus erythematosus, and 4.4% of patients with systemic lupus erythematosus may have chronic hepatitis or liver cirrhosis [9-12]. The relationships between the lupus-related advanced liver diseases and autoimmune hepatitis are controversial. However, the most common liver manifestation in patients with systemic lupus erythematosus is steatosis [13], and liver biopsy may be necessary for accurate diagnosis of the liver injury.

SHOCK OR HEART FAILURE

If the patient is in shock or has been in a condition with hemodynamic instability, liver injury may be so-called shock liver or ischemic hepatitis [14]. These patients usually show marked elevation of serum aminotransferase and lactate dehydrogenase (LDH) levels, and marked elevation of LDH (above the level of ALT) is one of the features that can distinguish ischemic hepatitis from acute viral hepatitis. Another feature of ischemic hepatitis is the rapid improvement of elevated aminotransferases and LDH after recovery from shock [15].

Liver congestion is another form of liver injury associated with cardiovascular diseases, and is caused by acute or chronic right-sided heart failure. Hepatomegaly and ascites in addition to the signs of heart failure, including peripheral edema and pleural effusion, are often seen in such cases [16, 17]. Serum bilirubin, mostly in the unconjugated form, is elevated to $1-5$ mg/dL depending on the severity of heart failure. Elevation of aminotransferase (AST > ALT) and ALP are often observed in patients with right-sided heart failure [16-18]. Longstanding liver congestion may lead to cardiac cirrhosis, but its incidence is relatively low.

HEMATOLOGICAL DISEASE (BENIGN)

Various hematological diseases, including polycythemia vera, myelodysplasia, sickle-cell disease, and thalassemia, are known to cause abnormal LFT results.

HORMONAL DISTURBANCES AND DIABETES MELLITUS

Thyroid Disease

The most common cause of abnormal LFT results secondary to hormonal disturbance is thyroid disease. Although both hyperthyroidism and hypothyroidism are known to cause liver injury, the former shows more prominent abnormalities in LFT results. Hyperthyroidism is thought to cause liver injury by increasing oxygen demand of hepatocytes without an associated increase in hepatic blood flow. Liver injury can be either cholestatic or hepatocellular, and up to 64% and 35% of patients show elevation of ALP and ALT, respectively. Interestingly, most of the increased ALP level is known to be bone-derived [19]. In contrast, only modest elevations of AST and ALT are seen in 84% and 60% of patients with hypothyroidism, respectively [20].

Adrenal Gland Disease

Hypercortisolism causes fatty infiltration of the liver, which may progress to non-alcoholic steatohepatitis (NASH) [21]. Elevated serum aminotransferase concentrations have been reported in patients with adrenal insufficiency [22, 23].

Diabetes Mellitus

Elevated serum aminotransferase, γ-GTP, or ALP levels are observed in 10% – 20% of patients with diabetes mellitus [24, 25], which are more common in type 2 diabetes mellitus. Non-alcoholic fatty liver disease is found in 32% - 78% of patients with type 2 diabetes mellitus, half of whom may have NASH [26, 27].

TOTAL PARENTERAL NUTRITION

Total parenteral nutrition (TPN) can cause steatosis or cholestasis. Elevation of serum aminotransferase level is common during the first 1 – 3 weeks of TPN [28-30], and bilirubin may also be elevated in some adults after 10 weeks or more of TPN. Chronic cholestasis may be induced by long-term TPN [31], which could lead to cholelithiasis or cholecystitis [32].

POSTOPERATIVE STATE

Jaundice often occurs after surgery, especially after cardiac surgery; of the latter, approximately 26.5% of cases show conjugated hyperbilirubinemia [33]. Postoperative jaundice usually occurs within 1 – 2 weeks after major surgery. Serum concentrations of mainly conjugated bilirubin may increase to 40 mg/dL, but these resolve within a few days to weeks without specific treatment [34]. If a patient with abnormal LFT results has had a recent operation, the abnormalities may be associated with surgery.

There are several possible causes of abnormal LFT results after surgery, including (1) liver congestion due to preexisting right-sided heart failure, (2) perioperative hypotension and hypoxia, (3) destruction of transfused red blood cells, (4) resorption of hematoma, (5) worsening of jaundice in Gilbert's syndrome, (6) total parenteral nutrition, (7) drug-induced liver injury, (8) postoperative infection, and (9) benign postoperative intrahepatic cholestasis. The frequency of abnormal LFT results is also known to depend on the type of operation, and jaundice is more common in patients undergoing valve surgery than coronary surgery.

GASTROENTEROLOGICAL DISEASE

Abnormal liver function test results are observed in over 50% of patients with inflammatory bowel diseases requiring surgery. Patients who undergoing jejunoileal bypass for treatment of severe obesity may experience liver damage [35]. The liver often shows NASH, leading to liver cirrhosis and liver failure. Similar liver injuries have been observed in patients undergoing gastrectomy *via* Billroth reconstruction. Bacterial overgrowth in the blind loop of the intestine can induce the production of endotoxin and intrinsic ethanol [36, 37], leading to Kupffer cell activation and hepatocyte damage.

GRANULOMA FORMATION IN THE LIVER

Several systemic diseases and drugs have been shown to induce granulomas in the liver, causing liver enlargement. The most consistently abnormal liver biochemistry result is elevated serum ALP. The diagnosis and causes of hepatic granulomas may be determined by histological examination of the liver. Granulomatous diseases that cause liver involvement include sarcoidosis, primary biliary cirrhosis, giant cell hepatitis, Wegener's granulomatosis, chronic granulomatous disease and allergic granulomatosis, hepatitis C virus, cytomegalovirus, Epstein–Barr virus infection, tuberculosis, *Mycobacterium avium-intracellulare* infection in patients with HIV infection, leprosy, brucellosis, typhoid fever, Whipple's disease, tularemia, yersiniosis, cat scratch disease, histoplasmosis, blastomycosis, coccidiomycosis, candidiasis, Q fever, leishmaniasis, toxoplasmosis, syphilis, and schistosomiasis drugs, such as penicillins, diphenylhydantoin, and allopurinol, neoplastic diseases, such as Hodgkin's disease and hypernephroma, and foreign bodies, such as beryllium, suture materials used in surgery, and thorotrast.

AMYLOIDOSIS

Hepatic involvement has been demonstrated in about one fifth of patients with amyloid type A (AA) amyloidosis and about half of those with the amyloid light chain (AL) type, and liver function tests can remain normal even in patients with substantial amyloid deposits and hepatomegaly. Elevated serum ALP and γ-GTP levels occur first in patients with massive amyloid deposits, followed by modest elevations of serum AST and ALT [38].

MESSAGES FROM HEPATOLOGISTS TO GENERAL PHYSICIANS

1. Bacteremia is the most common liver function abnormality caused by systemic disease. Patients with fever and signs of bacterial infection showing mild to moderate abnormal liver function test results only require treatment for the infection. The pattern of liver injury is mainly cholestasis, with frequent discordant elevation of T-Bil and ALP. It should be noted that isolated hyperbilirubinemia up to 10 mg/dL is not unusual in patients with bacteremia.

2. The other etiologies of abnormal liver function tests are connective tissue disease, shock, heart failure, and thyroid disease, and the common patterns of liver function test results for each condition should be taken into consideration. Among these, abnormal liver function tests in patients with connective tissue disease may be due to complication with connective tissue disease or concomitant autoimmune liver disease. Differentiation is often difficult, and liver biopsy may be required in such cases.

ACKNOWLEDGEMENTS

We are very thankful to Ms. Asma Ahmed, manager publications, Bentham Science Publishers, for her patience and long-term assistance.

CONFLICT OF INTEREST

The author confirms that he has no conflict of interest to declare for this publication.

REFERENCES

[1]   Shimizu Y. Liver in systemic disease. World J Gastroenterol 2008;14:4111-4119.
[2]   Chazouillères O, Housset C. Intrahepatic cholestasis. In: Rodés J, Benhaumou JP, Blei AT, Reichen J, Rizzetto M, editors. Textbook of Hepatology. 3rd ed, Oxford: Blackwell Publishing, 2007:1481-1500.
[3]   Kanai S, Honda T, Uehara T, Matsumoto T. Liver function tests in patients with bacteremia. J Clin Lab Anal 2008;22:66-69.
[4]   Ding Y, Zhao L, Mei H, Huang ZH, Zhang SL. Alterations of biliary biochemical constituents and cytokines in infantile hepatitis syndrome. World J Gastroenterol 2006;12:7038-7041.
[5]   Thiele DL. Hepatic manifestations of systemic disease and other disorders of the liver. In: Feldman M, Friedman LS, Sleisenger MH, editors. Sleisenger & Fordtran's Gastrointestinal and Liver Disease. 7th ed. Philadelphia: Elsevier Science, 2002: 1603-1619.

[6]   Fang MH, Ginsberg AL, Dobbins WO 3rd. Marked elevation in serum alkaline phosphatase activity as a manifestation of systemic infection. Gastroenterology 1980;78:592-597.
[7]   Miller DJ, Keeton DG, Webber BL, Pathol FF, Saunders SJ. Jaundice in severe bacterial infection. Gastroenterology 1976;71:94-97.
[8]   Neale G, Caughey DE, Mollin DL, Booth CC. Effects of intrahepatic and extrahepatic infection on liver function. Br Med J 1966;1:382-387.
[9]   Tojo J, Ohira H, Abe K, Yokokawa J, Takiguchi J, Rai T, Shishido S, Sato Y, Kasukawa R. Autoimmune hepatitis accompanied by systemic lupus erythematosus. Intern Med 2004;43:258-262.
[10]   Usta Y, Gurakan F, Akcoren Z, Ozen S. An overlap syndrome involving autoimmune hepatitis and systemic lupus erythematosus in childhood. World J Gastroenterol 2007;13:2764-2767.
[11]   Iwai M, Harada Y, Ishii M, Tanaka S, Muramatsu A, Mori T, Nakashima T, Okanoue T, Hirohata S. Autoimmune hepatitis in a patient with systemic lupus erythematosus. Clin Rheumatol 2003;22:234-236.
[12]   Lu MC, Li KJ, Hsieh SC, Wu CH, Yu CL. Lupus-related advanced liver involvement as the initial presentation of systemic lupus erythematosus. J Microbiol Immunol Infect 2006;39:471-475.
[13]   Ross A, Friedman LS. The liver in systemic disease. In: Bacon BR, O'Grady JG, Di Bisceglie AM, Lake JR, editors. Comprehensive Clinical Hepatology. 2nd ed. Philadelphia: Mosby Elsevier Ltd, 2006:537-547.
[14]   Kay PS, Keeffe EB. Cardiac disease and the liver. In: Gitlin N editor. The Liver and Systemic Disease. Hong Kong: Pearson Professional Limited, 1997: 1-16.
[15]   Gitlin N, Serio KM. Ischemic hepatitis: widening horizons. Am J Gastroenterol 1992;87:831-836.
[16]   Richman SM, Delman AJ, Grob D. Alterations in indices of liver function in congestive heart failure with particular reference to serum enzymes. Am J Med 1961;30:211-225.
[17]   Dunn GD, Hayes P, Breen KJ, Schenker S. The liver in congestive heart failure: a review. Am J Med Sci 1973;265:174-189.
[18]   Sherlock S. The liver in heart failure; relation of anatomical, functional, and circulatory changes. Br Heart J 1951;13:273-293.
[19]   Carithers RL. Endocrine disorders and the liver. In: Gitlin N, editor. The Liver and Systemic Disease. Hong Kong: Pearson Professional Limited, 1997:59-72.
[20]   Fong TL, McHutchison JG, Reynolds TB. Hyperthyroidism and hepatic dysfunction. A case series analysis. J Clin Gastroenterol 1992;14:240-244.
[21]   Sato T, Tajiri J, Shimada T, Hiramatsu R, Umeda T. Abnormal blood chemistry data in Cushing's syndrome: comparison with those for fatty liver. Endocrinol Jpn 1984;31:705-710.
[22]   Olsson RG, Lindgren A, Zettergren L. Liver involvement in Addison's disease. Am J Gastroenterol 1990;85:435-438.
[23]   Boulton R, Hamilton MI, Dhillon AP, Kinloch JD, Burroughs AK. Subclinical Addison's disease: a cause of persistent abnormalities in transaminase values. Gastroenterology 1995;109:1324-1327.
[24]   Salmela PI, Sotaniemi EA, Niemi M, Maentausta O. Liver function tests in diabetic patients. Diabetes Care 1984;7:248-254.
[25]   Foster KJ, Griffith AH, Dewbury K, Price CP, Wright R. Liver disease in patients with diabetes mellitus. Postgrad Med J 1980;56:767-772.
[26]   Silverman JF, O'Brien KF, Long S, Leggett N, Khazanie PG, Pories WJ, Norris HT, Caro JF. Liver pathology in morbidly obese patients with and without diabetes. Am J Gastroenterol 1990;85:1349-1355.
[27]   Marchesini G, Brizi M, Morselli-Labate AM, Bianchi G, Bugianesi E, McCullough AJ, Forlani G, Melchionda N. Association of nonalcoholic fatty liver disease with insulin resistance. Am J Med 1999;107:450-455.
[28]   Grant JP, Cox CE, Kleinman LM, Maher MM, Pittman MA, Tangrea JA, Brown JH, Gross E, Beazley RM, Jones RS. Serum hepatic enzyme and bilirubin elevations during parenteral nutrition. Surg Gynecol Obstet 1977;145:573-580.
[29]   Lindor KD, Fleming CR, Abrams A, Hirschkorn MA. Liver function values in adults receiving total parenteral nutrition. JAMA 1979;241:2398-2400.
[30]   Spiliotis JD, Kalfarentzos F. Total parenteral nutrition-associated liver dysfunction. Nutrition 1994;10:255-260.

[31]   Cavicchi M, Beau P, Crenn P, Degott C, Messing B. Prevalence of liver disease and contributing factors in patients receiving home parenteral nutrition for permanent intestinal failure. Ann Intern Med 2000;132:525-532.

[32]   Koppe SWP, Buchman AL. Total parenteral nutritionrelated liver disease. In Rodés J, Benhaumou JP, Blei AT, Reichen J, Rizzetto M, editors. Textbook of Hepatology. 3rd ed. Oxford: Blackwell Publishing, 2007:1634-1641.

[33]   Mastoraki A, Karatzis E, Mastoraki S, Kriaras I, Sfirakis P, Geroulanos S. Postoperative jaundice after cardiac surgery. Hepatobiliary Pancreat Dis Int 2007;6:383-387.

[34]   Schmid M, Hefti ML, Gattiker R, Kistler HJ, Senning A. Benign postoperative intrahepatic cholestasis. N Engl J Med 1965;272:545-550.

[35]   Chapman RW, Angus PW. The effect of gastrointestinal diseases on the liver and biliary tract. In: Rodés J, Benhaumou JP, Blei AT, Reichen J, Rizzetto M, editors. Textbook of Hepatology. 3rd ed. Oxford: Blackwell Publishing, 2007:1622-1633.

[36]   Peters RL. Patterns of hepatic morphology in jejunoileal bypass patients. Am J Clin Nutr 1977;30:53-57.

[37]   Baraona E, Julkunen R, Tannenbaum L, Lieber CS. Role of intestinal bacterial overgrowth in ethanol production and metabolism in rats. Gastroenterology 1986;90:103-110.

[38]   Hawkins PN. Amyloidosis. In: Rodés J, Benhaumou JP, Blei AT, Reichen J, Rizzetto M, editors. Textbook of Hepatology. 3rd ed. Oxford: Blackwell Publishing, 2007:1702-1708.

CHAPTER 7

Sytemic Abnormalities in Liver Disease

Yukihiro Shimizu[1,*] and Masami Minemura[2]

[1]*Gastroenterology Center, Nanto Municipal Hospital, Japan and* [2]*The Third Department of Internal Medicine, University of Toyama, Japan*

Abstract: Systemic abnormalities are often seen in patients with liver diseases. Especially, cardiopulmonary or renal diseases complicated by advanced liver disease are sometimes serious and may determine the quality of life and prognosis of patients. Therefore, both hepatologists and non-hepatologists should pay attention to these abnormalities in the management of patients with liver diseases.

Keywords: Cardiomyopathy, coronary heart disease, diabetes mellitus, liver injury, pulmonary disease, renal disease, thyroid disease.

KEY POINTS

1. Liver disease can induce abnormalities in various organs, and an understanding of these effects is important for the management of patients with liver disease.

2. Some systemic abnormalities are potentially life threatening.

Liver diseases can cause abnormalities in various organs [1]

CARDIOPULMONARY DISEASES

Cardiomyopathy

There have been reports of dilated hypertrophic cardiomyopathy associated with hepatitis C virus (HCV) infection [2, 3], and some human leukocyte antigen (HLA) haplotypes are associated with development of the disease [4], suggesting that a genetic predisposition may be involved. HCV core protein is thought to damage the myocardium through an immunological mechanism.

"Part of this chapter has been previously published in World J Gastroenterol. 2009 Jun 28; 15(24): 2960–2974. DOI: 10.3748/wjg.15.2960

*Corresponding author Yukihiro Shimizu: Gastroenterology Center, Nanto Municipal Hospital, Toyama, Japan; E-mail: rsf14240@nifty.com

In patients with cirrhosis, cardiac output and circulatory volumes are increased due to reduced vascular peripheral resistance and increased arteriovenous shunting [5, 6].

However, it is rare for the condition to lead to heart failure.

Coronary Artery Disease

Atherosclerotic coronary artery disease and acute myocardial infarction are less frequent in patients with liver cirrhosis than in non-cirrhotic patients [7-10]. In contrast, patients with non-alcoholic steatohepatitis (NASH)-related cirrhosis may have a higher incidence of coronary artery disease than those with other etiologies [11].

Pulmonary Disease

When a patient with advanced liver disease, mostly cirrhosis, complains of dyspnea in the absence of primary cardiopulmonary disease, the patient may have hepatopulmonary syndrome (HPS) or portopulmonary hypertension (PPHTN), with the prevalence being much higher in the former syndrome (11% – 32% *vs.* 2%, respectively) [12]. The clinical features, diagnostic strategy, and expected effectiveness of orthotopic liver transplantation are different between these two conditions, as summarized in Table **1**. Orthotopic liver transplantation is effective for patients with HPS [13], but is contraindicated in cases of severe PPHTN, indicating the necessity for differential diagnosis [14].

Moreover, the association of idiopathic pulmonary fibrosis (IPF) and HCV infection has been reported, and a report from Japan indicated that the cumulative rate of IPF development after 20 years of HCV infection is 0.9% [15].

ENDOCRINE DISEASES

Diabetes Mellitus

The prevalence of type 2 diabetes mellitus is higher in patients with chronic HCV infection than in those with hepatitis B virus (HBV) infection (21% and 12% in the USA, 23.6% and 9.4% in the UK, respectively) [16-19] and HCV core protein is associated with insulin resistance. Oral hypoglycemic drugs, such as biguanides, may be useful for the improvement of insulin resistance in such cases. Insulin therapy is recommended in patients with severely advanced liver disease.

Table 1. Difference between hepatopulmonary syndrome (HPS) and portopulmonary hypertension (PPHTN) [11].

	HPS		PPHTN
Prevalence	11-32% of patients with liver cirrhosis		2% of patients with portal hypertension
Pathogenesis	Increased intrapulmonary shunting		Unknown
Intrapulmonary vascular dilatations		(+)	(-)
Pulmonary arterial hypertension		(-)	(+)
Symptom	Dyspnea, Platypnea		Dyspnea on exertion , Syncope, Chest pain
Clinical manifestations	Cyanosis		No cyanosis
	Orthodeoxia		Accentuated pulmonic component of IIs
	Spider nevi		Systolic murmur, edema
ECG findings	None		RVH, RBBB, Right axis deviation
Arterial blood gas levels	Moderate-to-severe hypoxaemia (<60-80mmHg)		No/mild hypoxaemia
Chest radiography	Normal		Cardiomegaly, Hilar enlargement
CEE	Positive finding; left atrial opacification		Usually negative finding
	for 3–6 heart beats after right atrial opacification		
^{99m}TcMAA shunting index	≥6%		<6%
Pulmonary hemodynamics	Normal/low PVR		Elevated PVR
			mPAP>25mmHg at rest or >30mmHg with exercise
OLT	Indicated in severe stages		Only indicated in mild-to-moderate stages

RV: right ventricle, RVH: right ventricle hypertrophy, IIs: second heart sound, ECG: electrocardiography, RBBB: right bundle-branch block, AaPO2: alveolar arterial oxygen gradient, CEE: contrast-enhanced echocardiography, ^{99m}TcMAA: technetium-99m-labelled macroaggregated albumin, PVR: pulmonary vascular resistance, mPAP: mean pulmonary artery pressure, OLT: orthotopic liver transplantation.

Thyroid Disease

Thyroid disease and serum anti-thyroid autoantibodies are often found in patients with HCV infection, especially in infected women (13% and 15%, respectively) [20, 21]. Moreover, anti-HCV treatment with interferon-α is known to cause thyroid disorders. Therefore, thyroid function and anti-thyroid antibody should be monitored before and during the antiviral treatment.

RENAL DISEASES

Renal diseases in patients with liver diseases include hepatitis virus-associated nephropathy, including membranous nephropathy, membranoproliferative glomerulonephritis (MPGN), mesangioproliferative glomerulonephritis, and hepatorenal syndrome (HRS), which is a serious complication of advanced liver cirrhosis. Hepatitis virus-associated nephropathy should be considered in patients with chronic liver disease showing proteinuria and/or hematuria.

Hepatitis Virus-Associated Nephropathy

HBV infection is associated with a variety of renal diseases, including membranous nephropathy and MPGN [22, 23]. Diagnosis is based on assessment of the status of HBV replication (HBeAg/Ab and HBV DNA levels), laboratory findings (urinalysis and liver function test), and kidney biopsy, although it is sometimes difficult to detect the deposition of viral antigens in the kidney by routine immunohistochemical analysis. HBV-associated nephrotic syndrome due to membranous nephropathy is not uncommon in children, and spontaneous recovery has been reported, which is often associated with seroconversion of HBeAg to anti-HBe [24]. In adults, on the other hand, spontaneous resolution is relatively uncommon and antiviral therapy may be effective [25].

HBV-related MPGN has been reported to be improved by treatment with interferon or lamivudine.

HCV infection is more often associated with renal diseases, such as mixed cryoglobulinemia, MPGN, and membranous nephropathy, than is HBV infection [26]. Mixed cryoglobulinemia, which has been found in 35% – 90% of patients with HCV infection [27-29], is associated with systemic vasculitis and can frequently cause renal disease. The rate of MPGN in patients with mixed cryoglobulinemia is approximately 30% [26, 30, 31]. The clinical manifestations of renal diseases include hematuria, proteinuria, and renal insufficiency.

Improvements in both serum cryoglobulin levels and plasma creatinine concentration have been reported in patients who exhibited undetectable levels of serum HCV RNA after interferon therapy, with either interferon alone [32-34] or in combination with ribavirin [35, 36]. Recently, the effectiveness of anti-CD20 chimeric monoclonal antibody in the treatment of cryoglobulinemic glomerulonephritis has been reported [37].

Hepatorenal Syndrome

Hepatorenal syndrome (HRS) involves renal failure in patients with severe liver disease in the absence of any identifiable renal pathology [38, 39]. The incidences of HRS in patients with cirrhosis and ascites are 18% and 39% after 1 and 5 years of follow-up, respectively [40]. New criteria for a diagnosis of HRS were reported by the International Ascites Club in 2007 (Table **2**) [41]. HRS may be classified into two types: type-1 HRS is characterized by rapid progression of renal failure (within 2 weeks) and a mortality rate at 2 weeks of about 80%. In contrast, the degree of renal failure is less severe in patients with type-2 HRS, and median survival is around 4-6 months [39]. Type-1 HRS is often induced by a precipitating event, in particular spontaneous bacterial peritonitis. HRS is related to renal vasoconstriction following a reduction of effective circulating volume due to peripheral vasodilation. Orthotopic liver transplantation is the ideal treatment for cirrhotic patients with HRS, but the survival rate after orthotopic liver transplantation is lower in these patients than in those without HRS (60% *vs.* 70%-80%, respectively, at 3 years) [42]. The combined use of vasoconstrictors and albumin is one of the most useful options for treatment of patients with HRS [43].

Table 2. New diagnostic hepatorenal syndrome criteria in cirrhosis [41].

Cirrhosis with ascites.
Serum creatinine >133 µmol/l (1.5 mg/dl).
No improvement of serum creatinine (decrease to a level of ≤133 µmol/l) after at least 2 days with diuretic withdrawal and volume expansion with albumin. The recommended dose of albumin is 1 g/kg of body weight per day up to a maximum of 100 g/day.
Absence of shock.
No current or recent treatment with nephrotoxic drugs.

Other systemic manifestations include hematological abnormalities, bone diseases, neurological disorders, gastrointestinal diseases, and skin lesions, and are summarized in our previous review [1].

MESSAGES FROM HEPATOLOGISTS TO GENERAL PHYSICIANS

1. The most common problems seen in patients with liver diseases are hepatorenal syndrome and hepatic encephalopathy. The former often defines the prognosis of patients with advanced cirrhosis, while the latter is important for the quality of life of these patients.

2. The mechanisms of hepatorenal syndrome have not been clarified and there is no gold standard treatment. However, coadministration of vasoconstrictors, such as terlipressin, and albumin may be useful in the treatment of these patients.

3. Hepatopulmonary syndrome is a relatively common complication of liver cirrhosis, and can be a cause of hypoxemia in these patients.

ACKNOWLEDGEMENTS

We are very thankful to Ms. Asma Ahmed, manager publications, Bentham Science Publishers, for her patience and long-term assistance.

CONFLICT OF INTEREST

The author confirms that he has no conflict of interest to declare for this publication.

REFERENCES

[1]   Minemura M, Tajiri K, Shimizu Y. Systemic abnormalities in liver disease. World J Gastroenterol. 2009;15:2960-2974.
[2]   Matsumori A, Matoba Y, Sasayama S. Dilated cardiomyopathy associated with hepatitis C virus infection. Circulation 1995;92:2519-2525.
[3]   Teragaki M, Nishiguchi S, Takeuchi K, Yoshiyama M, Akioka K, Yoshikawa J. Prevalence of hepatitis C virus infection among patients with hypertrophic cardiomyopathy. Heart Vessels 2003;18:167-170.
[4]   Shichi D, Matsumori A, Naruse TK, Inoko H, Kimura A. HLA-DPbeta chain may confer the susceptibility to hepatitis C virus-associated hypertrophic cardiomyopathy. Int J Immunogenet 2008;35:37-43.
[5]   Kowalski HJ, Abelmann WH. The cardiac output at rest in Laennec's cirrhosis. J Clin Invest 1953;32:1025-1033.
[6]   Murray JF, Dawson AM, Sherlock S. Circulatory changes in chronic liver disease. Am J Med 1958;24:358-367.
[7]   Howell WL, Manion WC. The low incidence of myocardial infarction in patients with portal cirrhosis of the liver: A review of 639 cases of cirrhosis of the liver from 17,731 autopsies. Am Heart J 1960;60:341-344.
[8]   Vaněcek R. Atherosclerosis and cirrhosis of the liver. Bull World Health Organ 1976;53:567-570.
[9]   Marchesini G, Ronchi M, Forlani G, Bugianesi E, Bianchi G, Fabbri A, Zoli M, Melchionda N. Cardiovascular disease in cirrhosis--a point-prevalence study in relation to glucose tolerance. Am J Gastroenterol 1999;94 655-662
[10]   Berzigotti A, Bonfiglioli A, Muscari A, Bianchi G, Libassi S, Bernardi M, Zoli M. Reduced prevalence of ischemic events and abnormal supraortic flow patterns in patients with liver cirrhosis. Liver Int 2005;25:331-336.
[11]   Kadayifci A, Tan V, Ursell PC, Merriman RB, Bass NM. Clinical and pathologic risk factors for atherosclerosis in cirrhosis: a comparison between NASH-related cirrhosis and cirrhosis due to other aetiologies. J Hepatol 2008;49:595-599.
[12]   Rodríguez-Roisin R, Krowka MJ, Herve P, Fallon MB. Pulmonary-hepatic vascular disorders (PHD). Eur Respir J 2004;24:861-880.
[13]   Battaglia SE, Pretto JJ, Irving LB, Jones RM, Angus PW. Resolution of gas exchange abnormalities and intrapulmonary shunting following liver transplantation. Hepatology 1997;25:1228-1232.
[14]   Ramsay MA, Simpson BR, Nguyen AT, Ramsay KJ, East C, Klintmalm GB. Severe pulmonary hypertension in liver transplant candidates. Liver Transpl Surg 1997;3:494-500.
[15]   Arase Y, Suzuki F, Suzuki Y, Akuta N, Kobayashi M, Kawamura Y, Yatsuji H, Sezaki H, Hosaka T, Hirakawa M, Saito S, Ikeda K, Kumada H. Hepatitis C virus enhances incidence of idiopathic pulmonary fibrosis. World J Gastroenterol 2008;14:5880-5886.
[16]   Mason AL, Lau JY, Hoang N, Qian K, Alexander GJ, Xu L, Guo L, Jacob S, Regenstein FG, Zimmerman R, Everhart JE, Wasserfall C, Maclaren NK, Perrillo RP. Association of diabetes mellitus and chronic hepatitis C virus infection. Hepatology 1999;29:328-333.

[17]   Caronia S, Taylor K, Pagliaro L, Carr C, Palazzo U, Petrik J, O'Rahilly S, Shore S, Tom BD, Alexander GJ. Further evidence for an association between non-insulin-dependent diabetes mellitus and chronic hepatitis C virus infection. Hepatology 1999;30:1059-1063.

[18]   Mehta SH, Brancati FL, Sulkowski MS, Strathdee SA, Szklo M, Thomas DL. Prevalence of type 2 diabetes mellitus among persons with hepatitis C virus infection in the United States. Ann Intern Med 2000;133:592-599.

[19]   Mehta SH, Brancati FL, Strathdee SA, Pankow JS, Netski D, Coresh J, Szklo M, Thomas DL. Hepatitis C virus infection and incident type 2 diabetes. Hepatology 2003;38:50-56.

[20]   Preziati D, La Rosa L, Covini G, Marcelli R, Rescalli S, Persani L, Del Ninno E, Meroni PL, Colombo M, Beck-Peccoz P. Autoimmunity and thyroid function in patients with chronic active hepatitis treated with recombinant interferon alpha-2a. Eur J Endocrinol 1995;132:587-593.

[21]   Fernandez-Soto L, Gonzalez A, Escobar-Jimenez F, Vazquez R, Ocete E, Olea N, Salmeron J. Increased risk of autoimmune thyroid disease in hepatitis C *vs* hepatitis B before, during, and after discontinuing interferon therapy. Arch Intern Med 1998;158:1445-1448.

[22]   Johnson RJ, Couser WG. Hepatitis B infection and renal disease: clinical, immunopathogenetic and therapeutic considerations. Kidney Int 1990; 37: 663-676.

[23]   Levy M, Chen N. Worldwide perspective of hepatitis B-associated glomerulonephritis in the 80s. Kidney Int Suppl 1991;35:S24-S33.

[24]   Gilbert RD, Wiggelinkhuizen J. The clinical course of hepatitis B virus-associated nephropathy. Pediatr Nephrol 1994;8:11-14.

[25]   Lai KN, Li PK, Lui SF, Au TC, Tam JS, Tong KL, Lai FM. Membranous nephropathy related to hepatitis B virus in adults. N Engl J Med 1991;324:1457-1463.

[26]   Coccoli R, Esposito R, Cianciaruso B, Pota A, Visciano B, Annecchini R, Parrilli G. Hepatitis C and kidney disease. Dig Liver Dis 2007;39 Suppl 1:S83-S85.

[27]   Pawlotsky JM, Ben Yahia M, Andre C, Voisin MC, Intrator L, Roudot-Thoraval F, Deforges L, Duvoux C, Zafrani ES, Duval J. Immunological disorders in C virus chronic active hepatitis: a prospective case-control study. Hepatology 1994;19:841-848.

[28]   Tarantino A, Campise M, Banfi G, Confalonieri R, Bucci A, Montoli A, Colasanti G, Damilano I, D'Amico G, Minetti L. Long-term predictors of survival in essential mixed cryoglobulinemic glomerulonephritis. Kidney Int 1995;47:618-623.

[29]   D'Amico G. Renal involvement in hepatitis C infection: cryoglobulinemic glomerulonephritis. Kidney Int 1998;54:650-671.

[30]   Horikoshi S, Okada T, Shirato I, Inokuchi S, Ohmuro H, Tomino Y, Koide H. Diffuse proliferative glomerulonephritis with hepatitis C virus-like particles in paramesangial dense deposits in a patient with chronic hepatitis C virus hepatitis. Nephron 1993;64:462-464.

[31]   Arase Y, Ikeda K, Murashima N, Chayama K, Tsubota A, Koida I, Suzuki Y, Saitoh S, Kobayashi M, Kobayashi M, Kobayashi M, Kumada H. Glomerulonephritis in autopsy cases with hepatitis C virus infection. Intern Med 1998;37:836-840.

[32]   Johnson RJ, Gretch DR, Couser WG, Alpers CE, Wilson J, Chung M, Hart J, Willson R. Hepatitis C virus-associated glomerulonephritis. Effect of alpha-interferon therapy. Kidney Int 1994;46:1700-1704.

[33]   Fabrizi F, Lunghi G, Messa P, Martin P. Therapy of hepatitis C virus-associated glomerulonephritis: current approaches. J Nephrol 2008;21:813-825.

[34]   Casato M, Agnello V, Pucillo LP, Knight GB, Leoni M, Del Vecchio S, Mazzilli C, Antonelli G, Bonomo L. Predictors of long-term response to high-dose interferon therapy in type II cryoglobulinemia associated with hepatitis C virus infection. Blood 1997;90:3865-3873.

[35]   Loustaud-Ratti V, Liozon E, Karaaslan H, Alain S, Paraf F, Le Meur Y, Denis F, Vidal E. Interferon alpha and ribavirin for membranoproliferative glomerulonephritis and hepatitis C infection. Am J Med 2002;113:516-519.

[36]   Bruchfeld A, Lindahl K, Ståhle L, Söderberg M, Schvarcz R. Interferon and ribavirin treatment in patients with hepatitis C-associated renal disease and renal insufficiency. Nephrol Dial Transplant 2003;18:1573-1580.

[37]   Kamar N, Rostaing L, Alric L. Treatment of hepatitis C-virus-related glomerulonephritis. Kidney Int 2006;69:436-439.

[38]   Arroyo V, Guevara M, Ginès P. Hepatorenal syndrome in cirrhosis: pathogenesis and treatment. Gastroenterology 2002;122:1658-1676.

[39]   Ginès P, Guevara M, Arroyo V, Rodés J. Hepatorenal syndrome. Lancet 2003;362:1819-1827.

[40]   Ginès A, Escorsell A, Ginès P, Saló J, Jiménez W, Inglada L, Navasa M, Clària J, Rimola A, Arroyo V. Incidence, predictive factors, and prognosis of the hepatorenal syndrome in cirrhosis with ascites. Gastroenterology 1993;105:229-236.

[41]   Salerno F, Gerbes A, Ginès P, Wong F, Arroyo V. Diagnosis, prevention and treatment of hepatorenal syndrome in cirrhosis. Gut 2007;56:1310-1318.

[42]   Gonwa TA, Klintmalm GB, Levy M, Jennings LS, Goldstein RM, Husberg BS. Impact of pretransplant renal function on survival after liver transplantation. Transplantation 1995;59:361-365.

[43]   Alessandria C, Venon WD, Marzano A, Barletti C, Fadda M, Rizzetto M. Renal failure in cirrhotic patients: role of terlipressin in clinical approach to hepatorenal syndrome type 2. Eur J Gastroenterol Hepatol 2002;14:1363-1368.

CHAPTER 8

Infection and Liver

Kazuto Tajiri*

The Third Department of Internal Medicine, University of Toyama, Japan

Abstract: Various unique infections, including amebic and parasitic infections, are seen in the liver because of its characteristic anatomical features. History taking, including details of food, travel, and sexual behavior, is important for differential diagnosis. Imaging studies, such as X-ray, ultrasonography, and computed tomography, as well as serological tests are essential to make a definitive diagnosis. A delay in making a definitive diagnosis may adversely affect outcome, as specific therapy for each infection is required.

Keywords: History taking, liver abscess, paracyte, serological test.

INTRODUCTION

The liver has a unique anatomical location, receiving blood supplied directly from the gastrointestinal tract. Furthermore, the liver comes into a direct contact with the duodenum through the bile duct. Consequently, a number of unique infectious diseases are seen in the liver. In this chapter, we describe the practical points regarding infectious diseases involving the liver.

LIVER ABSCESS

Key Points (Fig. 1)

1. History taking, including travel and sexual behavior, is important.

2. Imaging studies are essential for diagnosis and management of liver abscesses.

3. Prompt treatment, including empirical antibacterial agents after collecting culture samples, is required.

4. Aspiration should be considered for large abscesses or those resistant to conservative therapy.

---

*Corresponding author Kazuto Tajiri: The Third Department of Internal Medicine, University of Toyama, Toyama, Japan; Email: tajikazu@med.u-toyama.ac.jp

The liver has the unique anatomical characteristics of being supplied by portal blood directly from the gastrointestinal tract and direct contact with the duodenum through the biliary tract. Consequently, many pathogens may gain entry into the liver resulting in abscess formation. Liver abscesses are divided into two types, pyogenic and amebic [1, 2], the differences between which are shown in Table **1**. Pyogenic liver abscess results from cellular necrosis due to microbial collection *via* direct spread from the biliary tract, portal circulation, hepatic artery, or direct spread.

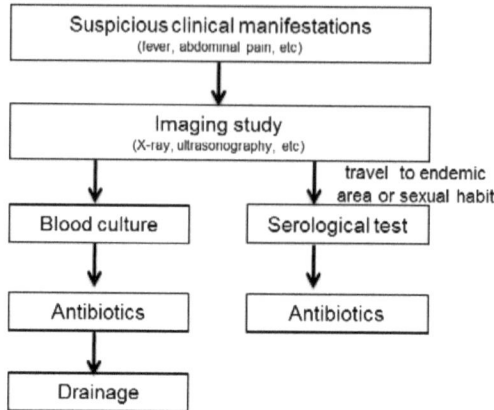

```
                    ┌─────────────────────────────────┐
                    │  Suspicious clinical manifestations │
                    │      (fever, abdominal pain, etc)   │
                    └─────────────────────────────────┘
                                    │
                    ┌─────────────────────────────────┐
                    │          Imaging study          │
                    │      (X-ray, ultrasonography, etc)  │
                    └─────────────────────────────────┘
                         │              │  travel to endemic
                         │              │  area or sexual habit
                 ┌──────────────┐   ┌──────────────┐
                 │ Blood culture │   │ Serological test │
                 └──────────────┘   └──────────────┘
                         │                 │
                 ┌──────────────┐   ┌──────────────┐
                 │  Antibiotics  │   │  Antibiotics  │
                 └──────────────┘   └──────────────┘
                         │
                 ┌──────────────┐
                 │   Drainage    │
                 └──────────────┘
```

Figure 1: Diagnosis and management of liver abscess.

Underlying biliary diseases, especially biliary malignancies, are the most frequent cause of hepatic abscess (about 60% of cases), and cryptogenic cases may be also seen (about 20% of cases).

The most common infectious agents involved in pyogenic abscess are the gram-negative bacteria *Escherichia coli*, *Streptococcus faecalis*, *Klebsiella*, and *Proteus vulgaris*. Recurrent pyogenic cholangitis may be due to *Salmonella typhi* [3]. Superinfection by anaerobes should be considered in cases resistant to antibiotic treatment. In amebiasis, trophozoites invade the wall of the intestine, and reach the liver *via* the portal circulation. Infection with *Entamoeba histolytica* affects 10% of the world's population. The prevalence rates are high in endemic areas and in some high-risk groups (Table **2**). The clinical manifestations of amebic liver abscess include fever and abdominal pain in both pyogenic and amebic abscess (Table **3**). In pyogenic abscess, fever and abdominal symptoms occur in about 90% and in more than 50% of patients, respectively. Diagnosis of liver abscess requires imaging studies, such as ultrasonography or computed tomography (CT), although such studies cannot differentiate between pyogenic and amebic abscess (Table **4**).

Table 1. Differences between pyogenic and amebic liver abscess.

	Pyogenic	Amebic
Background	Underlying biliary or intestinal disease, compromised host	Homosexual, traveler from endemic area
Symptoms	Fever, Abdominal pain, hepatomegaly, jaundice	Fever, Abdominal pain Diarrhea (<33%)
Laboratory findings	Increased inflammatory signs Increased biliary enzymes	Increased inflammatory signs Serum antibodies
Localization	Multiple	Solitary, mainly right lobe
Content	Pus like, rotten smell	Anochovy like, no smell
Infecting agents	*Escherichia coli* *Streptococcus faecalis* *Klebsiella* *Proteus vulgaris* etc.	Entamoeba histolytica
Diagnosis	Enhanced CT, US, MRI Culture of aspiration material Blood culture	US, CT, chest X-ray Serological test
Treatment	Drainage Antibiotics beta-lactam/beta-lactamase inhibitor, a third generation cephalosporin plus metronidazole etc.	Metronidazole

Table 2. Epidemiology of amebic liver abscess.

Prevalence	<1% in industrialized countries 50-80% in some tropical regions Men > women (3 to 10 times) Young adults > children or elderly
Spread	Poor sanitation Contamination of food by fries Unhygienic food handling Unclean water Use of human feces as fertilizer
High-risk group	Persons of lower socioeconomic status in endemic area Immigrants from endemic areas Institutionalized populations Men who have sex with men Travelers Persons who are immunosupressed, including those with AIDS

Table 3. Symptoms found in liver abscess.

High frequency (>66%)
Fever
Moderate frequency (33%< <66%)
Chills
Abdominal pain
Nausea
Low frequency but found (33%>)
Vomiting
Weight loss
Pleuritic chest pain
Cough
Dyspnea
Diarrhea
Abdominal distension

Table 4. Findings of imaging in liver abscess.

Chest X-p
Elevation of right hemidiaphragm
Blunting of right costphrenic angle
Atelectasis
Ultrasonography
Round or oval lesions
Lack of significant wall echoes
Hypoechoic appearance
CT scannig
Well-defined lesions, round or oval
Low density
Non-homogeous internal structure
MRI
T1 low T2 high

Aspiration and culture of abscess fluid are useful for determination of the infectious agents. As described above, pyogenic liver abscesses are frequently polymicrobial. Aspiration may be useful to distinguish between pyogenic and amebic abscess, because the gross appearance and smell are distinct between the two types. However, amebic abscess can be definitively diagnosed by serology [4]. Aspiration or drainage of pyogenic abscesses is suggested if the lesion is larger than 5 cm in diameter [5, 6]. Furthermore, empirical antibiotics covering gram-negative and anaerobic pathogens should be administered as follows [7]:

1. Monotherapy with a beta-lactam/beta-lactamase inhibitor, such as ampicillin/sulbactam (3 g IV every 6 hours), piperacillin/tazobactam (4.5 g IV every 6 hours), or ticarcillin/clavulanate (3.1 g IV every 6 hours).

2. A third-generation cephalosporin, such as ceftriaxone (1 g IV every 24 hours) plus metronidazole (500 mg IV every 8 – 12 hours).

For patients with beta-lactam intolerance, alternative empirical regimens are as follows:

1. A fluoroquinolone (such as ciprofloxacin 400 mg IV every 12 hours or levofloxacin 500 mg IV daily) plus metronidazole (500 mg IV every 8 – 12 hours).

2. Monotherapy with carbapenem, such as imipenem (500 mg IV every 6 hours), meropenem (1 g IV every 8 hours), or ertapenem (1 g IV/IM daily).

Antibiotic therapy is required for at least 4 to 6 weeks [8]. For amebic liver abscess, metronidazole (500 – 750 mg orally three times daily for 7 – 10 days) is commonly used, which results in a cure rate of more than 90% [9].

PARASITE IN THE LIVER (Table 5)

Key Points

1. History taking, including travel, pets, and food, are essential for diagnosis.

2. Serological or morphological tests are helpful to make a definitive diagnosis.

Parasite infections unique to the liver are occasionally seen, particularly in endemic areas. However, advances in global transportation networks have increased the possibility of infection in all parts of the world. Parasite infections usually require specific treatment, and delay in treatment may adversely affect the outcome with serious consequences for the patient. History taking, such as travel to endemic areas, may suggest the possibility of parasitic infection. To establish a definite diagnosis, imaging, serological, and morphological studies are required (Fig. **2**).

```
┌─────────────────────────────────────────────────┐
│       Suspicious clinical manifestations          │
│ (hepatomegaly, diarrhea, abdominal pain, eosinophilia, etc) │
└─────────────────────────────────────────────────┘
                        │
                        ▼
┌─────────────────────────────────────────────────┐
│                  History taking                    │
│  (recent travel to endemic area, food content, pet ) │
└─────────────────────────────────────────────────┘
                        │
                        ▼
┌─────────────────────────────────────────────────┐
│                  Imaging study                     │
│            (X-ray, ultrasonography, etc)           │
└─────────────────────────────────────────────────┘
                        │
                        ▼
┌─────────────────────────────────────────────────┐
│               Liver function test                  │
└─────────────────────────────────────────────────┘
                        │
                        ▼
┌─────────────────────────────────────────────────┐
│                Serological test                    │
└─────────────────────────────────────────────────┘
                        │
                        ▼
┌─────────────────────────────────────────────────┐
│               Morphological test                   │
│        (detection for eggs or body of parasites)   │
└─────────────────────────────────────────────────┘
```

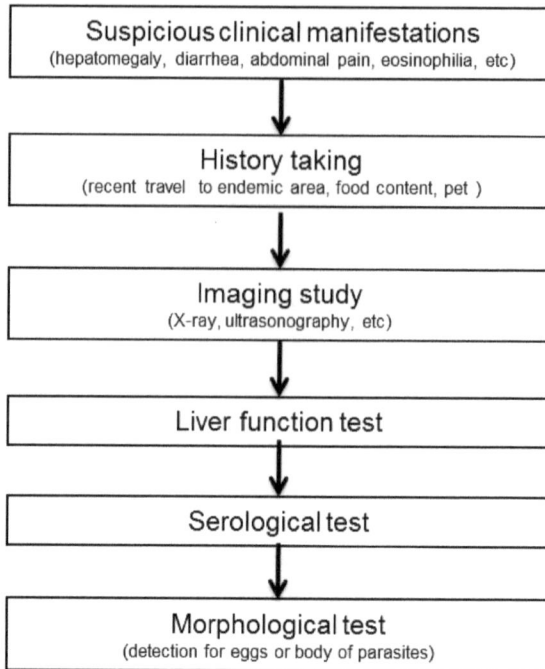

Figure 2: Management of patients with suspected parasite infection.

Schistosomiasis [10]

Schistosomiasis is caused by percutaneous infection by *Schistosoma japonicum* or *Schistosoma mansoni* [11]. *S. japonicum* is found in Japan, China, Indonesia, and the Philippines, whereas *S. mansoni* is found in Africa, the Middle East, the Caribbean, and Brazil. *S. japonicum* is more pathogenic than *S. mansoni* [12]. Eggs excreted in the feces release free-swimming embryos, which develop into fork-tailed cercariae in appropriate snails [3]. These pass through the skin of humans coming into contact with the infected water, leading to widespread hematogenous dissemination. Those reaching the mesenteric capillaries grow rapidly in the intrahepatic portal system [3]. The first clinical manifestation is itching at the site of entry of the cercariae through the skin. In the acute phase 3–4 weeks after infection, bloody diarrhea, abdominal discomfort, general fatigue, urticaria, appetite loss, or fever may be seen. Hepatomegaly is then found, and portal hypertension develops. For diagnosis, it is essential to ask whether the patient has traveled to, stayed in, or swum in an endemic area. Eosinophilia is found in some cases. For definitive diagnosis, detection of eggs in the feces or circulating schistosomal antigen is necessary. Praziquantel has high therapeutic efficacy against all species of *Schistosoma*, though early treatment is required.

Hydatid Disease [12, 13]

Hydatid disease is due to infection by *Echinococcus granulosus*, which causes cystic echinococcosis, or *Echinococcus multilocularis*, which causes alveolar echinococcosis [14]. The disease is common in sheep farming countries, such as South Australia, New Zealand, Africa, South America, Southern Europe, and the Middle and Far East, where dogs have access to infected offal [3, 15]. Patients are infected with the ova contained in the excreta of dogs as the definitive host. The ova have chitinous envelopes, which dissolve in gastric juice allowing the liberated ovum to burrow through the intestinal mucosa. From here, it is carried to the liver through the portal vein, where it develops into an adult cyst. Seventy percent of hydatid cysts are found in the liver, but a few cysts may be seen in the lung, spleen, brain, or bone [3]. The clinical manifestations may be silent unless the cysts develop to a large size. Rupture of the cyst may be serious, associated with anaphylaxis. Eosinophilia of > 7% is found in about 30% of patients. Imaging studies, such as ultrasonography or CT, indicate single or multiple cysts with thin or thick walls, and these findings are helpful for diagnosis. Serological tests for specific antigens are also useful for diagnosis [16]. Albendazole or mebendazole can be used for treatment [17], but the efficacy of these agents may be limited. Percutaneous drainage or resection may also be effective [18].

Ascariasis (Toxocariasis)

Ascaris infection occurs widely around the world, particularly in the Far East, India, and South Africa. Oral ingestion of *Toxocara canis* or *Toxocara cati* ova in the feces of dogs or cats, or larvae in the liver of chickens or cows as transient hosts, induce liver disease by retrograde flow in the bile ducts. The adult worm is 10–20 cm long, and may lodge in the common bile duct, causing obstruction [3]. Serological tests and imaging studies, such as ultrasonography or endoscopic retrograde cholangiopancreatography (ERCP), are useful for diagnosis. Ultrasonography demonstrates long linear echogenic structures or strips [3], which move in a characteristic manner. ERCP may be effective in treatment with endoscopic extraction of the worm(s). *Ascaris* is usually killed by the treatment with piperazine citrate, mebendazole, or albendazole [3], but the worms may occasionally remain in the bile duct. Treatment with these agents is generally required for 2 – 4 weeks.

Clonorchiasis [19]

Clonorchiasis is caused by ingestion of *Clonorchis sinensis* metacercariae in the skin or flesh of fresh water fish. Cases have been found in Eastern Asia, especially in

North East China, Southern Korea, Taiwan, Japan, Northern Vietnam, and the far eastern part of Russia [20]. In China, 15 million people were infected with *C. sinensis* in 2004 [21]. The cyst wall of metacercariae is destroyed by trypsin in the duodenum and the larvae enter the peripheral intrahepatic bile ducts where they grow into adult worms [3]. Clinical manifestations depend on the number of flukes, the duration of infestation, and the complications occurring as a result of infection [3]. With heavy infestation, patients may suffer weakness, epigastric discomfort, weight loss, and diarrhea. Jaundice can occur due to obstruction to the intrahepatic biliary tree by worms or inflammation. In uncomplicated cases, however, cirrhosis may develop silently. Cholangiocarcinoma may also be seen [22]. Eosinophilia and increased serum ALP levels are often recognized. Detection of ova in the stool or aspirated bile provides a definitive diagnosis, and praziquantel should be administered as treatment [23].

Table 5. Epidemiology of hepatic parasite infection.

Disease	Organism	Endemic area	Predisposition
Schistosomiasis	*S. mansoni* *S. japonicum*	Asia, Africa, South America Middle East, Caribbean	Exposure to fresh water
Echinococcus	*E. glanulosus* *E. multilocularis*	Oceania, Africa, South America Southern Europe, Middle East, etc	Ingestion of vegetables contaminated with dog feces
Toxocariasis	*T. canis* *T. cati*	Worldwide (Far East, India, South Africa)	Exposure to dogs or cats
Clonorchiasis	*C. sinensis*	Eastern Asia	Ingestion of fresh water
Opisthorchiasis	*O. viverrini* *O. felineus*	Eastern Europe Southeast Asia	Ingestion of fresh water
Fascioliasis	*F. Hepatica*	Worldwide	Ingestion of contaminated food
Cysticerosis	*T. solium*	Central and Latin America Africa, Asia	Contaminated pork

Opisthorchiasis [19]

Opisthorchiasis is caused by *Opisthorchis viverrini and Opisthorchis felineus*, and is very similar to clonorchiasis except in its geographical distribution [24]. Opisthorchiasis is found in Eastern Europe, especially in the Russian Federation, Siberia, the Ukraine, and Kazakhstan. *O. viverrini* is also endemic in Laos,

Thailand, Vietnam, and Cambodia, and approximately 6 million people are infected with this trematode parasite in Southeast Asia [23].

Fascioliasis [19]

Fascioliasis is a helminth disease caused by two trematodes, *Fasciola hepatica* or *Fasciola gigantica*. It is estimated that 17 million people are infected worldwide and 91.1 million people are at risk of infection [25]. Both species overlap in many areas of Africa and Asia [26], whereas *F. hepatica* is a major health concern in the Americas (especially Peru and Bolivia), Europe, and Oceania [27]. Women are affected at higher rates than men, and children are more affected than adults [27]. Infection occurs due to consumption of raw vegetables, alfalfa juice, salads, and contaminated water. The clinical manifestations of this disease reflect the worm burden, phase, and duration of infection. In the acute phase, which lasts from 3 to 5 months, prolonged fever, hepatomegaly with abdominal pain, mild eosinophilia, and multiple hypodense areas are recognized on CT. Other CT findings may include subcapsular hematomas, hepatic cysts, or residual hepatic calcifications [28]. Additional manifestations include anorexia, weight loss, nausea, vomiting, cough, diarrhea, urticaria, lymphadenopathy, and arthralgia. In the chronic phase, which begins after 6 months, half of all cases are asymptomatic. When symptoms appear, common bile duct obstruction, intermittent jaundice, intrahepatic cystic abscess, eosinophilic cholecystitis, and extrahepatic cholestasis may be involved. Eosinophilia may be absent in half of all chronic patients, and therefore the eosinophil count cannot be used for screening. Diagnosis can be confirmed by serological tests or by identification of ova in the feces (but cannot be detected in the early phase before worms have attained sexual maturity). Triclabendazole is effective for the treatment of both acute and chronic infections [28].

Cysticercosis (Taeniasis)[2]

Humans are the only definitive host of the tapeworm *Taenia solium*, and infection occurs due to ingestion of contaminated pork containing larval cysts. The disease is found in most developing countries (Central and Latin America, Africa, and large parts of Asia, including China). Cysticercosis may be seen in all tissues of the human host, especially the muscle, brain, eyes, heart, liver, lung, and peritoneum. Neurocysticercosis is serious, and is the most important cause of acquired epilepsy in developing countries. Serological tests in addition to imaging studies, such as CT, X-ray, and MRI, are helpful for diagnosis, and praziquantel or albendazole with steroids may be effective for treatment [29].

MESSAGES FROM HEPATOLOGISTS TO GENERAL PHYSICIANS

1. The possibility of liver abscess should be considered in patients with fever and abnormal liver function test results, which shows a cholestatic pattern of liver injury.

2. History taking, including travel history, food intake, and sexual habits, is important for the etiologic diagnosis of liver abscess.

3. Pyogenic liver abscesses larger than 5 cm in diameter sometimes require drainage in addition to antibiotics for good outcome. Antibiotics should be administered for 4 – 6 weeks, and should cover Escherichia coli, Klebsiella or anaerobes, especially Bacteroides fragilis. In contrast, amebic liver abscesses can be treated successfully only by 10-day administration of metronidazole. It is notable that half of all patients with amebic liver abscesses do not show accompanying diarrhea, mucous, or dysentery.

4. Cholangiocarcinoma sometimes resembles liver abscess with high fever and liver mass, but segmental or cuneiform enhancement around the lesion with reduced attenuation accompanying ring-like enhancement may be helpful for diagnosis. Aspiration or liver biopsy may finally be required for differentiation between these possibilities.

ACKNOWLEDGEMENTS

We are very thankful to Ms. Asma Ahmed, manager publications, Bentham Science Publishers, for her patience and long-term assistance.

CONFLICT OF INTEREST

The author confirms that he has no conflict of interest to declare for this publication.

REFERENCES

[1]   Huang CJ, Pitt HA, Lipsett PA, Osterman FA, Jr., Lillemoe KD, Cameron JL, Zuidema GD. Pyogenic hepatic abscess. Changing trends over 42 years. Ann Surg 1996;223:600-607; discussion 607-609.
[2]   Maltz G, Knauer CM. Amebic liver abscess: a 15-year experience. Am J Gastroenterol 1991;86:704-710.
[3]   Sherlock S. "The liver and Infections", Sherlock S, Dooley J. Diseases of the liver and biliary system. 11th ed. Oxford, UK ; Malden, MA: Blackwell Science, 2002

[4]   Kraoul L, Adjmi H, Lavarde V, Pays JF, Tourte-Schaefer C, Hennequin C. Evaluation of a rapid enzyme immunoassay for diagnosis of hepatic amoebiasis. J Clin Microbiol 1997;35:1530-1532.

[5]   Rajak CL, Gupta S, Jain S, Chawla Y, Gulati M, Suri S. Percutaneous treatment of liver abscesses: needle aspiration *versus* catheter drainage. AJR Am J Roentgenol 1998;170:1035-1039.

[6]   Yu SC, Ho SS, Lau WY, Yeung DT, Yuen EH, Lee PS, Metreweli C. Treatment of pyogenic liver abscess: prospective randomized comparison of catheter drainage and needle aspiration. Hepatology 2004;39:932-938.

[7]   Reddy KR. "Bacterial, Paracytic, Fungal, and Granulomatous Liver Diseases" Goldman L, Schafer AI. Goldman's Cecil Medicine, 24 th ed. Elsevier, 2012

[8]   Chen YW, Chen YS, Lee SS, Yen MY, Wann SR, Lin HH, Huang WK, *et al.* A pilot study of oral fleroxacin once daily compared with conventional therapy in patients with pyogenic liver abscess. J Microbiol Immunol Infect 2002;35:179-183.

[9]   Li E, Stanley SL, Jr. Protozoa. Amebiasis. Gastroenterol Clin North Am 1996;25:471-492.

[10]   Burke ML, Jones MK, Gobert GN, Li YS, Ellis MK, McManus DP. Immunopathogenesis of human schistosomiasis. Parasite Immunol 2009;31:163-176.

[11]   Gryseels B, Polman K, Clerinx J, Kestens L. Human schistosomiasis. Lancet 2006;368:1106-1118.

[12]   Garcia HH, Moro PL, Schantz PM. Zoonotic helminth infections of humans: echinococcosis, cysticercosis and fascioliasis. Curr Opin Infect Dis 2007;20:489-494.

[13]   Moro P, Schantz PM. Echinococcosis: a review. Int J Infect Dis 2009;13:125-133.

[14]   Schantz PM. Progress in diagnosis, treatment and elimination of echinococcosis and cysticercosis. Parasitol Int 2006;55 Suppl:S7-S13.

[15]   Romig T, Dinkel A, Mackenstedt U. The present situation of echinococcosis in Europe. Parasitol Int 2006;55 Suppl:S187-191.

[16]   Zhang W, McManus DP. Recent advances in the immunology and diagnosis of echinococcosis. FEMS Immunol Med Microbiol 2006;47:24-41.

[17]   Smego RA, Jr., Sebanego P. Treatment options for hepatic cystic echinococcosis. Int J Infect Dis 2005;9:69-76.

[18]   Smego RA, Jr., Bhatti S, Khaliq AA, Beg MA. Percutaneous aspiration-injection-reaspiration drainage plus albendazole or mebendazole for hepatic cystic echinococcosis: a meta-analysis. Clin Infect Dis 2003;37:1073-1083.

[19]   Marcos LA, Terashima A, Gotuzzo E. Update on hepatobiliary flukes: fascioliasis, opisthorchiasis and clonorchiasis. Curr Opin Infect Dis 2008;21:523-530.

[20]   Rim HJ. Clonorchiasis: an update. J Helminthol 2005;79:269-281.

[21]   Lun ZR, Gasser RB, Lai DH, Li AX, Zhu XQ, Yu XB, Fang YY. Clonorchiasis: a key foodborne zoonosis in China. Lancet Infect Dis 2005;5:31-41.

[22]   Choi D, Lim JH, Lee KT, Lee JK, Choi SH, Heo JS, Jang KT, *et al.* Cholangiocarcinoma and Clonorchis sinensis infection: a case-control study in Korea. J Hepatol 2006;44:1066-1073.

[23]   Kaewpitoon N, Kaewpitoon SJ, Pengsaa P. Opisthorchiasis in Thailand: review and current status. World J Gastroenterol 2008;14:2297-2302.

[24]   Park GM. Genetic comparison of liver flukes, Clonorchis sinensis and Opisthorchis viverrini, based on rDNA and mtDNA gene sequences. Parasitol Res 2007;100:351-357.

[25]   Keiser J, Utzinger J. Emerging foodborne trematodiasis. Emerg Infect Dis 2005;11:1507-1514.

[26]   Mas-Coma S, Bargues MD, Valero MA. Fascioliasis and other plant-borne trematode zoonoses. Int J Parasitol 2005;35:1255-1278.

[27]   Marcos LA, Terashima A, Leguia G, Canales M, Espinoza JR, Gotuzzo E. [Fasciola hepatica infection in Peru: an emergent disease]. Rev Gastroenterol Peru 2007;27:389-396.

[28]   Marcos LA, Tagle M, Terashima A, Bussalleu A, Ramirez C, Carrasco C, Valdez L, *et al.* Natural history, clinicoradiologic correlates, and response to triclabendazole in acute massive fascioliasis. Am J Trop Med Hyg 2008;78:222-227.

[29]   Garg RK, Potluri N, Kar AM, Singh MK, Shukla R, Agrawal A, Verma R. Short course of prednisolone in patients with solitary cysticercus granuloma: a double blind placebo controlled study. J Infect 2006;53:65-69.

CHAPTER 9

Approach to Liver Injury Caused by Drugs and Toxins

Kazuto Tajiri[1,*] and Yukihiro Shimizu[2]

[1]The Third Department of Internal Medicine, University of Toyama, Japan and [2]Gastroenterology Center, Nanto Municipal Hospital, Japan

Abstract: The liver is an essential organ involved in elimination of drugs and toxins. Any drug, including herbal remedies or dietary supplements, can be a causative agent for drug-induced liver injury (DILI). An aging society or requirement for advanced medical care with multiple medications may complicate the management of DILI, especially in developed countries. The possibility of developing DILI should always be considered when starting new drugs. The classification of DILI—hepatocellular, cholestatic, or mixed—is useful for management. Discontinuation of the causative drug is usually sufficient to manage patients with DILI, but liver injury may persist or progress even after the drug has been stopped, especially in cholestatic type DILI.

Keywords: Causality assessment, DILI, liver function, Toxic liver injury.

KEY POINTS

1. As any drugs can induce drug-induced liver injury (DILI), we should always consider the possibility of DILI when starting a new drug.

2. As DILI may develop to severe hepatitis, cases of hepatocellular injury with jaundice should be managed carefully.

3. Determination of the epidemiology of DILI may help in its management.

MANAGEMANT of DILI (Fig. 1)

Cases in Which DILI Should be Suspected

Many drugs can cause liver injury without any symptoms [1]. In patients with abnormal liver function test results, careful history taking, including not only hospital medications but also herbal remedies or dietary supplements, should always be performed.

> *"Part of this chapter has been previously published in World J Gastroenterol. 2008 Nov 28; 14(44): 6774–6785. doi: 10.3748/wjg.14.6774".*

---

*Corresponding author Kazuto Tajiri:** The Third Department of Internal Medicine, University of Toyama, Toyama, Japan; Email: tajikazu@med.u-toyama.ac.jp

Drug dosage, administration route, previous administration, concomitant drugs, alcohol consumption, and underlying chronic liver disease should be assessed. During physical examination, presence of fever, rash, or jaundice is carefully checked. Especially, jaundice is a sign of severe liver injury indicating the necessity of prompt cessation of the suspected drug. Liver function tests, including serum transaminase, ALP, γ-GTP, and bilirubin, and hematological tests, including eosinophil count and coagulation tests, should be performed. Classification of the pattern of liver injury should be done first because clinical course and causative drugs are different for each pattern [2]. Other etiologies, such as viral infection, autoimmune liver disease, and biliary disease, autoimmune liver disease, and biliary disease, should be excluded by serological tests or imaging studies if necessary.

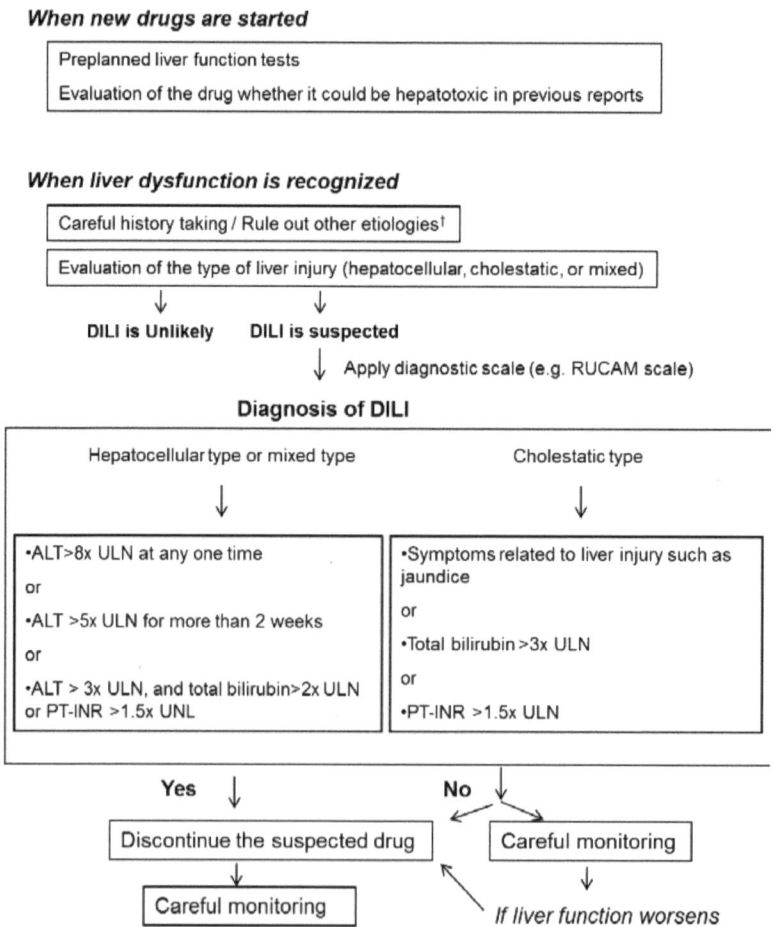

When new drugs are started

Preplanned liver function tests

Evaluation of the drug whether it could be hepatotoxic in previous reports

When liver dysfunction is recognized

Careful history taking / Rule out other etiologies[†]

Evaluation of the type of liver injury (hepatocellular, cholestatic, or mixed)

↓	↓
DILI is Unlikely	**DILI is suspected**

↓ Apply diagnostic scale (e.g. RUCAM scale)

Diagnosis of DILI

Hepatocellular type or mixed type	Cholestatic type
↓	↓
•ALT>8x ULN at any one time or •ALT >5x ULN for more than 2 weeks or •ALT > 3x ULN, and total bilirubin>2x ULN or PT-INR >1.5x UNL	•Symptoms related to liver injury such as jaundice or •Total bilirubin >3x ULN or •PT-INR >1.5x ULN

Yes ↓   **No** ↓

Discontinue the suspected drug	Careful monitoring
↓	↓
Careful monitoring	*If liver function worsens*

Figure 1: Algorithm for management of DILI.

Situations in Which DILI Should be Suspected

In daily clinical practice, DILI should be always considered as a cause of liver injury whenever patients are taking medications. Although fever, rash, arthralgia, and eosinophilia are symptoms and signs of an immunoallergic reaction to a drug, there are few clinical features associated specifically with DILI, and the frequencies of these symptoms are not particularly high. However, there are some situations in which DILI should be particularly suspected as follows [3]: 1) starting a new drug in the past 3 months; 2) presence of rash or eosinophilia; 3) mixed type with hepatocellular and cholestatic liver injury; 4) cholestatic liver injury with normal hepatobiliary imaging; and 5) acute or chronic liver injury without autoantibodies or hypergammaglobulinemia.

Epidemiology and Causative Drug of DILI

Any drug can cause DILI, and the possibility of DILI should be considered in patients with liver injury of unknown origin. Thus, it is important to know the epidemiology of causative drugs of DILI. The database of the World Health Organization (WHO) indicated that the frequencies of DILI has been increasing since the 1990s [4]. Thirteen to thirty percent of cases with fulminant liver failure has been reported to be caused by DILI [5-7] Acetaminophen, drugs against human immunodeficiency virus (HIV), troglitazone, anticonvulsants (such as valproate), analgesics, antibiotics, and anticancer drugs are common causative agents of DILI with fatalities in the WHO database [4].

The risk of liver injury for most drugs is estimated to be $1 - 10/100000$ people exposed [1]. DILI was reported to occur in 1/100 patients hospitalized in the departments of internal medicine [8]. In another analysis with 461 cases from Spain, amoxicillin/clavulanate was the most common drug as a cause of DILI (59/461 cases, 12.8%) [9]. Moreover, bentazepam, atorvastatin, and captopril were frequent causative drugs often leading to chronic liver damage [10]. On the other hand, a report from Italy demonstrated that hydroxymethylglutaryl-CoA reductase inhibitors were the most frequent causative drugs among 1069 cases of DILI (4.5% of cases of adverse drug reactions) [11]. Other drugs responsible for DILI include acetaminophen, anti-retroviral therapy, antibiotics, lipid-lowering drugs, and anticonvulsants [12-18]. In recent analyses in Asia, traditional alternative medicines were reported to be the most common causes of DILI [19]. Table **1** summarizes the drugs suspected to be responsible for DILI and the types of liver injury reported in the literature from various regions [7-10, 12, 17-19]. In general, frequent causative drugs of DILI are antibiotics, non-steroidal anti-inflammatory drugs, and anticonvulsants. Although not shown in Table **1**, about 10% of cases of DILI were suspected to be due to two or more drugs. Furthermore, it should be noted that the incidence rates of DILI caused by herbal remedies or traditional medicines have been increasing over the last decade [1].

Table 1. Main drugs associated with DILI from recent summarized reports.

Category	Drugs	Hepatocellular	Cholestatic	Mixed
Anti-microbe	Amoxicillin-clavulanate	28	25	23
	Azithromycin	0	8	0
	Trovafloxacin	5	0	1
	Erythromycin	2	4	3
	Clindamycin	2	0	0
	Nitrofurantoin	1	1	0
	Levofloxacin	0	0	1
	Ciprofloxacin	2	1	1
	Flucloxacillin	0	7	1
	Sulfasalazine	1	0	1
	Isoniazid/pyrazinamide/rifampin	24	6	32
	HAART	4	1	1
	Dapsone	2	0	0
Anti-inflammatory	Acetaminophen	40	0	0
	Diclofenac	18	8	3
	Nimesulide	7	2	0
	Ibuprofen	8	3	9
Anti-convulsant	Carbamazepine	6	1	3
	Valproic acid	4	1	3
For psychiatric	Bentazepam	5	0	2
	Paroxetine	4	1	2
	Disulfiram	2	0	0
Anti-cancer	Tetrabamate	6	1	0
	Flutamide	12	1	5
	Methotrexate	3	0	0
Lipid-lowering	Atorvastatin	6	2	2
	Fenofibrate	1	0	2
For Gastrointestinal	Ebrotidine	23	0	2
Anti-hypertensive	Captopril	1	0	1
Anti-coagulant	Ticlopidine	8	5	1
For endocrine	Thiamazole	1	4	0
Immunosuppressant	Azathioprine	5	4	2
Others	Medical herbs	26	3	2
	OTC health supplements	3	0	0
		285	170	103

Risk Factors of DILI

Recognition of risk factors is important for the diagnosis of DILI, and some scoring systems include these elements. Age, gender, pregnancy, and alcohol consumption are estimated as risk factors on the host side, and these risk factors are thought to be related with increased incidence of liver injury [20]. In an analysis, age was found to be the most important factor in the development of amoxicillin/clavulanate hepatotoxicity, probably because of the decreased drug elimination related to aging [21]. In contrast, adverse events associated with valproate or erythromycin are more common in children [22]. On the other hand, female predominancy has been reported in patients with drug-induced acute liver failure undergoing liver transplantation [23]. Thus, age and female gender could predispose the development of DILI. However, based on an evaluation of recent cases, Shapiro and Lewis suggest that factors such as age (over 55 years old), gender (female dominant), or a history of alcohol consumption may not be specific for DILI [24]. Moreover, genetic factors for drug metabolism, such as polymorphisms of cytochrome P (CYP) 450 or deficiency of N-acetyltransferase, are closely related with the development of DILI [25, 26]. Interestingly, a recent report suggested that the daily dose of drug ingestion is associated with idiosyncratic DILI, and the number of cases and poor outcome of DILI were reported to increase in a dose-dependent manner [27]. Furthermore, underlying liver disease, viral hepatitis or systemic infection may increase susceptibility to DILI, and the frequency of DILI caused by antituberculous therapy is relatively high in patients with hepatitis B or C virus infection [28]. Antiretroviral therapy in HIV infection was reported to induce severe hepatitis and may lead to acute liver failure [29]. Moreover, hepatic steatosis is known to increases the risk of DILI [30].

> **# *Whenever a new drug, be it herbal remedy or traditional medicine, is started, we should consider the possibility of the patient developing DILI.***

Diagnosis of DILI

DILI cases with elevation of serum bilirubin to more than 3×ULN may lead to liver failure, and should be referred to the hepatologist after discontinuing all suspected drugs. Although readministration of the causative drug may be helpful for diagnosis of DILI, it is not recommended because of the possibility of the development of severe liver injury. The probability of DILI can be evaluated using a diagnostic scoring system, such as the Roussel Uclaf Causality Assessment Method (RUCAM) criteria (Table **2**) [20]. However, there is no gold standard set of diagnostic criteria for DILI. After making diagnosis of DILI, the initial management is withdrawal of the suspected drug. However, the causative drug is hard to be discontinued if the patient is receiving many drugs and the causative drug cannot be determined, or the underlying disease is serious. Medications may be continued with careful monitoring in such cases.

Table 2. Axes and score of RUCAM scales.

Axes			Score
Chronologic criteria	Hepatocellular	Cholestatic / mixed	
From drug intake until onset	5 to 90 days (1 to 15 days)*	5 to 90 days (1 to 90 days)	+2
	<5 or >90 days (> 15 days)	<5 or > 90 days (> 90 days)	+1
From cessation of the drug	≤ 15 days	≤ 30 days	+1
Course of the reaction	Decrease ≥ 50% within 8 days	N.A.**	+3
	Decrease ≥ 50% within 30 days	Decrease ≥ 50% within 180 days	+2
	N.A.	Decrease < 50% within 180 days	+1
	No improvement or lack of information		0
	Worsening or <50% improvement within 30 days	N.A.	-1
Risk factors	Age ≥ 55 years		+1
	Alcohol	Alcohol or pregnancy	+1
Concomitant therapy	None or no information		0
	Concomitant drug with compatible or suggestive time to onset		-1
	Concomitant drug known as hepatotoxin		-2
	Concomitant drug with evidence for its role		-3
Exclusion of other causes	All causes rule out		+2
Group1:HAV(anti-HAV IgM), HBV(anti-HBc IgM),	The 6 causes of group1 ruled out		+1
HCV(anti-HCV and circumstantial arguments),	5 or 4 causes of group1 ruled out		0
Biliary obstruction(ultrasonography), Shock liver	Less than 4 causes of group1 ruled out		-2
Group2: complications of underlying disease,	Non drug cause highly probable		-3
CMV, EBV, herpes virus infection			
Previous information	Reaction labelled in the product characteristics		+2
	Reaction published but unlabelled		+1
	Reaction unknown		0
Rechallenge (with the drug alone)	ALT ≥ x2	ALP(or T-Bil) ≥ x2	+3
(with the drug already given at the time of the 1st reaction)	ALT ≥ x2	ALP(or T-Bil) ≥ x2	+1
(Increase but less than normal limit in the same conditions			
as for the first administartion)	ALT	ALP(or T-Bil)	-2
Other situations			0
Total		Definitive	> 8
		Probable	6 to 8
		Possible	3 to 5
		Unlikely	1 to 2
		Excluded	< or = 0

* (in the second treatment), **N.A.: not applicable

Initial Management of DILI

DILI shows a variety of manifestations, ranging from asymptomatic mild biochemical abnormalities to hepatic failure. As there are many causes of liver injury including viral hepatitis (hepatitis A virus, hepatitis B virus, hepatitis C virus, hepatitis E virus, EB virus, cytomegalovirus, human herpes virus-6, parvovirus B19, *etc.*), biliary diseases, such as cholelithiasis, alcohol abuse, nonalcoholic fatty liver disease, autoimmune liver diseases, and hereditary diseases, such as hemochromatosis, α1-antitrypsin deficiency, and Wilson's disease, exclusion of those etiologies is required in the diagnosis of DILI. Among those, differential diagnosis of acute onset autoimmune hepatitis (AIH) is sometimes difficult, because serum IgG levels or antinuclear antibody titers are often low in acute AIH [31]. Histological examination of the liver may be useful and liver biopsy should be considered for the differential diagnosis.

Taken together, a low threshold of suspicion, thorough history of drug exposure, exclusion of other possible etiologies, or occupational hazards with exposure to potential toxins, are important to make an accurate diagnosis of DILI [3, 6]. Some clinical scales, such as the RUCAM scale [20, 32], Clinical Diagnostic Scale [33] method, or Naranjo Adverse Drug Reaction Probability Scale [34], are available for the diagnosis of DILI. Among these, the RUCAM scale has been mostly used, and seems to be the standard method for diagnosis of DILI [1] (Table **2**). However, most patients are taking more than one drug, and identification of a single drug as a causative agent is difficult even with these scales. Moreover, patients with underlying liver or systemic diseases that also affect the liver biochemical tests complicate the situation for diagnosis of DILI.

DILI is divided into three types, *i.e.*, hepatocellular, cholestatic, and mixed, according to the Councils for International Organizations of Medical Sciences [20, 32]. Hepatocellular type is defined by ALT > 2×ULN (upper limit of normal) or R ≥ 5, where R is the ratio of serum activity of ALT/serum activity of ALP. Liver injury is likely to be more severe in hepatocellular type than in cholestatic/mixed type.Cholestatic type is defined by ALP > 2×ULN or R ≤ 2 and mixed type is defined by ALT > 2×ULN and 2 < R < 5. Patients with cholestatic/mixed type are likely to develop chronic disease more frequently than those with hepatocellular type [10].

It is of note that some DILI patients may show resolution of liver injury without discontinuation of the drug. Therefore, it should be necessary to carefully evaluate whether the suspected drug should be discontinued with adequate consideration of the importance of the medication. Although there are no definitive criteria for cessation of the suspected causative drug, some textbooks suggest that ALT < 5×ULN and no symptoms allow continuation of the suspected drug with close observation, whereas ALT > 8×ULN indicates the need to discontinue the suspected drug [35, 36]. Zimmerman reported as Hy's rule for monitoring DILI that elevation of liver enzymes (AST or ALT > 3×ULN or ALP > 1.5×ULN) in combination with elevated bilirubin (> 3×ULN) at any time after starting a new drug may suggest serious liver injury and the suspected drug should be stopped [37]. As many drugs can induce mild and transient elevation of liver enzyme levels without severe hepatotoxicity, elevation of transaminase levels does not always require withdrawal of the causative drug. Based on these observations, the FDA recently proposed draft guidelines (http://www.fda.gov/cder/guidance/7507dft.htm) in which ALT > 8×ULN, ALT > 5×ULN for two weeks, ALT > 3×ULN in association with serum bilirubin > 2×ULN, PT-INR > 1.5, or symptoms of liver injury should be used to predict severe hepatotoxicity and recommend discontinuing the drug. Hepatocellular liver injury with jaundice requires prompt referral to a center with hepatologists. On the other hand, cholestatic DILI cases could be observed with continuation of the suspected causative drug except if jaundice, elevation of serum bilirubin (> 3×ULN), or prolongation of PT-INR (> 1.5) is recognized.

Management of DILI involves prompt withdrawal of the drug suspected to be responsible. There have been no reports regarding specific therapies except the use of N-acetylcysteine for acetaminophen hepatotoxicity. Corticosteroid may be administered in DILI cases with evident hypersensitivity, but the significant benefits have not been proved [38]. A positive de-challenge is a more than 50% decrease in serum ALT within 8 days of discontinuation of the suspected drug in the hepatocellular type [32]. On the other hand, improvement of biliary enzymes after cessation of the suspected drug may require a longer period in cases of cholestatic type DILI.

> *# Classification of DILI case by type of liver injury is required for diagnosis and management of DILI.*
>
> *# DILI cases with jaundice or PT prolongation should be managed carefully because such cases may develop to fulminant hepatitis.*
>
> *# Essential treatment for DILI involves cessation of the causative drug. However, cessation of the drug should be done with careful consideration to severity of disease and necessity of the drug.*

SUMMARY

DILI is a common liver disease that generally occurs between 5 and 90 days after drug ingestion. Any drug can induce DILI. The clinical picture of DILI is variable, ranging from transient mild elevation of liver enzymes to fulminant liver failure leading to death. The first step in diagnosis is suspicion of DILI based on careful consideration of recent comprehensive reports on the disease. Exclusion of other possible etiologies is essential for the diagnosis. Early management of DILI involves prompt withdrawal of the drug suspected to be responsible.

TOXINS AND LIVER INJURY (Table 3)

Key Points

1. Toxin-induced liver injury frequently induces severe liver injury with fatalities, and sometimes leads to liver cancer.

2. The possibility of toxin poisoning should be considered in patients with liver injury without any obvious cause.

Table 3. Toxic liver injury.

Agent	Cause	Symptoms
Poisonous mushroom	Amateur mushroom hunting	Diarrhea and vomiting about 12h after eating
Aflatoxins	Contaminated food Warm and moist environment	Hepatocellular carcinoma Acute hepatic injury
Pyrrolizidine Alkaloids	Some plant	Hepatic venoocculsive disease
Paraquat	Suicide	Severe gastrointestinal injury related
DDT	Suicide	Fatty necrosis of hepatocytes
CCl4	Industrial exposure	Drowsiness followed by abdominal pain, diarrhea or vomitting
Phosphrous	Industrial exposure	Similar to that of CCl4
Diaminodiphenylmethane	Industrial exposure	Abdominal pain, fever, jaundice
Vinyl Chloride	Industrial exposure	Raynaud's phenomenon, hepatic tumor
Arsenic	Industrial exposure	Hepatocelluar necrosis, hepatic tumor

One of the essential functions of the liver is the elimination of foreign materials, such as toxins as well as drugs. Acute episodes of poisoning induce liver injury immediately. Mild to serious changes such as fatty liver to diffuse hepatocellular necrosis are seen in cases of liver poisoning. Chronic exposure involves a risk of carcinogenesis [39]. Here, we describe hepatic injury due to poisoning.

Plant Poisoning

Destroying Angel Poisoning (Poisonous Mushroom)

Poisoning by the mushroom destroying angel (*Amanita bisporigera*) is still an important cause of acute liver injury in some parts of the world, and has an extremely high mortality rate with roughly one third to half of all cases being fatal. A single toadstool of *A. phalloides* and related species, in which phallotoxins and amatoxins are responsible for poisoning, is sufficient to cause serious poisoning. Clinical manifestations, such as diarrhea and vomiting with increases of serum transaminases due to phallotoxins, are observed after a latent period of 8 – 12 hours. A few days later, the clinical features of acute liver failure, such as deepening jaundice, hemorrhagic manifestations, and encephalopathy, are found, following centrizonal hepatocellular fat necrosis by amatoxins. Treatment involves symptomatic therapy, but liver transplantation may be considered in severe cases [39].

Aflatoxins

Aflatoxins are mycotoxins that grow on foodstuffs, such as peanuts, rice, maize, wheat, and soybeans, in hot and humid tropical climates. Acute poisoning may induce severe toxic hepatitis with jaundice caused by hepatocellular necrosis, centrilobular fibrosis, and massive bile duct proliferation. Aflatoxins have a carcinogenic effect, and are known to be a risk factor for hepatocellular carcinoma, and may also be responsible for Reye's syndrome.

Pyrrolizidine Alkaloids

Pyrrolizidine is an alkaloid found in several plants, such as *Senecio*, *Crotalaria fulva*, and *Heliotropium*. Pyrrolizidine is metabolized to toxic pyrrole derivatives and induces pericentral hepatocellular necrosis followed by the development of veno-occlusive disease.

Disinfectants

Paraquat

Paraquat is a highly toxic chemical containing dimethyl bipyridylium dichloride. Paraquat affects the mucosa, liver, and kidneys, and a teaspoonful is sufficient to kill a man. The first manifestations are burning sensations in the tongue and difficulty in swallowing followed by gastrointestinal symptoms, such as vomiting, colicky pain, and diarrhea. Thereafter, hepatorenal syndrome with jaundice of cholestatic type, oliguria, proteinuria, and finally anuria occur. The liver damage is characterized by moderate elevation of transaminase (from 200 to 800 IU) and hyperbilirubinemia (usually lower than 10 mg/dL). Lung fibrosis is the main cause of death. Removal of the toxin by gastrointestinal washing is the only established therapy.

DDT (Dichlorodiphenyltrichloroethane)

DDT is a highly potent enzyme inducer and may cause hepatocellular fatty changes or necrosis. DDT is stored in the adipose tissue of the body with its enzyme-inducing effect as a permanent threat.

Industrial and Trade Poisons

Carbon Tetrachloride (CCl4) Poisoning

CCl_4 was once widely used in many cleaning compounds, in fire extinguishers, and as a solvent, and is the classical example of a poison that induces toxic liver damage. It has largely been replaced by other chemicals because of its toxicity. The first clinical manifestations after exposure to CCl_4 are drowsiness leading to loss of consciousness, headache, and dizziness. After a short symptom-free interval of $1 - 2$ days, intestinal symptoms such as abdominal pain, vomiting, and diarrhea followed by jaundice are seen. Renal damage is then seen around day 3 after onset. Serum values of transaminase may reach astronomical levels (> 10000 IU), while levels of ALP are usually only slightly elevated. Most deaths caused by liver failure occur during the first week, while deaths by renal failure usually occur during the second week. Renal failure is responsible for about 75% of fatal cases, and the introduction of hemodialysis markedly reduces the fatality rate. Acetylcysteine administration is effective to trap toxic metabolites. This treatment is also effective in trichloroethylene poisoning. Hypoxia enhances conversion of CCl_4 to the toxic free radical $\cdot CCl_3$. Hyperbaric oxygen is an effective therapeutic option for patients with known exposure to CCl_4. These treatments should be started within the first 24 hours after exposure.

Phosphorus

Phosphorous poisoning shows a syndrome somewhat similar to that of CCl_4 poisoning. The clinical course consists of three phases: a severely symptomatic phase, a quiescent phase, and a hepatic and renal failure phase. The clinical manifestations are characterized by more severe gastrointestinal symptoms and shock than those seen in CCl_4 poisoning and by phosphorescence and garlic-like odor of excreta and vomitus. The fully developed clinical picture is fulminant hepatic and renal failure. Early administration of atropine and pralidoxime methiodide is the only established therapeutic regimen.

4,4'-Diaminodiphenylmethane Poisoning

4,4'-Diaminodiphenylmethane is a hardener used for the plastic material epoxy resin, and may cause jaundice, histologically resembling jaundice with cholestasis caused by chlorpromazine, cholangitis, and eosinophil infiltration. The first clinical manifestation is abdominal pain during the first 1 – 2 days. After an interval of 2 – 3 days, pain in the limbs is accompanied by fever with shivering. This is followed by jaundice with generalized pruritus. Serum aminotransferase levels are only moderately increased, while ALP is greatly elevated. The symptoms and signs may usually recover after one to several weeks.

Vinyl Chloride Disease

After a variable period of exposure (usually several years), patients (autoclave cleaners in the plastics industry) develop a peculiar disease characterized by Raynaud's syndrome, scleroderma, thrombocytopenia, and liver damage. Some patients show portal hypertension. Hemangioendothelioma may develop several years after exposure, and hepatomegaly and splenomegaly may be seen. The pattern of laboratory findings is nonspecific. Slight increases in aminotransferase activity together with elevated ALP levels are found.

Arsenic Poisoning

Arsenic is used as a pesticide and for the production of dyes, ceramics, paint, petroleum, and semiconductors. Acute poisoning may result in hepatocellular necrosis, while chronic poisoning may lead to either hepatic cirrhosis or to portal hypertension. Hemangioendothelioma and primary hepatocellular carcinoma have been described in cases of chronic arsenic poisoning.

MESSAGES FROM HEPATOLOGISTS TO GENERAL PHYSICIANS

1. Any drug can cause liver injury in certain subjects due to allergic reactions, and most causative drugs are started within 3 months before liver injury. For diagnosis, it is essential to exclude other competing etiologies. Antimicrobials are the most common agents responsible for

DILI. History taking, including over-the-counter medications and herbal remedies, is also necessary.

2. Older age, female gender, polypharmacy, alcoholism, and genetic polymorphisms may affect or exacerbate DILI.

3. Some scores are useful for diagnosis of DILI, but a possible diagnosis of DILI with hepatocellular type can be suspected based on a decrease in serum ALT level to lower than 50% of the initial level within 8 days after cessation of the causative drug. ALT levels do not show elevation after cessation of the causative drug. On the other hand, DILI with cholestatic type is sometimes complex, and some patients continue to show elevation of biliary enzyme levels even after cessation of the causative drug.

4. For prediction of severe clinical course, Hy's rule, which is defined as ALT > 3× the upper limit of normal plus serum total bilirubin levels > 2× the upper limit of normal may be applicable.

5. In cholestatic type DILI, T-Bil is exclusively elevated after long-term elevation of biliary enzymes, whereas acute bile duct obstruction caused by stones shows simultaneous elevation of T-Bil and biliary enzymes usually accompanied by AST-predominant aminotransferase elevation.

6. It is not always necessary to stop the possible causative drugs. Cessation or continuation of the causative drugs should be determined by taking the balance between severity of liver injury and therapeutic importance of the drugs into consideration. In patients with severe liver injury, however, all drugs started within the last 6 months should be discontinued.

ACKNOWLEDGEMENTS

We are very thankful to Ms. Asma Ahmed, manager publications, Bentham Science Publishers, for her patience and long-term assistance.

CONFLICT OF INTEREST

The author confirms that he has no conflict of interest to declare for this publication.

REFERENCES

[1] Tajiri K, Shimizu Y. Practical guidelines for diagnosis and early management of drug-induced liver injury. World J Gastroenterol 2008;14:6774-6785.

[2] Bleibel W, Kim S, D'Silva K, Lemmer ER. Drug-induced liver injury: review article. Dig Dis Sci 2007;52:2463-2471.

[3] Schiff ER, Sorrell MF, Maddrey WC. Schiff's diseases of the liver. 10th ed. Philadelphia: Lippincott Williams & Wilkins, 2007: 2 v. (xxxiv, 1576, I-1548 p, 735-742.)

[4] Bjornsson E, Olsson R. Suspected drug-induced liver fatalities reported to the WHO database. Dig Liver Dis 2006;38:33-38.

[5] Hussaini SH, Farrington EA. Idiosyncratic drug-induced liver injury: an overview. Expert Opin Drug Saf 2007;6:673-684.

[6] Norris W, Paredes AH, Lewis JH. Drug-induced liver injury in 2007. Curr Opin Gastroenterol 2008;24:287-297.

[7] Carey EJ, Vargas HE, Douglas DD, Balan V, Byrne TJ, Harrison ME, Rakela J. Inpatient admissions for drug-induced liver injury: results from a single center. Dig Dis Sci 2008;53:1977-1982.

[8] Meier Y, Cavallaro M, Roos M, Pauli-Magnus C, Folkers G, Meier PJ, Fattinger K. Incidence of drug-induced liver injury in medical inpatients. Eur J Clin Pharmacol 2005;61:135-143.

[9] Andrade RJ, Lucena MI, Fernandez MC, Pelaez G, Pachkoria K, Garcia-Ruiz E, Garcia-Munoz B, *et al*. Drug-induced liver injury: an analysis of 461 incidences submitted to the Spanish registry over a 10-year period. Gastroenterology 2005;129:512-521.

[10] Andrade RJ, Lucena MI, Kaplowitz N, Garcia-Munoz B, Borraz Y, Pachkoria K, Garcia-Cortes M, *et al*. Outcome of acute idiosyncratic drug-induced liver injury: Long-term follow-up in a hepatotoxicity registry. Hepatology 2006;44:1581-1588.

[11] Motola D, Vargiu A, Leone R, Cocci A, Salvo F, Ros B, Meneghelli I, *et al*. Hepatic adverse drug reactions: a case/non-case study in Italy. Eur J Clin Pharmacol 2007;63:73-79.

[12] Vuppalanchi R, Liangpunsakul S, Chalasani N. Etiology of new-onset jaundice: how often is it caused by idiosyncratic drug-induced liver injury in the United States? Am J Gastroenterol 2007;102:558-562; quiz 693.

[13] Jinjuvadia K, Kwan W, Fontana RJ. Searching for a needle in a haystack: use of ICD-9-CM codes in drug-induced liver injury. Am J Gastroenterol 2007;102:2437-2443.

[14] Hussaini SH, O'Brien CS, Despott EJ, Dalton HR. Antibiotic therapy: a major cause of drug-induced jaundice in southwest England. Eur J Gastroenterol Hepatol 2007;19:15-20.

[15] Bower WA, Johns M, Margolis HS, Williams IT, Bell BP. Population-based surveillance for acute liver failure. Am J Gastroenterol 2007;102:2459-2463.

[16] Akhtar AJ, Shaheen M. Jaundice in African-American and Hispanic patients with AIDS. J Natl Med Assoc 2007;99:1381-1385.

[17] Sgro C, Clinard F, Ouazir K, Chanay H, Allard C, Guilleminet C, Lenoir C, *et al*. Incidence of drug-induced hepatic injuries: a French population-based study. Hepatology 2002;36:451-455.

[18] De Valle MB, Av Klinteberg V, Alem N, Olsson R, Bjornsson E. Drug-induced liver injury in a Swedish University hospital out-patient hepatology clinic. Aliment Pharmacol Ther 2006;24:1187-1195.

[19] Wai CT, Tan BH, Chan CL, Sutedja DS, Lee YM, Khor C, Lim SG. Drug-induced liver injury at an Asian center: a prospective study. Liver Int 2007;27:465-474.

[20] Danan G. Causality assessment of drug-induced liver injury. Hepatology Working Group. J Hepatol 1988;7:132-136.

[21] Lucena MI, Andrade RJ, Fernandez MC, Pachkoria K, Pelaez G, Duran JA, Villar M, *et al*. Determinants of the clinical expression of amoxicillin-clavulanate hepatotoxicity: a prospective series from Spain. Hepatology 2006;44:850-856.

[22] Maddrey WC. Drug-induced hepatotoxicity: 2005. J Clin Gastroenterol 2005;39:S83-89.

[23] Russo MW, Galanko JA, Shrestha R, Fried MW, Watkins P. Liver transplantation for acute liver failure from drug induced liver injury in the United States. Liver Transpl 2004;10:1018-1023.

[24] Shapiro MA, Lewis JH. Causality assessment of drug-induced hepatotoxicity: promises and pitfalls. Clin Liver Dis 2007;11:477-505, v.

[25]   Huang YS, Chern HD, Su WJ, Wu JC, Chang SC, Chiang CH, Chang FY, *et al*. Cytochrome P450 2E1 genotype and the susceptibility to antituberculosis drug-induced hepatitis. Hepatology 2003;37:924-930.

[26]   Huang YS, Su WJ, Huang YH, Chen CY, Chang FY, Lin HC, Lee SD. Genetic polymorphisms of manganese superoxide dismutase, NAD(P)H:quinone oxidoreductase, glutathione S-transferase M1 and T1, and the susceptibility to drug-induced liver injury. J Hepatol 2007;47:128-134.

[27]   Lammert C, Einarsson S, Saha C, Niklasson A, Bjornsson E, Chalasani N. Relationship between daily dose of oral medications and idiosyncratic drug-induced liver injury: search for signals. Hepatology 2008;47:2003-2009.

[28]   Lee BH, Koh WJ, Choi MS, Suh GY, Chung MP, Kim H, Kwon OJ. Inactive hepatitis B surface antigen carrier state and hepatotoxicity during antituberculosis chemotherapy. Chest 2005;127:1304-1311.

[29]   Nunez M. Hepatotoxicity of antiretrovirals: incidence, mechanisms and management. J Hepatol 2006;44:S132-139.

[30]   Tarantino G, Conca P, Basile V, Gentile A, Capone D, Polichetti G, Leo E. A prospective study of acute drug-induced liver injury in patients suffering from non-alcoholic fatty liver disease. Hepatol Res 2007;37:410-415.

[31]   Zachou K, Muratori P, Koukoulis GK, *et al*. Review article: autoimmune hepatitis - current management and challenges. Aliment Pharmacol Ther 2013;38:887-913.

[32]   Danan G, Benichou C. Causality assessment of adverse reactions to drugs--I. A novel method based on the conclusions of international consensus meetings: application to drug-induced liver injuries. J Clin Epidemiol 1993;46:1323-1330.

[33]   Maria VA, Victorino RM. Development and validation of a clinical scale for the diagnosis of drug-induced hepatitis. Hepatology 1997;26:664-669.

[34]   Naranjo CA, Busto U, Sellers EM, Sandor P, Ruiz I, Roberts EA, Janecek E, *et al*. A method for estimating the probability of adverse drug reactions. Clin Pharmacol Ther 1981;30:239-245.

[35]   Kaplowitz N, DeLeve LD. Drug-induced liver disease. 2nd ed. New York: Informa Healthcare, 2007: xv, 808 p.

[36]   Zimmerman HJ. Hepatotoxicity : the adverse effects of drugs and other chemicals on the liver. 2nd ed. Philadelphia: Lippincott Williams & Wilkins, 1999: ix, 789 p., [716] pages of plates.

[37]   Vuppalanchi R, Teal E, Chalasani N. Patients with elevated baseline liver enzymes do not have higher frequency of hepatotoxicity from lovastatin than those with normal baseline liver enzymes. Am J Med Sci 2005;329:62-65.

[38]   Lee WM. Drug-induced hepatotoxicity. N Engl J Med 1995;333:1118-1127.

[39]   M. Schmid. Liver damage caused by environmental factors. In Clinical Hepatology. Ed. Géza Csomós and Heribert Thaler M.D. Pub. Springer-Verlag Berlin Heidelberg. DOI 10.1007/978-3-642-68748-8_27 (1983, pp374-387)

CHAPTER 10

Risk of Surgery and Drug Therapy in Patients with Liver Disease

Yukihiro Shimizu*

Gastroenterology Center, Nanto Municipal Hospital, Japan

Abstract: Patients with severe or advanced liver diseases have greater risks during surgery than healthy subjects, which must be assessed by hepatologists. Decreases in hepatic blood flow during anesthesia or surgery are associated with postoperative liver damage. The risk of surgery in patients with liver cirrhosis is assessed by the Child–Pugh grade or the Model for End-Stage Liver Disease score. The type of surgery is another factor affecting the risk of patients with liver disease, and cardiac surgery is associated with higher mortality in patients with cirrhosis than other type of operations.

The liver is the main organ of metabolism and elimination of drugs. Thus, decreased liver function may result in abnormally high concentrations of drugs in the body. Drug elimination by the liver could be afftected by the first-pass effect, hepatic metabolism, and biliary extraction, and decreased haptic blood flow or cytochrome P 450 enzyme activities may affect drug metabolism in patients with advanced liver cirrhosis.

Keywords: Cardiac surgery, Child-Pugh (C-P) grade, dosage adjustment of drug, first-pass effect of drug, liver cirrhosis, liver disease, Model for End-Stage Liver Disease (MELD) score, risk assessment, surgery.

RISK OF SURGERY IN PATIENTS WITH LIVER DISEASE

Key Points

1. The risks of surgery in patients with liver diseases must be assessed by hepatologists before surgery.

2. The risks differ according to the severity of liver disease and the type of surgery.

"Part of this chapter has been previously published in World J Gastroenterol. 2009 Jun 28; 15(24): 2960–2974. DOI: 10.3748/wjg.15.2960".

*Corresponding author Yukihiro Shimizu: Gastroenterology Center, Nanto Municipal Hospital, Toyama, Japan; Email: rsf14240@nifty.com

INTRODUCTION

Some patients with liver diseases have high risks during surgery, and these risks are increased according to the severity of liver disease [1]. Decreases in hepatic blood flow during anesthesia or surgery are associated with postoperative liver damage, and Cowan *et al.* reported that a major reduction in hepatic blood flow is observed after the induction of anesthesia, but not during or after surgery [2]. The type of surgery is another factor affecting the risk of patients with liver disease.

Liver Disease

The risks of surgery may be extremely high in patients with acute viral hepatitis, as well as in those with alcoholic hepatitis [3]. Therefore, surgery in these patients should be avoided if the patient is in a serious condition. In contrast, surgery in patients with chronic hepatitis can be safely performed [4], and no deaths or complications have been reported in patients with chronic hepatitis C undergoing laparoscopic cholecystectomy [5]. The complications and mortality rates for surgery are high in patients with liver cirrhosis [6], especially in those with one or more of the following factors: elevated bilirubin, prolonged prothrombin time (PT), ascites, decreased albumin, encephalopathy, portal hypertension, elevated creatinine concentration, intraoperative hypotension, and emergent surgery [7]. The progression of liver cirrhosis can be assessed by the Model for End-Stage Liver Disease (MELD) score or the Child–Pugh (C–P) grade [8]. Both scores are useful for assessing the risk of surgery, and C–P grade is useful for predicting the risk of death: Patients in class A, B and C had mortality rates of about 10%, 30% and above 70%, respectively [9, 10]. Another study in Italy also indicated similar mortality rates of surgery for patients with liver cirrhosis (C–P grade A; 7.1%, C–P grade B; 23%, C–P grade C; 84%) [11]. Moreover, MELD score, age and American Society of Anesthesiologists class were shown to be useful for the prediction of the risk of postoperative mortality in patients with cirrhosis [12]. Operation risks increase in accordance with the MELD score, and one report showed that poor outcomes are associated with a MELD score of 14 or more or plasma hemoglobin levels below 10 g/dL in patients undergoing abdominal surgery, excluding hepatic surgery [13]. For patients undergoing laparoscopic cholecystectomy, a preoperative MELD score of 8 or more was associated with high morbidity [14], and this could be the cutoff value for indication of the operation in patients with liver cirrhosis. However, Schiff *et al.* reported that preoperative platelet counts and PT-INR are more important as the risk factors for cholecystectomy than C–P grade [15].

Patients with obstructive jaundice are at high risk of perioperative complications, including infections, stress ulcer, disseminated intravascular coagulation, wound dehiscence, and renal failure, with several reports indicating perioperative mortality rates ranging from 8% to 28%.

Type of Surgery

The risk of surgery depends on the invasiveness or duration of the operation. Laparotomy is associated with significant reduction in hepatic arterial blood flow, and large amounts of blood loss during surgery increase the risk of ischemic hepatic injury. Cholecystectomy, gastric surgery, and colectomy have been reported associated with high mortality rates in patients with decompensated cirrhosis.

Cardiac surgery, especially cardiopulmonary bypass surgery, shows increased mortality in patients with cirrhosis compared to other surgical procedures. [16]. The mortality rate of cirrhotic patients with C–P grade A is low, but high in patients with C–P grade B being for a long period and all patients with C–P grade C, especially for open-heart surgery. Therefore, open-heart surgery should be avoided in patients with C–P grade C, and off-pump cardiac operation is recommended for patients with C–P grade B [17]. Another study recommended that cardiac surgery with cardiopulmonary bypass should be avoided in patients with a C–P score greater than 7 [18].

In summary, surgery should be avoided in patients with acute hepatitis. On the other hand, surgery is generally safe for most patients with chronic hepatitis and cirrhotic patients with C–P grade A. The risks are elevated for cirrhotic patients with C–P grade B or C, or patients with a MELD score of 8 or more, though this may vary according to the type of surgery performed. Other predictive factors for safe surgery are platelet count and PT-INR, which are the markers of bleeding tendency and advanced liver disease.

DOSAGE ADJUSTMENT OF DRUGS IN LIVER DISEASE

The liver is the main organ responsible for metabolism and elimination of drugs. Thus, advanced liver diseases with decreased liver functions could affect drug metabolism resulting in high serum concentrations of drugs [1]. Drug elimination by the liver is mainly affected by the first-pass effect, hepatic metabolism, and biliary extraction. Moreover, as the liver produces most plasma proteins, decreased liver function with low plasma proteins could influence the binding of drugs to plasma proteins, leading to changes in the action and metabolism of the drugs [19].

The first-pass effect of each drug is variable, and drugs with high first-pass effects are shown in Table 1 [20]. The serum concentrations of these drugs could easily be elevated by decreases in hepatic blood flow (especially portal blood flow) or total hepatocyte mass. It is therefore recommended that initial and maintenance dose of drugs with a high first-pass effect should be reduced in cirrhotic patients especially if the drug is administered orally.

Table 1. Drugs that may need to be administered at reduced doses in patients with liver cirrhosis [20, 22].

Drugs with high first-pass effect	Drugs metabolized mainly by		
	CYP 1A2	CYP3A4	CYP2C9
Amitriptyline	Acetaminophen	Quinidine	Diclofenac
Bromocriptine	Phenacetin	Amiodarone	Ibuprophen
Diltiazem	Mexitilene	Lidocaine	Mephenam
Flumazenil	(R)-Warfarin	Mitazaolam	Tolbutamide
Fluorouracil	Imipramine	Diazepam Phenytoin	Phenobarbital
Imipramine	Theophyline	Amitriptyline	(S)-Warfarin
Isosorbide dinitrate	Propranolol	Imipramine	Rosartan
Labetalol	Tamoxiphen	Carbamazepine	Pyroxicam
Lidocaine	Estradiol	(R)-Warfarin	
Morphine	Cafeine	Erythromycin	
Nifedipine	Clarythromicin		
Pentazocin			
Propranolol			
Verapamil			

Drug metabolism in the liver mainly depends on the activities of the cytochrome P (CYP) 450 enzymes, which are known to be affected in patients with cirrhosis. The activities of CYP 1A, 3A, and 2C19 are considerably reduced, whereas those of CYP 2D6, 2C9, 2B, and 2E1 are also reduced, but to a lesser extent in cirrhotic patients [21]. The severity of liver cirrhosis is assessed by the C–P classification, and patients with C–P grade A show mild to moderate decrease in CYP activities. In contrast, patients with C–P grade B or C have marked reduction in CYP activity. Therefore, it may be necessary to reduce the doses of drugs mainly metabolized by CYP 1A, 3A, or 2C19 in such patients [22]. Moreover, patients with advanced cirrhosis often show decreased renal function, despite a normal serum creatinine level [23]. Therefore, creatinine clearance in addition to liver function should be taken into consideration to determine the appropriate doses of drugs showing predominantly renal excretion in those patients.

MESSAGES FROM HEPATOLOGISTS TO GENERAL PHYSICIANS

1. The risks of surgery may be extremely high in patients with acute viral hepatitis and alcoholic hepatitis, and surgery should be avoided in such cases.

2. Patients with chronic hepatitis and with Child–Pugh grade A liver cirrhosis have low surgical risks and can undergo any type of surgery with careful perioperative management.

3. The risk of surgery in patients with Child–Pugh grade B – C liver cirrhosis cannot be ignored, however, and the indication should be considered based on the balance between the risks and importance of the surgery.

4. Surgery with the highest risk in patients with advanced liver cirrhosis is cardiac surgery.

5. Most drug therapies are feasible in patients with chronic hepatitis and liver cirrhosis Child–Pugh grade A. However, the doses of drugs that are mainly metabolized in the liver should be reduced in liver cirrhosis Child-Pugh grade B – C.

ACKNOWLEDGEMENTS

We are very thankful to Ms. Asma Ahmed, manager publications, Bentham Science Publishers, for her patience and long-term assistance.

CONFLICT OF INTEREST

The author confirms that he has no conflict of interest to declare for this publication.

REFERENCES

[1]   Minemura M, Tajiri K, Shimizu Y. Systemic abnormalities in liver disease. World J Gastroenterol. 2009; 15: 2960-74.
[2]   Cowan RE, Jackson BT, Grainger SL, Thompson RP. Effects of anesthetic agents and abdominal surgery on liver blood flow. Hepatology 1991; 14: 1161-66.
[3]   Powell-Jackson P, Greenway B, Williams R. Adverse effects of exploratory laparotomy in patients with unsuspected liver disease. Br J Surg 1982; 69: 449-51

[4]   Runyon BA. Surgical procedures are well tolerated by patients with asymptomatic chronic hepatitis. J Clin Gastroenterol 1986; 8: 542-44.

[5]   O'Sullivan MJ, Evoy D, O'Donnell C, Rajpal PK, Cannon B, Kenny-Walsh L, Whelton MJ, Redmond HP, Kirwan WO. Gallstones and laparoscopic cholecystectomy in hepatitis C patients. Ir Med J 2001; 94: 114-7

[6]   Suman A, Carey WD. Assessing the risk of surgery in patients with liver disease. Cleve Clin J Med 2006; 73: 398-404.

[7]   Ziser A, Plevak DJ, Wiesner RH, Rakela J, Offord KP, Brown DL. Morbidity and mortality in cirrhotic patients undergoing anesthesia and surgery. Anesthesiology 1999; 90: 42-53.

[8]   Durand F, Valla D. Assessment of prognosis of cirrhosis. Semin Liver Dis 2008; 28: 110-22.

[9]   Mansour A, Watson W, Shayani V, Pickleman J. Abdominal operations in patients with cirrhosis: still a major surgical challenge. Surgery 1997; 122: 730-735; discussion 735-6.

[10]   Garrison RN, Cryer HM, Howard DA, Polk HC Jr. Clarification of risk factors for abdominal operations in patients with hepatic cirrhosis. Ann Surg 1984; 199: 648-55.

[11]   Franzetta M, Raimondo D, Giammanco M, *et al.* Prognostic factors of cirrhotic patients in extra-hepatic surgery. Minerva Chir 2003; 58: 541-544.

[12]   Teh SH, Nagorney DM, Stevens SR, *et al.* Risk factors for mortality after surgery in patients with cirrhosis. Gastroenterology 2007; 132: 1261-1269.

[13]   Befeler AS, Palmer DE, Hoffman M, Longo W, Solomon H, Di Bisceglie AM. The safety of intra-abdominal surgery in patients with cirrhosis: model for end-stage liver disease score is superior to Child-Turcotte-Pugh classification in predicting outcome. Arch Surg 2005; 140: 650-654.

[14]   Perkins L, Jeffries M, Patel T. Utility of preoperative scores for predicting morbidity after cholecystectomy in patients with cirrhosis. Clin Gastroenterol Hepatol 2004; 2: 1123-1128.

[15]   Schiff J, Misra M, Rendon G, Rothschild J, Schwaitzberg S. Laparoscopic cholecystectomy in cirrhotic patients. Surg Endosc 2005; 19: 1278-1281.

[16]   An Y, Xiao YB, Zhong QJ. Open-heart surgery in patients with liver cirrhosis: indications, risk factors, and clinical outcomes. Eur Surg Res 2007; 39: 67-74.

[17]   Kaplan M, Cimen S, Kut MS, Demirtas MM. Cardiac operations for patients with chronic liver disease. Heart Surg Forum 2002; 5: 60-65.

[18]   Suman A, Barnes DS, Zein NN, Levinthal GN, Connor JT, Carey WD. Predicting outcome after cardiac surgery in patients with cirrhosis: a comparison of Child-Pugh and MELD scores. Clin Gastroenterol Hepatol 2004; 2: 719-723.

[19]   Verbeeck RK. Pharmacokinetics and dosage adjustment in patients with hepatic dysfunction. Eur J Clin Pharmacol 2008; 64: 1147-1161.

[20]   Larrey D, Pageaux GP. Prescribibg drugs in liver disease. In: Rodés J, Benhaumou JP, Blei AT, Reichen J, Rizzetto M, eds. Textbook of Hepatology. 3rd ed. Oxford: Blackwell Sci Pub, 2007: 1912-1921.

[21]   Villeneuve JP, Pichette V. Cytochrome P450 and liver diseases. Curr Drug Metab 2004; 5: 273-282.

[22]   Spray JW, Willett K, Chase D, Sindelar R, Connelly S. Dosage adjustment for hepatic dysfunction based on Child-Pugh scores. Am J Health Syst Pharm 2007; 64: 690, 692-693.

[23]   Orlando R, Mussap M, Plebani M, Piccoli P, De Martin S, Floreani M, Padrini R, Palatini P. Diagnostic value of plasma cystatin C as a glomerular filtration marker in decompensated liver cirrhosis. Clin Chem 2002; 48: 850-858.

Approach to Children with Abnormal Liver Function Tests Results

Masami Minemura[*]

The Third Department of Internal Medicine, University of Toyama, Japan

Abstract: Although the incidence of acquired liver diseases such as viral hepatitis or fatty liver is lower during infancy and childhood than in adults, congenital or metabolic disorders should be suspected in children with liver dysfunction. It should be noted that normal ranges of biochemical liver tests in children are different from those of adult subjects. Pediatric liver diseases may cause a life threatening event, such as kernicterus, intracranial hemorrhage, or metabolic derangements.

Keywords: Children, congenital disease, fatty liver, liver dysfunction, metabolic disease, viral hepatitis.

KEY POINTS

1. The incidence of acquired liver diseases is lower in infants and children than in adults, but congenital or metabolic disorders should be considered when a child has liver dysfunction.

2. Normal ranges of biochemical liver tests (*e.g.* serum concentrations of alkaline phosphatase (ALP), aminotransferases (AST, ALT), and bile acids) differ during the neonatal period, puberty and adulthood.

3. Liver disease may present as jaundice, stool color change, hepatomegaly, or metabolic derangement.

4. Pediatric liver diseases may cause a life threatening event, such as kernicterus, intracranial hemorrhage, or metabolic derangements.

INTRODUCTION

The incidence of acquired liver diseases such as viral hepatitis or fatty liver is lower during infancy and childhood than in adults, but congenital or metabolic

[*]**Corresponding author Masami Minemura:** The Third Department of Internal Medicine, University of Toyama, Toyama, Japan; Email: minemura@med.u-toyama.ac.jp

disorders should be suspected in children with liver dysfunction. Metabolism and clearance of endogenous and exogenous toxic compounds differ in children and adults, as do normal ranges of biochemical liver tests (*e.g.* serum concentrations of ALP and aminotransferases) (Table **1**). Jaundice is one of the most common symptoms suggesting liver disease in children, but physiological jaundice is frequently observed in newborns [1]. Abnormalities in liver function tests (LFTs) should be carefully evaluated because pediatric liver diseases sometimes may cause life threatening events, such as kernicterus, intracranial hemorrhage, or metabolic derangements. LFTs should therefore be performed as soon as possible in children showing signs of liver diseases, including jaundice, color changes in stool or urine, hepatomegaly, or disturbed consciousness (Fig. **1**).

Table 1. Physiological changes in liver function tests in infancy and childhood.

Tests	Normal ranges
Bilirubin	Physiological jaundice, peaking 2-5 days after birth and disappearing within 2 weeks
Aminotransferases	About 2-fold higher than the level in normal adults during the first month of life
Alkaline phosphatase	Increased during the first month of life and around puberty; About twice the normal adult level due to bone ALP in response to normal growth during adolescence.
Serum bile acids	Increased
α-fetoprotein	Increased in infants, remaining from the fetal period.

JAUNDICE

Almost all newborn infants have a total serum bilirubin level higher than 1 mg/dL (17 μmol/L), with jaundice observed in up to one third of newborns within the first week of life. This jaundice usually resolves spontaneously within 2 weeks and is regarded as "physiological jaundice". This condition has been associated with increased production of bilirubin by large red cells in newborns, with a shorter half-life and immature hepatic conjugating and transport systems for bilirubin [2]. Bilirubinemia is not physiological if its concentration exceeds 5 mg/dl on the first day or 10 mg/dl on the second day of life, if total bilirubin exceeds 15 mg/dl of total bilirubin at any time, or if conjugated bilirubin concentration exceeds 2 mg/dl at any time. The initial laboratory evaluation of a child presenting with jaundice should begin by measuring total bilirubin with fractionation (unconjugated and conjugated bilirubin) [3].

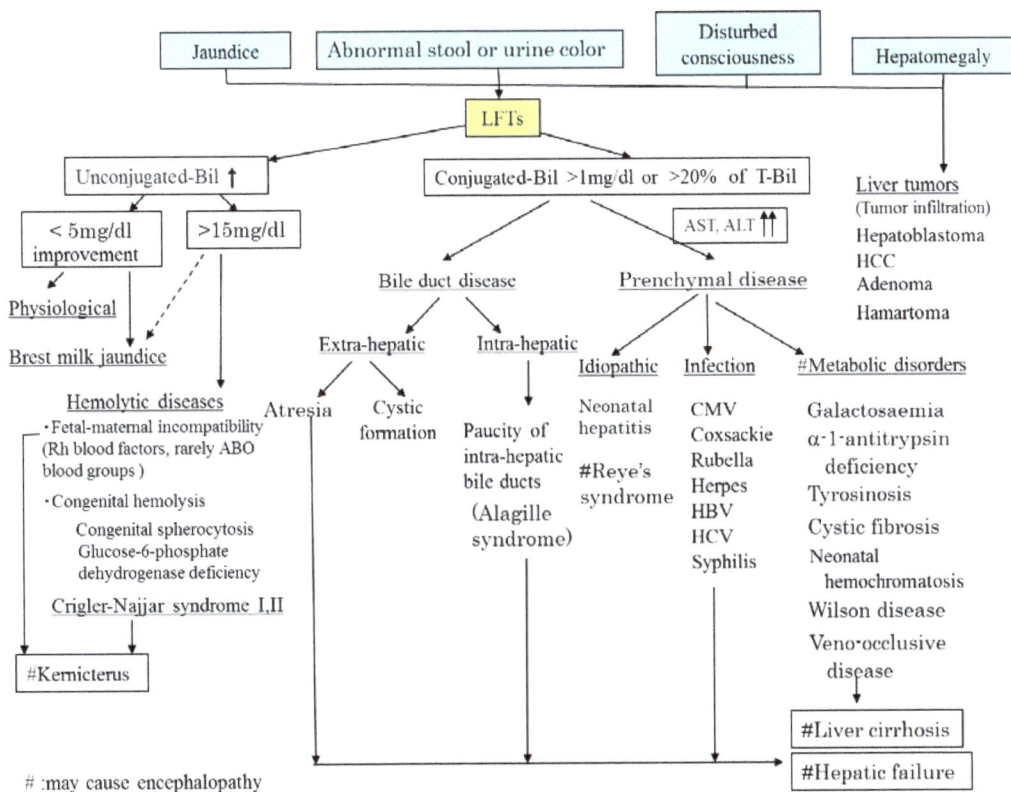

Figure 1: Liver diseases in infancy. LFTs; liver function tests, HCC; hepatocellular carcinoma, CMV; cytomegalovirus.

Unconjugated Hyperbilirubinemia

Disorders causing unconjugated hyperbilirubinemia are more common in children than in adults, and can be classified by their pathophysiologic mechanisms into three groups; (1) bilirubin overproduction, (2) impaired hepatic bilirubin uptake, and (3) impaired hepatic bilirubin conjugation [4].

i.   Bilirubin overproduction mainly results from increased breakdown of hemoglobin due to extravascular and intravascular hemolysis.

- Hemolysis due to Rh incompatibility or, rarely, ABO incompatibility [5-7] may be suspected following antenatal examination of the mother's blood for specific antibodies and confirmed by a positive Coombs' test in the infant and by blood typing.

- Congenital hemolytic disorders include deficiencies in red cell enzymes (glucose-6-phosphate dehydrogenase and pyruvate kinase) [8], congenital spherocytosis, and pyknocytosis.

- Enclosed hematoma – Hemorrhage may increase bilirubin load and exacerbate jaundice and may be associated with cephalohematoma [9-10].

2) Impaired hepatic bilirubin uptake may be caused by several mechanisms.

- Pituitary or adrenal dysfunction

- Hypothyroidism [11], which can result in reduced bilirubin uptake into hepatocytes, because thyroxine is important for hepatocyte plasma membrane function.

- Hypoalbuminemia – A decreased amount of protein-bound bilirubin may reduce bilirubin uptake by hepatocytes.

- Reduced hepatic blood flow – Heart failure or portosystemic shunts may reduce hepatic blood flow and delivery of bilirubin to hepatocytes.

3) Impaired hepatic bilirubin conjugation

Bilirubin is conjugated to glucuronic acid by uridine diphosphogluconurate glucuronyl transferase (UGT) in hepatocytes to produce bilirubin diglucronides and monoglucronides. Gilbert's syndrome is the most common inherited disorder of bilirubin glucuronidation [12]. A mutation in the promoter region of the UGT1A1 gene reduces UGT production, resulting in unconjugated hyperbilirubinemia. Crigler-Najjar syndrome type I, in which UGT activity is essentially absent, is the most severe form of inherited UGT disorders leading to severe unconjugated hyperbilirubinemia. In Crigler-Najjar syndrome type II, UGT activity is very low but detectable, making this type less severe than type I [13, 14].

Neonatal Cholestasis (Conjugated Hyperbilirubinemia)

Conjugated hyperbilirubinemia is defined as a serum concentration of conjugated bilirubin greater than 1 mg/dl when total bilirubin concentration is < 5 mg/dl or as more than 20 % of total bilirubin when the latter concentration is > 5 mg/dl [15]. Infants with neonatal cholestasis are usually detected by their primary care physicians, who note prolonged jaundice and abnormal stool/urine color. Conjugated hyperbilirubinemia may be caused not only by bile duct obstruction but by hepatitis and metabolic diseases. This condition can be broadly classified as extrahepatic and intrahepatic conjugated hyperbilirubinemia. The former includes biliary atresia and choledochal cyst, and the latter is subdivided into neonatal hepatitis and paucity of the bile ducts. Biliary atresia should be differentiated from other causes of cholestasis, because early surgical intervention (within 2 months of birth, ideally within 4 weeks) results in better patient prognosis [16-18]. Prompt diagnosis is also necessary to initiate effective therapy in infants with metabolic disorders (tyrosinemia and galactosemia) and infections. The evaluation of neonatal cholestasis is complicated because there are many potential diagnoses and few specific tests. However, physicians should know the most common causes of neonatal cholestasis (Table **2**).

Neonatal hepatitis and biliary atresia account for 70% to 80 % of infants with cholestasis, with α1-antitrypsin deficiency accounting for another 5% to 15 %. Total parenteral nutrition (TPN) and sepsis are among the most common causes in premature infants.

Table 2. Common causes of neonatal cholestasis.

Diseases	Clinical features
Extrahepatic biliary atresia	One in 10,000 to 20,000 births Jaundice, hepatosplenomegaly and acholic stools
Idiopathic neonatal hepatitis	Fluctuating jaundice during the first 2 weeks up to 4 months of life, elevated aminotransferases, hepatosplenomegaly
Infectious hepatitis	Common pathogens are Hepatitis A, Hepatitis B, and CMV
α1-antitrypsin deficiency	Accumulation of abnormal proteins within the endoplasmic reticulum
Alagille syndrome	Peripheral pulmonary arterial stenosis, butterfly vertebrae, characteristic facial features
Progressive familial intrahepatic cholestasis	Defects in members of the ATP-binding cassette transport superfamily
Parenteral nutrition-associated cholestasis	Usually occurs two weeks after starting parenteral nutrition

Biliary Atresia

Cholestasis is a common presentation of extrahepatic biliary obstruction. Extrahepatic biliary atresia is characterized by inflammation and fibrosis of the bile ducts leading to progressive obliteration of the extrahepatic biliary tract. The incidence of extrahepatic biliary atresia is approximately one in 10,000 to 20,000 births. Infants with biliary atresia usually present with icteric sclera and jaundice, hepatosplenomegaly and acholic stools. Liver function tests show elevations in serum concentrations of bilirubin, aminotransferases and γ-GTP. Ultrasound imaging results supporting a diagnosis of biliary atresia includes absence or abnormal size of the gallbladder, the "triangular cord" sign, and absence of the common bile duct. The primary treatment for biliary atresia is surgical intervention such as hepatoportoenterostomy (the Kasai procedure), which often delays the progression of disease [19]. End-stage liver disease caused by biliary atresia is the most common reason for orthotopic liver transplantation in children [20].

Other, less common extrahepatic causes of biliary obstruction include choledochal cysts, cystic fibrosis [21], gallstones, biliary sludge, and tumors. Imaging examinations are useful for differential diagnosis.

Intrahepatic Cholestasis

A paucity of intrahepatic bile ducts causes intrahepatic cholestasis, with these patients showing a reduced ratio of interlobular bile ducts to portal tracts (normal 0.9 – 1.8 *vs* paucity < 0.5). Paucity of bile ducts may be due to Alagille syndrome (arterio-hepatic dysplasia) [22, 23], which has been associated with peripheral pulmonary arterial stenosis; butterfly vertebrae; and characteristic facial features, including a broad nasal bridge, triangular face, and deep set eyes.

Genetic cholestatic syndromes related to defects in members of the ATP-binding cassette (ABC) transport superfamily include progressive familial intra-hepatic cholestasis types 1 (PFIC 1; Byler's disease), 2 (PFIC 2), and 3 (PFIC 3); benign recurrent intra-hepatic cholestasis (BRIC), and Dubin-Johnson syndrome. The incidence of these genetic cholestatic syndromes is very low, but they are being increasingly identified [24-27]. Patients with intrahepatic cholestasis of unknown etiology should be referred to specialists.

Liver Injury with Parenchymal Damage (Neonatal Hepatitis)

Several infections and metabolic disorders may cause liver parenchymal injury, usually with conjugated hyperbilirubinemia. Reactions of the neonatal liver to different insults include the proliferation of giant cells because of the high regenerative ability of these organs [28, 29]. For example, metabolic disturbances such as galactosemia can cause a giant cell reaction. Therefore, the etiology of liver injury accompanied by conjugated hyperbilirubinemia is difficult to determine histologically by examination of liver biopsy specimens.

Viral Hepatitis and Other Infections

Immunity is reduced in the neonate and viral infections are frequent. The most common causes of viral hepatitis are hepatitis A and B viruses. Hepatitis A, which is transmitted by the fecal-oral route, is often asymptomatic (75% to 95 %) in children but is more commonly symptomatic in adults [30]. Hepatitis B infection in infants is usually transmitted from the mother's blood during delivery or later during her care of the infant. Clinically the disease is mild, with high viral titers and fulminant hepatitis being rare, although hepatitis B infection is a frequent cause of chronic hepatitis [31]. Liver biopsy shows giant cell hepatitis during the acute stage of the disease. HBV infection rarely causes immune complex-mediated extrahepatic disease, such as membranous glomerulonephritis or papular acrodermatitis of childhood (Gianotti-Crosti syndrome) [32, 33].

Antibody to hepatitis C virus (HCV) is positive for the first 6 months in infants whose mothers have anti-HCV antibody. Mothers who have HCV-RNA can transmit HCV to their babies, but the possibility is low. The histology of liver biopsy in infants is similar to that in adults [34, 35].

Other types of infectious pathogens can also result in cholestasis. Common congenitally acquired pathogens include cytomegalovirus (CMV), herpes, rubella, toxoplasmosis, and syphilis. CMV infection is very common, with an incidence of 5% to 10 % in small children in good hygienic conditions [36]. Herpes simplex infection in infants occurs at birth from maternal genital herpes [37]. Rubella infection during the first trimester of pregnancy may cause fetal malformations, since infection with this virus involves not only the liver but also other organs, including the brain, lungs, heart, and eyes [38]. These infants show hepatosplenomegaly and jaundice within 1 or 2 days of birth. Congenital toxoplasmosis and congenital syphilis are very rare [39]. Bacterial infection may also contribute to cholestasis in infants with a urinary tract infection.

Metabolic and Genetic Disorders

Galactosemia is the most common disorder of carbohydrate metabolism that may cause neonatal cholestasis [40]. Galactosemia is due galactose 1-phosphate uridyltransferase deficiency, and confirmed by assays of enzyme activity in erythrocytes, leukocytes, or the liver. Treatment involves the removal of lactose (and galactose) from the diet, because lactose is broken down to glucose and galactose [41]. Tyrosinemia is a disorder of amino acid metabolism that causes progressive liver disease, renal tubular acidosis, and neurologic impairment [42, 43].

Individuals with inherited disorders of bile acid synthesis usually present with severe cholestatic jaundice at birth and later show progressive liver failure. Patients with disorders of lipid metabolism, including Wolman [44], Niemann-Pick [45], and Gaucher [46, 47] diseases, may occasionally present with cholestasis.

α-1 antitrypsin is an antiprotease and the natural inhibitor of the serine proteases released by activated neutrophils. A deficiency in α-1 antitrypsin causes abnormal proteins to accumulate within the endoplasmic reticulum resulting in liver injury including neonatal cholestasis [48].

Neonatal hemochromatosis is a rare disorder characterized by extrahepatic iron accumulation and hepatic failure with conjugated and unconjugated hyperbilirubinemia. The prognosis of infants with hepatic failure due to neonatal hemochromatosis is very poor, with a survival rate of about 10 % in the absence of liver transplantation [49-51].

Idiopathic Neonatal Hepatitis

Idiopathic neonatal hepatitis is defined as prolonged conjugated hyperbilirubinemia after exclusion of known causes including identifiable infections and metabolic/genetic disorders [28, 52]. Fluctuating jaundice may occur during the first 2 weeks of life or for up to 4 months. Hepatosplenomegaly is usually observed, and serum levels of aminotransferases may be above 800 IU/L. Multinucleated giant cells, variable inflammation with infiltration of lymphocytes, neutrophils, and eosinophils, and minimal bile duct proliferation may be observed on liver biopsy, but these findings are not specific. Most cases resolve slowly over months. A 10-year follow-up study reported that 2 of 29 patients diagnosed with this condition had died.

Reye's Syndrome

Reye's syndrome is a rare type of fulminant hepatic failure in children, which may be associated with aspirin administration during a febrile episode such as an upper respiratory tract infection [53]. Serum aminotransferase levels are typically more than three to four fold higher than normal. Liver biopsies show microvesicular fat in hepatocytes, and electron microscopy may show swelling and distortion of the mitochondria.

Parenteral Nutrition-Associated Cholestasis

Some premature infants who depend upon parenteral nutrition to treat intestinal failure may develop cholestasis. They are diagnosed by exclusion of other specific causes of cholestasis. This disorder, called parenteral nutrition-associated cholestasis (PNAC), usually occurs two weeks after starting parenteral nutrition, and continues as long as the latter is administered. Cholestasis is thought to be related to a loss of enterohepatic circulation of bile acids and reduced bile formation. Laboratory findings are non-specific, and may include conjugated hyperbilirubinemia with mild elevations of aminotransferases and γ-GTP. Conjugated hyperbilirubinemia (> 2mg/dL) has been reported in 67 % of infants receiving parenteral nutrition after intestinal resection [54-56].

HEPATOMEGALY

Hepatomegaly is a physical sign on abdominal examination in infants, suggesting liver disorders. Among the pathogenic causes of hepatomegaly are inflammatory cell infiltration [57], venous congestion, the accumulation of fat and metabolic substances, and tumor infiltration (Table **3**). Hepatomegaly with marked elevations in serum aminotransferases may suggest viral hepatitis. Congenital metabolic disorders with abnormal accumulation of metabolic substances are very rare, and deficiencies of specific enzymes should be assessed in diagnosing these diseases [58, 59]. Fat accumulation with hepatomegaly is rather common and has been associated with obesity [60, 61], diabetes mellitus, and malnutrition. Although imaging modalities, including ultrasonography and CT scanning, are very useful for the diagnosis of fatty infiltration of the liver, liver biopsy is needed for a precise diagnosis.

Tumor infiltration of the liver can induce hepatomegaly. Primary tumors in infants and children are rare, with two-thirds of these patients diagnosed within the first two years of life. Imaging examinations using ultrasonography are very useful for detecting liver tumors in infants with hepatomegaly, because general biochemical liver tests are usually non-specific. Hamartoma, adenoma, and infantile hemangioendothelioma are usually benign. In contrast, hepatoblastoma and hepatocellular carcinoma are malignant; the former usually presents before age 3 years, whereas the latter presents after 5 years of age [62, 63]. Elevated serum α-fetoprotein concentrations may be seen in patients with both types of these malignant tumors [64]. Secondary tumor infiltration is usually associated with a neuroblastoma of the adrenal glands, but its incidence is very low [65].

Table 3. Causes of hepatomegaly in infants.

Mechanism	Diseases
Inflammation	Viral hepatitis, Autoimmune hepatitis, Juvenile rheumatoid arthritis
Accumulation of Metabolic Substances	
• Triglycerides (chronic)	Fatty liver, Obesity, DM, Mauriac's syndrome Malnutrition
• Triglycerides (acute)	Reye's syndrome
• Cholesterol	Wolman's disease
• Glycogen	Glycogen storage disease types I and IV
• Sphingolipid	Gaucher's disease
• Sphingomyelin	Niemann-Pick disease
• Copper	Wilson disease, Indian childhood cirrhosis
• Abnormal alpha-1 antitrypsin	Alpha-1 antitrypsin deficiency
Biliary Tract Disorders	
Venous Congestion	Heart failure (*e.g.* congenital heart diseases)
Tumor Infiltration	
• Primary tumors	Hepatoblastoma, hamartoma
• Secondary tumor infiltration	Lymphoma, neuroblastoma of the adrenals, Wilm's tumor

ENCEPHALOPATHY

Several pathogeneses should be considered in the differential diagnosis of infants presenting with abnormalities in consciousness, reflexes, respiration, or feeding [66-68]. Abnormalities in consciousness plus hyperbilirubinemia may suggest kernicterus (bilirubin encephalopathy) or hepatic failure, regardless of their low incidence. Kernicterus results from elevated levels of unconjugated bilirubin (>30 mg/dL) [69], which may occur in individuals with Crigler-Najjar syndrome type I or hemolytic disorders due to fetal-maternal incompatibility. An infant with kernicterus becomes restless or lethargic within the first 5 days of life, later developing stiffness of the neck and limbs. Seventy percent of affected infants may die within 7 days of onset, and the remaining 30 % may have cerebral palsy or athetosis.

Reye's syndrome is a rare cause of acute hepatic failure in children (described above), and may be accompanied by neurologic deterioration seizures and coma.

Generally neonatal encephalopathy is characterized by signs of central nervous dysfunction. Although hypoxic-ischemic brain injury is thought to contribute to neonatal encephalopathy, some metabolic and genetic abnormalities may cause neonatal encephalopathy:

1) Neonatal hypoglycemia [70, 71]

   - Glycogen storage disease (GSD) types I and IV

   - Fatty acid oxidation defect (medium-chain acyl-CoA dehydrogenase deficiency; LCAD) [72]

2) Hyperammonemia: urea cycle defects (Citrullinemia), congenital porto-systemic shunt [73]

3) Disorders of amino acid metabolism: Maple syrup urine disease [74], phenylketonuria [75], nonketotic hyperglycinemia.

4) Other causes: mitochondrial disorders, severe peroxisomal disorders (*e.g.* Zellweger syndrome [76])

MESSAGES FROM HEPATOLOGISTS TO GENERAL PHYSICIANS

1. It is very important to distinguish between "physiological" and "pathological" jaundice in newborn infants, because early intervention can improve prognosis, especially in patients with kernicterus or biliary atresia. The serum bilirubin level is the key point for differentiation between these two types of jaundice.

2. The causes of liver cirrhosis in children include hepatitis B or C infection, autoimmune hepatitis (especially type II), glycogen storage disease (especially type IV), or Wilson's disease.

3. Liver dysfunction of unknown etiology and neurological symptoms may suggest metabolic disorders, such as galactosemia or tyrosinemia. As early diagnosis is sometimes difficult, and screening tests are recommended for early therapeutic intervention.

4. For differential diagnosis of neonatal encephalopathy, it is important to check for the presence of jaundice. Encephalopathy with jaundice suggests kernicterus or hepatic failure rather than metabolic diseases, such as citrullinemia.

ACKNOWLEDGEMENTS

We are very thankful to Ms. Asma Ahmed, manager publications, Bentham Science Publishers, for her patience and long-term assistance.

CONFLICT OF INTEREST

The author confirms that he has no conflict of interest to declare for this publication.

REFERENCES

[1]   Rosenthal P. Assessing liver function and hyperbilirubinemia in the newborn. National Academy of Clinical Biochemistry. Clin Chem 1997;43:228-234.
[2]   Bhutani VK, Johnson L, Sivieri EM. Predictive ability of a predischarge hour-specific serum bilirubin for subsequent significant hyperbilirubinemia in healthy term and near-term newborns. Pediatrics 1999;103:6-14.
[3]   Dennery PA, Seidman DS, Stevenson DK. Neonatal hyperbilirubinemia. N Engl J Med 2001;344:581-590.
[4]   Huang MJ, Kua KE, Teng HC, Tang KS, Weng HW, Huang CS. Risk factors for severe hyperbilirubinemia in neonates. Pediatr Res 2004;56:682-689.
[5]   Bhat YR, Kumar CG. Morbidity of ABO haemolytic disease in the newborn. Paediatr Int Child Health 2012;32:93-96.
[6]   Hadley AG. Laboratory assays for predicting the severity of haemolytic of the fetus and newborn. Transpl Immunol 2002;10:191-198.
[7]   Mundy CA. Intravenous immunoglobulin in the management of hemolytic disease of the newborn. Neonatal Netw 2005;24:17-24.
[8]   Keitt AS. Hemolytic anemia with impaired hexokinase activity. J Clin Invest 1969;48:1997-2007.
[9]   Bansal A, Bothra GC, Verma CR. Hyperbilirubinemia due to massive cephalhematoma. Indian Pediatr 1985;22:619-621.
[10]   Miyao M, Abiru H, Ozeki M, Kotani H, Tsuruyama T, Kobayashi N, Omae T, Osamura T, Tamaki K. Subdural hemorrhage: A unique case involving secondary vitamin K deficiency bleeding due to biliary atresia. Forensic Sci Int 2012;221:e25-e29.
[11]   Rastogi MV, LaFranchi SH. Congenital hypothyroidism. Orphanet J Rare Dis 2010;5:17.
[12]   Watson KJ, Gollan JL. Gilbert's syndrome. Baillieres Clin Gastroenterol 1989;3:337-355.
[13]   Bartlett MG, Gourley GR. Assessment of UGT polymorphisms and neonatal jaundice. Semin Perinatol 2011;35:127-133.
[14]   Costa E. Hematologically important mutations: bilirubin UDP-glucuronosyltransferase gene mutations in Gilbert and Crigler-Najjar syndromes. Blood Cells Mol Dis 2006;36:77-80.
[15]   Moyer V, Freese DK, Whitington PF, Olson AD, Brewer F, Colletti RB, Heyman MB. Guideline for the evaluation of cholestatic jaundice in infants: recommendations of the North American Society for Pediatric Gastroenterology, Hepatology and Nutrition. J Pediatr Gastroenterol Nutr 2004;39:115-128.
[16]   Hartley JL, Davenport M, Kelly DA. Biliary atresia. Lancet 2009;374:1704-1713.
[17]   Davenport M. Biliary atresia: clinical aspects. Semin Pediatr Surg 2012;21:175-184.
[18]   Jimenez-Rivera C, Jolin-Dahel KS, Fortinsky KJ, Gozdyra P, Benchimol EI. International incidence and outcomes of biliary atresia. J Pediatr Gastroenterol Nutr 2013;56:344-354.

[19]   Bijl EJ, Bharwani KD, Houwen RH, de Man RA. The long-term outcome of the Kasai operation in patients with biliary atresia: a systematic review. Neth J Med 2013;71:170-173.

[20]   Karnsakul W, Intihar P, Konewko R, Roy A, Colombani PM, Lau H, Schwarz KB. Living donor liver transplantation in children: a single North American center experience over two decades. Pediatr Transplant 2012;16:486-495.

[21]   Singhavejsakul J, Ukarapol N. Choledochal cysts in children: epidemiology and outcomes. World J Surg 2008;32:1385-1388.

[22]   Lee CN, Tiao MM, Chen HJ, Concejero A, Chen CL, Huang YH. Characteristics and outcome of liver transplantation in children with Alagille syndrome: A single-center experience. Pediatr Neonatol 2014;55:135-138.

[23]   Hartley JL, Gissen P, Kelly DA. Alagille syndrome and other hereditary causes of cholestasis. Clin Liver Dis 2013;17:279-300.

[24]   Hirschfield GM. Genetic determinants of cholestasis. Clin Liver Dis 2013;17:147-159.

[25]   Jacquemin E. Progressive familial intrahepatic cholestasis. Clin Res Hepatol Gastroenterol 36 Suppl 2012;1:S26-S35.

[26]   Davit-Spraul A, Fabre M, Branchereau S, Baussan C, Gonzales E, Stieger B, Bernard O, Jacquemin E. ATP8B1 and ABCB11 analysis in 62 children with normal gamma-glutamyl transferase progressive familial intrahepatic cholestasis (PFIC): phenotypic differences between PFIC1 and PFIC2 and natural history. Hepatology 2010;51:1645-1655.

[27]   Davit-Spraul A, Gonzales E, Baussan C, Jacquemin E. Progressive familial intrahepatic cholestasis. Orphanet J Rare Dis 2009;4:1.

[28]   Torbenson M, Hart J, Westerhoff M, Azzam RK, Elgendi A, Mziray-Andrew HC, Kim GE, Scheimann A. Neonatal giant cell hepatitis: histological and etiological findings. Am J Surg Pathol 2010;34:1498-1503.

[29]   Roberts EA. Neonatal hepatitis syndrome. Semin Neonatol 2003;8:357-374.

[30]   Nwachuku N, Gerba CP. Health risks of enteric viral infections in children. Rev Environ Contam Toxicol 2006;186:1-56.

[31]   Wong F, Pai R, Van Schalkwyk J, Yoshida EM. Hepatitis B in pregnancy: a concise review of neonatal vertical transmission and antiviral prophylaxis. Ann Hepatol 2014;13:187-195.

[32]   Baig S, Alamgir M. The extrahepatic manifestations of hepatitis B virus. J Coll Physicians Surg Pak 2008;18:451-457.

[33]   Dikici B, Uzun H, Konca C, Kocamaz H, Yel S. A case of Gianotti Crosti syndrome with HBV infection. Adv Med Sci 2008;53:338-340.

[34]   Floreani A. Hepatitis C and pregnancy. World J Gastroenterol 2013;19:6714-6720.

[35]   Cottrell EB, Chou R, Wasson N, Rahman B, Guise JM. Reducing risk for mother-to-infant transmission of hepatitis C virus: a systematic review for the U.S. Preventive Services Task Force. Ann Intern Med 2013;158:109-113.

[36]   Shibata Y, Kitajima N, Kawada J, Sugaya N, Nishikawa K, Morishima T, Kimura H. Association of cytomegalovirus with infantile hepatitis. Microbiol Immunol 2005;49:771-777.

[37]   McGoogan KE, Haafiz AB, Gonzalez Peralta RP. Herpes simplex virus hepatitis in infants: clinical outcomes and correlates of disease severity. J Pediatr 2011;159:608-611.

[38]   Papania MJ, Wallace GS, Rota PA, Icenogle JP, Fiebelkorn AP, Armstrong GL, Reef SE, Redd SB, Abernathy ES, Barskey AE, Hao L, McLean HQ, Rota JS, Bellini WJ, Seward JF. Elimination of endemic measles, rubella, and congenital rubella syndrome from the Western hemisphere: the US experience. JAMA Pediatr 2014;168:148-155.

[39]   Rodriguez-Cerdeira C, Silami-Lopes VG. Congenital syphilis in the 21st century. Actas Dermosifiliogr 2012;103:679-693.

[40]   Berry GT. Galactosemia: when is it a newborn screening emergency? Mol Genet Metab 2012;106:7-11.

[41]   Naito E, Ito M, Matsuura S, Yokota, Saijo T, Ogawa Y, Kitamura S, Kobayashi K, Saheki T, Nishimura Y, Sakura N, Kuroda Y. Type II citrullinaemia (citrin deficiency) in a neonate with hypergalactosaemia detected by mass screening. J Inherit Metab Dis 2002;25:71-76.

[42]   Ameen VZ, Powell GK, Rassin DK. Cholestasis and hypermethioninemia during dietary management of hereditary tyrosinemia type 1. J Pediatr 1986;108:949-952.

[43]   Tannuri AC, Gibelli NE, Ricardi LR, Santos MM, Maksoud-Filho JG, Pinho-Apezzato ML, Silva MM, Velhote MC, Ayoub AA, Andrade WC, Leal AJ, Miyatani HT, Tannuri U. Living related donor liver transplantation in children. Transplant Proc 2011;43:161-164.

[44]   Wolman M. Wolman disease and its treatment. Clin Pediatr (Phila) 1995;34:207-212.

[45]   Yerushalmi B, Sokol RJ, Narkewicz MR, Smith D, Ashmead JW, Wenger DA. Niemann-pick disease type C in neonatal cholestasis at a North American Center. J Pediatr Gastroenterol Nutr 2002;35:44-50.

[46]   vom Dahl S, Mengel E. Lysosomal storage diseases as differential diagnosis of hepatosplenomegaly. Best Pract Res Clin Gastroenterol 2010;24:619-628.

[47]   Elias AF, Johnson MR, Boitnott JK, Valle D. Neonatal cholestasis as initial manifestation of type 2 Gaucher disease: a continuum in the spectrum of early onset Gaucher disease. JIMD Rep 2012;5:95-98.

[48]   Topic A, Prokic D, Stankovic I. Alpha-1-antitrypsin deficiency in early childhood. Fetal Pediatr Pathol 2011;30:312-319.

[49]   Siafakas CG, Jonas MM, Perez-Atayde AR. Abnormal bile acid metabolism and neonatal hemochromatosis: a subset with poor prognosis. J Pediatr Gastroenterol Nutr 1997;25:321-326.

[50]   Rand EB, Karpen SJ, Kelly S, Mack CL, Malatack JJ, Sokol RJ, Whitington PF. Treatment of neonatal hemochromatosis with exchange transfusion and intravenous immunoglobulin. J Pediatr 2009;155:566-571.

[51]   Vohra P, Haller C, Emre S, Magid M, Holzman I, Ye MQ, Iofel E, Shneider BL. Neonatal hemochromatosis: the importance of early recognition of liver failure. J Pediatr 2000;136:537-541.

[52]   Crig JM, Landing BH. Form of hepatitis in neonatal period simulating biliary atresia. AMA Arch Pathol 1952;54:321-333.

[53]   Belay ED, Bresee JS, Holman RC, Khan AS, Shahriari A, Schonberger LB. Reye's syndrome in the United States from 1981 through 1997. N Engl J Med 1999;340:1377-1382.

[54]   Rangel SJ, Calkins CM, Cowles RA, Barnhart DC, Huang EY, Abdullah F, Arca MJ, Teitelbaum DH. Parenteral nutrition-associated cholestasis: an American Pediatric Surgical Association Outcomes and Clinical Trials Committee systematic review. J Pediatr Surg 2012;47:225-240.

[55]   Sondheimer JM, Asturias E, Cadnapaphornchai M. Infection and cholestasis in neonates with intestinal resection and long-term parenteral nutrition. J Pediatr Gastroenterol Nutr 1998;27:131-137.

[56]   Kelly DA. Liver complications of pediatric parenteral nutrition--epidemiology. Nutrition 1998;14:153-157.

[57]   Maggiore G, Sciveres M, Fabre M, Gori L, Pacifico L, Resti M, Choulot JJ, Jacquemin E, Bernard O. Giant cell hepatitis with autoimmune hemolytic anemia in early childhood: long-term outcome in 16 children. J Pediatr 2011;159:127-132.e1.

[58]   Matern D, Starzl TE, Arnaout W, Barnard J, Bynon JS, Dhawan A, Emond J, Haagsma EB, Hug G, Lachaux A, Smit GP, Chen YT. Liver transplantation for glycogen storage disease types I, III, and IV. Eur J Pediatr 158 Suppl 1999;2:S43-S48.

[59]   Manolaki N, Nikolopoulou G, Daikos GL, Panagiotakaki E, Tzetis M, Roma E, Kanavakis E, Syriopoulou VP. Wilson disease in children: analysis of 57 cases. J Pediatr Gastroenterol Nutr 2009;48:72-77.

[60]   el-Karaksy HM, el-Koofy NM, Anwar GM, el-Mougy FM, el-Hennawy A, Fahmy ME. Predictors of non-alcoholic fatty liver disease in obese and overweight Egyptian children: single center study. Saudi J Gastroenterol 2011;17:40-46.

[61]   Nanda K. Non-alcoholic steatohepatitis in children. Pediatr Transplant 2004;8:613-618.

[62]   Kremer N, Walther AE, Tiao GM. Management of hepatoblastoma: an update. Curr Opin Pediatr 2014;26:362-369.

[63]   Zen Y, Vara R, Portmann B, Hadzic N. Childhood hepatocellular carcinoma: a clinicopathological study of 12 cases with special reference to EpCAM. Histopathology 2014;64:671-682.

[64]   Ishiguro T, Tsuchida Y. Clinical significance of serum alpha-fetoprotein subfractionation in pediatric diseases. Acta Paediatr 1994;83:709-713.

[65]   Yasmeen N, Ashraf S. Childhood acute lymphoblastic leukaemia; epidemiology and clinicopathological features. J Pak Med Assoc 2009;59:150-153.

[66]   Stromme P, Kanavin OJ, Abdelnoor M, Woldseth B, Rootwelt T, Diderichsen J, Bjurulf B, Sommer F, Magnus P. Incidence rates of progressive childhood encephalopathy in Oslo, Norway: a population based study. BMC Pediatr 2007;7:25.

[67]   Stromme P, Magnus P, Kanavin OJ, Rootwelt T, Woldseth B, Abdelnoor M. Mortality in childhood progressive encephalopathy from 1985 to 2004 in Oslo, Norway: a population-based study. Acta Paediatr 2008;97:35-40.

[68]   Stromme P, Suren P, Kanavin OJ, Rootwelt T, Woldseth B, Abdelnoor M, Magnus P. Parental consanguinity is associated with a seven-fold increased risk of progressive encephalopathy: a cohort study from Oslo, Norway. Eur J Paediatr Neurol 2010;14:138-145.

[69]   Watchko JF, Tiribelli C. Bilirubin-induced neurologic damage--mechanisms and management approaches. N Engl J Med 2013;369:2021-2030.

[70]   Lang TF, Hussain K. Pediatric hypoglycemia. Adv Clin Chem 2014;63:211-245.

[71]   Park E, Pearson NM, Pillow MT, Toledo A. Neonatal Endocrine Emergencies: A Primer for the Emergency Physician. Emerg Med Clin North Am 2014;32:421-435.

[72]   Coman D, Bhattacharya K. Extended newborn screening: an update for the general paediatrician. J Paediatr Child Health 2012;48:E68-E72.

[73]   Sokollik C, Bandsma RH, Gana JC, van den Heuvel M, Ling SC. Congenital portosystemic shunt: characterization of a multisystem disease. J Pediatr Gastroenterol Nutr 2013;56:675-681.

[74]   Lee JY, Chiong MA, Estrada SC, Cutiongco-De la Paz EM, Silao CL, Padilla CD. Maple syrup urine disease (MSUD)--clinical profile of 47 Filipino patients. J Inherit Metab Dis 31 Suppl 2008;2:S281-S285.

[75]   Greene CL, Longo N. National Institutes of Health (NIH) review of evidence in phenylalanine hydroxylase deficiency (phenylketonuria) and recommendations/guidelines for therapy from the American College of Medical Genetics (ACMG) and Genetics Metabolic Dietitians International (GMDI). 10.1016/j.ymgme.2014.03.005 2014.

[76]   Lee PR, Raymond GV. Child neurology: Zellweger syndrome. Neurology 2013;80:e207-e210.

Comprehensive Practical Hepatology, 2016, 215-220

CHAPTER 12

Practical Management of Elderly Patients with Liver Injury

Kazuto Tajiri*

The Third Department of Internal Medicine, University of Toyama, Japan

Abstract: The population of elderly individuals is increasing, especially in developed countries. Reductions in organ function are more frequent in the elderly, complicating treatment of various conditions. Elderly individuals are more susceptible to severe liver injury, show a decrease in drug metabolism and are at greater risk of developing malignancies.

Keywords: Blood flow, carcinogenesis, drug metabolism, immune function, liver size.

KEY POINTS (FIG. 1)

1. Some morphological changes in the liver are seen in the elderly, but liver function is almost completely conserved.

2. Elderly individuals show decreases in the ability to metabolize drugs due to age-related reductions in liver size, hepatic blood flow, and hepatic regenerative capacity, affecting the management of liver injury in the elderly.

3. The incidence of hepatic malignancy increases with age.

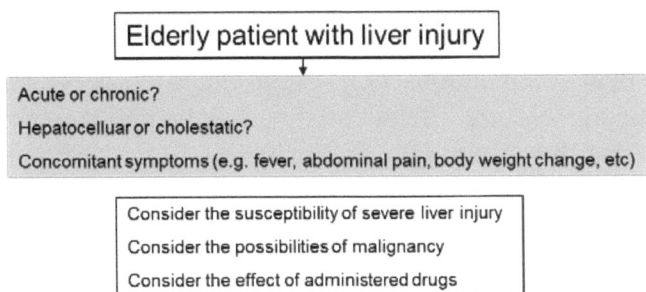

Elderly patient with liver injury

Acute or chronic?
Hepatocelluar or cholestatic?
Concomitant symptoms (e.g. fever, abdominal pain, body weight change, etc)

Consider the susceptibility of severe liver injury
Consider the possibilities of malignancy
Consider the effect of administered drugs

Figure 1: Management of liver injury in elderly patients.

***Corresponding author Kazuto Tajiri:** The Third Department of Internal Medicine, University of Toyama, Toyama, Japan; Email: tajikazu@med.u-toyama.ac.jp

Yukihiro Shimizu (Ed)

LIVER FUNCTION AND AGING

Most studies on age-related changes in liver morphology have been performed in rodents, with fewer reports in humans. Liver weight and volume have been found to decrease by 40%, and liver blood flow by 50%, during aging [1]. The number of hepatocytes decreases, whereas their size and multinucleation increase with age [2, 3]. Subcellular compartments in most hepatocytes undergo few or no changes in volume or distribution during aging, but a few organelles or cytoplasmic inclusions exhibit age-associated changes in appearance or density [4]. Hepatocyte lysosomes show accumulation of the aging pigment lipofuscin, which consists of the end products of lipid peroxidation. However, aging does not appear to affect hepatic functions [5]. Although many studies have assessed age-associated changes in hepatic functions, their results have been conflicting. The liver seems to be relatively spared from the age-related changes in mitochondrial activity and mitochondrial DNA that occur in other tissues [6], although impaired liver mitochondrial enzyme activity and defects in the respiratory chain have been reported [7, 8]. Aging in the liver was recently reported associated with pseudocapillarization of the sinusoidal endothelium, which is characterized by thickening of the endothelium, basement membrane formation and defenestration [9]. Those age-related changes in sinusoidal epithelium may be associated with impaired clearance of chylomicron remnants, postprandial hypertriglyceridemia and atherosclerosis [10].

Age was found to have a minor effect on liver function tests [11]. Bilirubin levels seem to decline with age, which may reflect reductions in whole body muscle mass and hemoglobin concentrations. However, bile acid synthesis and cholesterol secretion decline in elderly subjects [12], which may contribute to increases in the cholesterol saturation of bile, leading to increases in the frequency of gallstones and in the incidence of coronary heart disease in elderly subjects [4].

Decreased drug clearance in elderly people, especially reduced phase I hepatic metabolism, has practical ramifications [13, 14]. Reduced drug clearance may predispose elderly patients, who are often treated with polypharmacy regimens, to increased rates of adverse drug reactions. This reduction in first-pass metabolism may be due to reduced liver mass and hepatic blood flow rather than to alterations in the relevant enzyme systems.

LIVER INJURY IN THE ELDERLY (TABLE 1)

Fundamentally, hepatic function is relatively preserved in elderly individuals, suggesting that these patients be managed similar to younger adults with acute or chronic liver injury. However, age-related features of liver diseases should be considered in the management of elderly patients.

Table 1. Changes with aging found in liver disease.

Etiology	Findings	Treatment
Hepatitis A	Mortality↑	Symptomatic therapy
Hepatitis B	Frequency↓, HCC ↑, Mortality↑	Anti-viral treatment*
Hepatitis C	HCC↑	Anti-viral treatment**
Autoimmune	Frequency↑	Corticosteroid***
Alcoholic	Disease severity↑	Stop drinking, symptomatic therapy
Drug-induced	Frequency↑(especially Cholestatic)	Cessation of causative drug

HCC: hepatocellular carcinoma, * anti-viral treatment such as nucleot(s)ide analogs are available. **Direct anti-viral drugs are now available. ***Prophylaxis for osteoporosis is important.

In viral hepatitis, symptoms and diagnostic strategies are similar in elderly and younger patients. Residents of nursing homes have been reported infected with hepatitis B (HBV) or hepatitis C virus (HCV) [15, 16], indicating that risk factors, including sharing bath brushes, non-disposable syringes and shaving blades, as well as sexual contact, should be avoided. Elderly individuals who plan to travel to areas in which hepatitis A is endemic should be vaccinated because mortality from acute hepatitis A increases with advancing age [17]. The efficacy of treatment regimens for viral hepatitis is similar in elderly and younger patients [18, 19], although the frequency of side effects of treatment, especially with interferon, is higher in older patients [20]. Furthermore, the course of viral hepatitis may be more prolonged, severe, and indolent in elderly than in younger patients, possibly because of age-related reductions in immune functions (Fig. **2**).

The incidence of hepatocellular carcinoma (HCC) in patients infected with HBV and HCV increases with age [21, 22], indicating that the development of HCC should be monitored closely in elderly patients, even after antiviral treatment [23]. The prevalence of autoimmune liver diseases, such as autoimmune hepatitis, primary biliary cirrhosis, and primary sclerosing cholangitis, are higher in older than in younger subjects [24-26], but no significant age-related differences in laboratory test results have been observed. Treatment strategies are thus identical for all adult patients.

Elderly individuals with alcoholic liver disease were reported to have more advanced disease than younger patients [27]. Furthermore, the adverse effects of benzodiazepines, which are used to treat withdrawal symptoms, such as drowsiness, fatigue, confusion, ataxia, falls, and incontinence, are more frequent with increasing age [28].

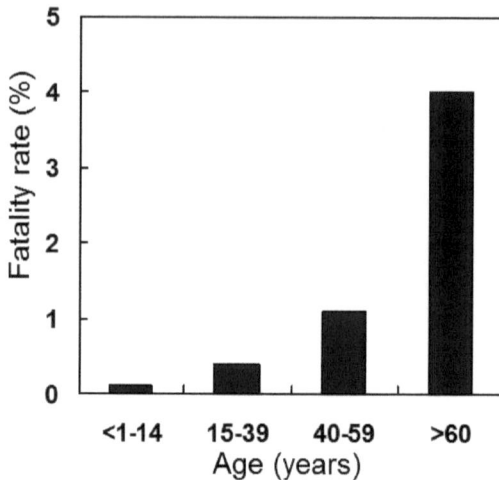

Figure 2: Age-dependent fatality rates from hepatitis A.

Elderly people are more susceptible to adverse drug reaction, making older age a risk factor for drug-induced liver injury (DILI) [29]. Many elderly patients take several drugs for multiple concomitant diseases and are therefore susceptible to the adverse effects of individual drugs and combinations of drugs, which may interact synergistically. Older age was recently reported associated with the cholestatic type of liver injury, but is not a predisposing factor to DILI [30].

Collectively, the prevalence of liver diseases increases with aging. Clinical manifestations and treatments of liver diseases are generally identical in elderly and younger patients, but the adverse effects of treatment should be especially considered in the management of elderly patients.

SUMMARY

The proportion of the world's population over age 60 years is increasing, especially in developed countries. Aging is associated with reductions in liver weight and volume, and in liver blood flow. Alterations in the function of the liver and other organs may require special management of liver diseases in elderly patients.

MESSAGES FROM HEPATOLOGISTS TO GENERAL PHYSICIANS

1. Liver volume is reduced by 20% – 40% in the elderly, which may alter its morphology to that resembling a chronically damaged liver.

2. The course of acute viral hepatitis may be more prolonged, severe, or indolent than in younger patients. The risks of DILI and alcoholic liver disease are increased in elderly patients compared to younger counterparts.

3. Reduced hepatic metabolism and derangement of immune homeostasis are predisposing factors in the elderly for increased incidence of DILI, autoimmune liver disease, and hepatocarcinogenesis. Especially, aged patients with HCV infection show greater risks of hepatocarcinogenesis even after eradication of HCV, indicating a need for long-term careful follow-up in such cases.

ACKNOWLEDGEMENTS

We are very thankful to Ms. Asma Ahmed, manager publications, Bentham Science Publishers, for her patience and long-term assistance.

CONFLICT OF INTEREST

The author confirms that he has no conflict of interest to declare for this publication.

REFERENCES

[1]   Wynne HA, Cope LH, Mutch E, Rawlins MD, Woodhouse KW, James OF. The effect of age upon liver volume and apparent liver blood flow in healthy man. Hepatology 1989;9:297-301.
[2]   Watanabe T, Tanaka Y. Age-related alterations in the size of human hepatocytes. A study of mononuclear and binucleate cells. Virchows Arch B Cell Pathol Incl Mol Pathol 1982;39:9-20.
[3]   Barz H, Kunze KD, Voss K, Simon H. Image processing in pathology. IV. Age dependent changes of morphometric features of liver cell nuclei in biopsies. Exp Pathol (Jena) 1977;14:55-64.
[4]   Schmucker DL. Aging and the liver: an update. J Gerontol A Biol Sci Med Sci 1998;53:B315-20.
[5]   Schmucker DL. Liver function and phase I drug metabolism in the elderly: a paradox. Drugs Aging 2001;18:837-851.
[6]   Barazzoni R, Short KR, Nair KS. Effects of aging on mitochondrial DNA copy number and cytochrome c oxidase gene expression in rat skeletal muscle, liver, and heart. J Biol Chem 2000;275:3343-7.
[7]   Sastre J, Pallardo FV, Pla R, Pellin A, Juan G, O'Connor JE, Estrela JM, *et al.* Aging of the liver: age-associated mitochondrial damage in intact hepatocytes. Hepatology 1996;24:1199-1205.
[8]   Muller-Hocker J, Aust D, Rohrbach H, *et al.* Defects of the respiratory chain in the normal human liver and in cirrhosis during aging. Hepatology 1997;26:709-19.

[9]   Yokomori H, Yoshimura K, Ohshima S, *et al*. The endothelin-1 receptor-mediated pathway is not involved in the endothelin-1-induced defenestration of liver sinusoidal endothelial cells. Liver int. 2006; 26: 1268-76.

[10]   Le Couteur DG, Fraser R, Cogger VC, *et al*. Hepatic pseudocapillarisation and atherosclerosis in ageing. Lacet 2002; 359: 1612-5.

[11]   Tietz NW, Shuey DF, Wekstein DR. Laboratory values in fit aging individuals--sexagenarians through centenarians. Clin Chem 1992;38:1167-1185.

[12]   Einarsson K, Nilsell K, Leijd B, Angelin B. Influence of age on secretion of cholesterol and synthesis of bile acids by the liver. N Engl J Med 1985;313:277-282.

[13]   Durnas C, Loi CM, Cusack BJ. Hepatic drug metabolism and aging. Clin Pharmacokinet 1990;19:359-389.

[14]   McLean AJ, Le Couteur DG. Aging biology and geriatric clinical pharmacology. Pharmacol Rev 2004;56:163-184.

[15]   Sugauchi F, Mizokami M, Orito E, Ohno T, Kato H, Maki M, Suzuki H, *et al*. Hepatitis B virus infection among residents of a nursing home for the elderly: seroepidemiological study and molecular evolutionary analysis. J Med Virol 2000;62:456-462.

[16]   Chien NT, Dundoo G, Horani MH, Osmack P, Morley JH, Di Bisceglie AM. Seroprevalence of viral hepatitis in an older nursing home population. J Am Geriatr Soc 1999;47:1110-1113.

[17]   Mahon MM, James OF. Liver disease in the elderly. J Clin Gastroenterol 1994;18:330-334.

[18]   Kawaoka T, Suzuki F, Akuta N, Suzuki Y, Arase Y, Sezaki H, Kawamura Y, *et al*. Efficacy of lamivudine therapy in elderly patients with chronic hepatitis B infection. J Gastroenterol 2007;42:395-401.

[19]   Bresci G, Del Corso L, Romanelli AM, Giuliano G, Pentimone F. The use of recombinant interferon alfa-2b in elderly patients with anti-HCV-positive chronic active hepatitis. J Am Geriatr Soc 1993;41:857-862.

[20]   Honda T, Katano Y, Urano F, Murayama M, Hayashi K, Ishigami M, Nakano I, *et al*. Efficacy of ribavirin plus interferon-alpha in patients aged >or=60 years with chronic hepatitis C. J Gastroenterol Hepatol 2007;22:989-995.

[21]   Beasley RP. Hepatitis B virus. The major etiology of hepatocellular carcinoma. Cancer 1988;61:1942-1956.

[22]   Hamada H, Yatsuhashi H, Yano K, Daikoku M, Arisawa K, Inoue O, Koga M, *et al*. Impact of aging on the development of hepatocellular carcinoma in patients with posttransfusion chronic hepatitis C. Cancer 2002;95:331-339.

[23]   Asahina Y, Tsuchiya K, Tamaki N, Hirayama I, Tanaka T, Sato M, Yasui Y, *et al*. Effect of aging on risk for hepatocellular carcinoma in chronic hepatitis C virus infection. Hepatology 2010;52:518-527.

[24]   Al-Chalabi T, Boccato S, Portmann BC, McFarlane IG, Heneghan MA. Autoimmune hepatitis (AIH) in the elderly: a systematic retrospective analysis of a large group of consecutive patients with definite AIH followed at a tertiary referral centre. J Hepatol 2006;45:575-583.

[25]   Talwalkar JA, Lindor KD. Primary biliary cirrhosis. Lancet 2003;362:53-61.

[26]   Wiesner RH, Grambsch PM, Dickson ER, Ludwig J, MacCarty RL, Hunter EB, Fleming TR, *et al*. Primary sclerosing cholangitis: natural history, prognostic factors and survival analysis. Hepatology 1989;10:430-436.

[27]   Potter JF, James OF. Clinical features and prognosis of alcoholic liver disease in respect of advancing age. Gerontology 1987;33:380-387.

[28]   Kruse WH. Problems and pitfalls in the use of benzodiazepines in the elderly. Drug Saf 1990;5:328-344.

[29]   Danan G, Benichou C. Causality assessment of adverse reactions to drugs--I. A novel method based on the conclusions of international consensus meetings: application to drug-induced liver injuries. J Clin Epidemiol 1993;46:1323-1330.

[30]   Lucena MI, Andrade RJ, Kaplowitz N, Garcia-Cortes M, Fernandez MC, Romero-Gomez M, Bruguera M, *et al*. Phenotypic characterization of idiosyncratic drug-induced liver injury: the influence of age and sex. Hepatology 2009;49:2001-2009.

CHAPTER 13

Practical Management of Pregnant Women with Liver Injury

Kazuto Tajiri*

The Third Department of Internal Medicine, University of Toyama, Japan

Abstract: Several specific liver diseases, which may be serious and require specific therapy including immediate delivery, are incidentally found in pregnant women. Since some of these diseases may be serious or even fatal, prompt diagnosis and treatment are important to save both mother and baby. The effect on the fetus of drugs administered to pregnant women must be considered. Moreover, if the mother has an infectious disease, prophylactic procedures are needed to protect the fetus.

Keywords: AFLP, eclampsia, HELLP syndrome, Hyperemesis gravidarum, prophylaxis, trimester.

KEY POINTS [1, 2]

1. Characteristic symptoms and timing of disease onset are important for diagnosis.

2. In managing pregnant patients, it is important to consider the effects of the disease itself and of its treatment on the fetus

Most normal pregnant women show almost no abnormalities on liver function tests, including tests of transaminase, γ-GTP and bilirubin concentrations [3] (Table **1**).

Therefore, abnormalities in these values suggest the possibility of liver disease. Liver injuries in pregnancy fall into three patterns: (1) diseases unique to pregnancy, (2) diseases coincidental with pregnancy, and (3) underlying chronic liver disease. Liver diseases unique to pregnancy have a characteristic timing dependent on the trimesters of pregnancy (Table **2**). Hyperemesis gravidarum (HG) occurs during the first trimester; intrahepatic cholestasis of pregnancy (ICP) during the second half of pregnancy; and other diseases, such as HELLP

---

*Corresponding author Kazuto Tajiri: The Third Department of Internal Medicine, University of Toyama, Toyama, Japan; Email: tajikazu@med.u-toyama.ac.jp

syndrome, acute fatty liver in pregnancy (AFLP) and preeclampsia, during the third trimester. Liver diseases coincidental with pregnancy involve viral hepatitis, gallstones and drug-induced liver injury. Management of liver diseases during pregnancy should consider the effects of both the disease and treatment on the fetus (Table **3**).

Table 1. Physiological changes in liver function tests during normal pregnancy.

Test	Changes during pregnancy
Bilirubin	Unchanged or slightly increased
Transaminase	Unchanged
Alkaline phosphatase	Increased to 2 to 4-fold
Cholesterol	Increased to 2-fold
Triglyceride	Increased
Prothrombin time	Unchanged
Fibrinogen	Increased by 50%
Globulin	Increased in α and β globulins, decreases in γ globulin
Alpha-fetoprotein	Moderately increased, especially in twins
Ceruloplasmin	Increased
White blood cell	Increased
Hemoglobin	Decreased in later pregnancy

Table 2. Distinguished features of liver diseases unique to pregnancy.

	HG	ICP	HELLP	AFLP	Preeclampsia
Onset/trimester	1 (typically 4 to 8 wk)	2, 3 (typically 25-32 wk)	3 or postpartum	3 or postpartum	2, 3 trimester
% pregnancies	0.3%	0.1%	0.2-0.6%	0.005-0.01%	5-10%
Preeclampsia	(-)	(-)	(+)	(++) 50%	(+)
Clinical features	Vomiting	Pruritus Mild jaundice Elevated bile acids Decreased Vitamin K	Hemolysis Thrombocytopenia	Liver failure with coagulopathy, Encephalopathy, Hypoglycemia, DIC	Hyperytension Edema Proteinuria
Aminotransferases	Mild to 2-fold elevation	Mild to 20-fold elevation	Mild to 20-fold elevation	300-500 typical	Mild to 20-fold elevation
Bilirubin	Occasional jaundice	<5 mg/dL	<5 mg/dL	<5 mg/dL, higher if severe	<5 mg/dL
Hepatic imaging	Normal	Normal	Hepatic infarct Hematomas, rupture	Fatty infiltration	
Histology	Normal Bland cholestasis	Normal Mild cholestasis	Patchy/extensive necrosis and hemorrhage	Macrovesicular fat in zone 3	Macrovesicular fat Fibrin deposition
Maternal mortality	Rare	0%	1-25%	7-18%	Rare
Fetal mortality	Rare	0.4-1.4%	11%	9-23%	1-2%
Recurrence	Often	45-70%	4-19%	20-70% in LCHAD mutation	
Treatment	Rehydration Nutritional support Steroid occasionally	UDCA(10-15 mg/kg.bw) Delivery	Immediate delivery	Immediate delivery	Immediate delivery Calcium channel blockers Magnesium sulfate

HG; Hyperemesis gravidarum, ICP; intrahepatic cholestasis of pregnancy, HELLP; hemolysis, elevated liver tests and low platelets, AFLP; acute fatty liver of pregnancy, DIC; Disseminated intravascular coagulation, LCHAD; Long-chain 3-hydroxyacyl-CoA dehydrogenase, UDCA; Ursodeoxycholic acid

DIAGNOSIS OF LIVER DISEASES DURING PREGNANCY

Pregnant patients who show evidence of liver dysfunction should be first suspected of having the same liver diseases as nonpregnant patients. Viral hepatitis, due to hepatitis A, B, C, D, and E viruses; herpes simplex virus; cytomegalovirus; and Epstein-Barr virus, accounts for 40% of jaundice in pregnant women [4]. The development of hepatitis A, B, and C occurs in the same frequency between pregnant and nonpregnant populations during each of the 3 trimesters of pregnancy. Furthermore, the clinical and serological course of acute hepatitis in pregnant women is not different from that seen in nonpregnant patients [4]. Hepatitis E during the third trimester of pregnancy can lead to fulminant hepatitis, which has a high mortality rate (up to 25%). Pregnant patients with jaundice should be assessed for viral hepatitis by detailed history taking and serological tests. Furthermore, biliary sludge or gallstones has been observed in 5% to 12% of pregnant women, and symptomatic gallstones in 0.1% to 0.3%, suggesting that pregnancy may predispose to biliary sludge and gallstone formation. Increased estrogen levels, especially during the second and third trimesters, cause increased cholesterol secretion and supersaturation of bile, and increased progesterone levels reduce small intestinal motility [1]. Moreover, the volumes of fasting and postprandial gallbladders are large and the increased residual volume of supersaturated bile in pregnant women thus leads to the formation of biliary sludge and gallstones [1]. A high body mass index, high serum leptin levels, low high-density lipoprotein levels, and insulin resistance are risk factors for the development of gallstones [1]. Thus, pregnant women who present with liver dysfunction and right upper quadrant pain should be examined by ultrasonography to determine whether these symptoms are associated with gallstones.

Liver diseases unique to pregnancy can be characterized by their timing in relation to the trimesters of pregnancy. During the first trimester, typically between 4 and 10 weeks' gestation, liver dysfunction accompanied by intractable vomiting may suggest HG. Immunological, hormonal, and psychological factors associated with pregnancy may be involved in the etiology of HG. Risk factors for HG include hyperthyroidism, psychiatric illness, molar pregnancy, preexisting diabetes, and multiple pregnancies. During the second and third trimesters, typically around 25 to 32 weeks' gestation, liver dysfunction with pruritus may suggest ICP. Hormonal, genetic, and exogenous factors may be associated with the etiology of ICP. During the third trimester, preeclampsia, HELLP syndrome and AFLP may occur. These diseases are fairly uncommon, but they should be carefully diagnosed and managed due to their severity and mortality. Liver dysfunction with hypertension, edema, and proteinuria may suggest preeclampsia. Hypertension is defined as a systolic pressure >140 mmHg and a diastolic blood pressure >90 mmHg on at least two occasions at least 4 to 6 hours apart in a previously normotensive patient, and proteinuria is defined as ≥300 mg protein in a 24 hour urine collection or ≥1+ protein on urine dipstick testing of two random urine samples collected at least 4 to 6 hours apart [1]. The main pathophysiology of preeclampsia involves procoagulant and proinflammatory states that induce glomerular endotheliosis, increased vascular permeability, and a systemic inflammatory response. [1]. About 2% to 12% of women with preeclampsia (0.2-0.6% of all pregnancies) experience severe preeclampsia, which is characterized by hemolysis, elevated liver tests, and low platelet counts, called HELLP syndrome. The pathogenesis of HELLP syndrome is a microangiopathic hemolytic anemia, fibrin deposition in blood vessels, and platelet consumption, resulting in intrahepatic and intraperitoneal bleeding. There are no practical criteria to distinguish HELLP syndrome from preeclampsia. Most patients with HELLP present with upper abdominal pain and tenderness, nausea and vomiting, malaise, headache, edema, weight gain, hypertension, and proteinuria. Most patients present between 27 and 36 weeks' gestation, although 25% initially present during the postpartum period. Increased lactate dehydrogenase levels (>600 IU/L), elevated indirect bilirubin, abnormal blood smear, or low platelet counts may suggest HELLP syndrome. Unlike patients with HELLP, 40% to 50% of those with AFLP present during nulliparous and twin pregnancies. AFLP, which is characterized by abnormalities in fatty acid oxidation in the mitochondria, usually occurs during the third trimester of pregnancy (28 to 40 weeks' gestation). In a few patients, it presents as jaundice during the postpartum period. Common symptoms and signs include 1 to 2 weeks of anorexia, nausea and vomiting, headache, right upper quadrant pain, jaundice, hypertension, edema, ascites, and hepatic encephalopathy. About 50% of patients with AFLP have preeclampsia, and some overlap is observed with HELLP syndrome [5].

TREATMENT OF LIVER DISEAES DURING PREGNANCY

In managing pregnant patients with liver disease, the effect of medications on the fetus should always be considered (Table **3**). Acute viral hepatitis is not an indication for termination of pregnancy, caesarean section, or refrain of breastfeeding. However, it should be of note that congenital malformations in the fetus can occur in patients with early cytomegalovirus infection [6]. The administration of anti-viral drugs may be considered for patients with severe and viral hepatitis, such as fulminant hepatitis or acute exacerbation of chronic hepatitis B. Lamivudine appears relatively safe in pregnant women with a severe form of hepatitis B (Table **3**). Recently tenofovir was shown to be safe in pregnancy and effective for prevention of perinatal transmission of HBV [7].

Table 3. Risks and safety of drugs used during pregnancy.

Drug	FDA pregnancy category	Risk and Safety
Antimetics		
Promethazine	C	Impair neonatal platelet aggregation
Metoclopramide	B	Relatively low risk
Ondansetron	B	Few data
Prochlorperazine	C	Possibilities of congenital abnormalities
Antihypertensives		
ACE inhibitors	C/D	Probable congenital abnormalities
Beta blockers	C/D	Fatal bradycardia, hypotension, growth retardation
Calcium blockers	C	Teratogenic and embryotoxic effects in animals
Anticoagulation		
Aspirin	C/D	Fatal adverse effects (e.g. growth retardation, bleeding)
Enoxaparin	B	Possible congenital abnormalities and fatal death
Heparin	C	Does not cross the placenta, few data
Intrahepatic cholestasis		
Ursodeoxycholic acid	B	Relatively low risk
S-adenosyl-L-methionine	n.e	Relatively low risk
Cholestylamine	C	May interfere with vitamin absorption
Prednisone	C	Intrauterine growth retardation, cleft palate, adrenal insufficiency
Azathioprine	D	Lymphopenia, hypogammaglobulinemia, thymic hypoplasia
Cyclosporine	C	Premature labout, low birthweight, neonatal hyperkalemia
Tacrolimus	C	Similar side effects to cyclosporine, neonatal malformation
Mycophenylate mofetil	D	First trimester loss, microtia, congenital malformation
Sirolimus	C	Not recommended
Lamivudine	C	Low risk
Adefovir	C	Few data
Entecavir	C	Few data
Interferon	C	Not recommended
Ribavirin	X	Contraindicated-severe fatal toxicity
Penicillamine	D	Embryopathy but needed to treat for Wilson disease
Trientine	C	Limited data-potential toxicity
Octreotide	B	Probably safe-limited data
Vasopressin	X	Contraindicated, uterine ischemia

FDA, United States Food and Drug Administration; Category B: Animal reproduction studies failed to show a risk to the fetus, and there are no adequate studies in pregnant women. Category C: Animal reproduction studies have shown an adverse effect on the fetus, and there are no adequate studies in humans. Category D: There is evidence of human fatal risk based on data from investigational or marketing experience or studies in humans. Category X: Data have demonstrated fetal abnormalities in animals and humans, and/or there is positive evidence of human fatal risk based on data from investigational or marketing experience. n.e, not evaluated by FDA

Despite pregnancy, women with intractable biliary colic or severe acute cholecystitis not responding to conventional conservative treatments should be considered for cholecystectomy [8]. However, when possible, surgery should be avoided during the first and third trimesters because anesthesia carries a risk of spontaneous abortion during the first trimester and surgery is associated with an increased risk of premature labor during the third trimester. Therefore, symptomatic pregnant patients with gallstones should undergo cholecystectomy, ideally laparoscopically, during the second trimester, if possible [8]. The urgency and possibility for delivery in women with liver diseases unique to pregnancy differ for each disease. HG during the first trimester does not usually require specific treatment.

Rehydration or nutritional support is often required, and antiemetic drugs, occasionally steroids, may be used. ICP during the second trimester is generally treated with UDCA (usually 10 to 15 mg/kg body weight, occasionally 1.5 to 2.0 g/day). UDCA provides relief of pruritus with improvements in liver functions tests and with no adverse effects on mother or fetus. In ICP, the main risk is to the fetus, and it may be necessary to refer the patient to a specialist. Fetal monitoring is essential but fetal deaths from acute anoxia can be prevented only by delivery as soon as the fetal lungs become mature [2, 3]. During the third trimester, liver diseases unique to pregnancy often require immediate delivery. There is no specific treatment for preeclampsia, and immediate delivery may be considered to avoid eclampsia, hepatic rupture or necrosis [2, 3]. In HELLP syndrome, delivery is also the only definitive therapy. Immediate delivery is recommended at later than 34 weeks' gestation or if there is any evidence of multiorgan dysfunction, DIC, renal failure, abruptio placentae, or fetal distress [2, 3]. Most patients experience rapid resolution of HELLP after delivery, with normalization of platelets within 5 days, but some patients may experience persistent thrombocytopenia or hemolysis, worsening hepatic or renal failure, or life-threatening complications. In patients with AFLP, immediate termination of pregnancy is essential for maternal survival. These pregnancy-specific liver diseases, especially AFLP, HELLP, and preeclampsia-associated liver disease, are associated with high morbidity and mortality rates. MELD score, total bilirubin concentration and INR are closely associated with mortality [9].

PROPHYLAXIS FOR LIVER DISEASES IN THE FETUS

All pregnant women should be tested for hepatitis B on the first antenatal visit. Those who do not have anti-HBs antibodies but are at high risk for HBV infection during pregnancy (e.g., women with multiple sex partners or who use intravenous drugs) should be vaccinated during pregnancy. Perinatal transmission of hepatitis B is high in mothers with chronic hepatitis B with hepatitis B e antigen during the third trimester. Most of these babies lead to persistent positivity for hepatitis B surface antigen. Transplacental transmission of hepatitis B is rare and most of the transmission is thought to occur at delivery. Therefore, it is preventable in more than 95% of cases by passive-active immunoprophylaxis of the babies at birth with hyperimmune B immunoglobulin and hepatitis B virus vaccine (3 doses: the first during the first 2 days after birth, and the second and third at 1, and 6 months, respectively) [10]. Antiviral treatment during the third trimester may reduce vertical transmission from mothers with a high viral load [11]. Vertical transmission of hepatitis A and D viruses is rare and occurs only in mothers with high viral loads at the time of delivery. The mother-to-infant transmission rate of hepatitis C is 1% to 5% and the maternal risk factors for the transmission include co-infection with human immunodeficiency virus, history of intravenous drug abuse, and maternal viremia of greater than 10^6 copies/mL [4]. Transmission, however, is unaffected by mode of delivery or breastfeeding. Hepatitis C viral load should therefore be checked in the third trimester.

MESSAGES FROM HEPATOLOGISTS TO GENERAL PHYSICIANS

1. Specific diseases may be found in pregnant women according to the trimesters of pregnancy. The time of gestation when abnormal liver test results are found, the occurrence of multiple births, a history of past pregnancies, and family history provide clues to the possible causes of pregnancy-associated liver disease.

2. Symptoms and physical findings, such as pruritus, hypertension, edema, and abdominal pain, are particularly important for diagnosis. Laboratory findings, such as proteinuria, hyperuricemia, elevated serum bile acid levels, thrombocytopenia, and anemia, are also important.

3. Prompt management, including the cessation of pregnancy, may be required in cases with severe preeclampsia/eclampsia, and HELLP syndrome, which usually do not occur in the first trimester of pregnancy.

ACKNOWLEDGEMENTS

We are very thankful to Ms. Asma Ahmed, manager publications, Bentham Science Publishers, for her patience and long-term assistance.

CONFLICT OF INTEREST

The author confirms that he has no conflict of interest to declare for this publication.

REFERENCES

[1]   Lee NM, Brady CW. Liver disease in pregnancy. World J Gastroenterol 2009;15:897-906.

[2]   Hay JE. Liver disease in pregnancy. Hepatology 2008;47:1067-1076.

[3]   Joshi D, James A, Quaglia A, Westbrook RH, Heneghan MA. Liver disease in pregnancy. Lancet 2010;375:594-605.

[4]   Hay JE. "Liver disease and pregnancy" Mayo Clinic Gastroenterology and Hepatology Board Review. 3rd ed. 2008

[5]   Goel A, Jamwal KD, Ramachandran A, Barasubramanian KA, Eapen CE. Pregnancy-related liver disorders. J Clin Exp Hepatol 2014;4:151-62.

[6]   Licata A, Ingrassia D, Serruto A, *et al.* Clinical course and management of acute and chronic viral hepatitis during pregnancy. J Viral Hepat. 2015;22:515-23.

[7]   Greenup AJ, Tan PK, Nguyen V, Glass A, Davison S, Chatterjee U, Holdaway S, Samarasinghe D, Jackson K, Locarnini SA, Levy MT. Efficacy and safety of tenofovir disoproxil fumarate in pregnancy to prevent perinatal transmission of hepatitis B virus. J Hepatol. 2014;61:502-507.

[8]   Gurusamy KS, Davidson C, Gluud C, Davidson CR. Cochrane Database Syst Rev. 2013 Jun 30;6;CD005440.

[9]   Murali AR, Devarbhavi H, Venkatachala PR, Singh R, Sheth KA. Factors that predict 1-month mortality in patients with pregnancy-specific liver disease. Clin Gastroenterol Hepatol. 2014;12:109-113.

[10]   Zhang L, Gui XE, Teter C, *et al.* Effects of hepatitis B immunization on prevention of mother-to-infant transmission of hepatitis B virus and on the immune response of infants towards hepatitis B vaccine. Vaccine 2014;32:6091-7.

[11]   Lu YP, Liang XJ, Xiao XM, *et al.* Telbivudine during the second and third trimester of pregnancy interrupts HBV intrauterine transmission: a systematic review and meta-analysis. ClinLab 2014;60:571-86.

CHAPTER 14

Lifestyle Recommendation for Patients with Liver Diseases

Kazuto Tajiri*

The Third Department of Internal Medicine, University of Toyama, Japan

Abstract: Excess body weight has become a problem, especially in most developed countries. Excess nutrition is harmful to the liver and causes liver diseases including nonalcoholic fatty liver disease and hepatic malignancies. A well balanced diet and adequate exercise can help maintain a healthy liver and prevent liver diseases induced by metabolic abnormalities. In contrast, infectious liver diseases such as viral hepatitis and their consequent cirrhosis and hepatocellular carcinoma can be prevented by prophylaxis, including adequate vaccination against viruses and patient education.

Keywords: Exercise, lifestyle, liver, nutrition, prophylaxis.

KEY POINTS

1. Excess nutrition can exacerbate various liver diseases.

2. Adequate exercise should be considered for most patients with liver injury.

3. Education is important in avoiding the risk of liver diseases and in managing these conditions.

In recent years, obesity and overweight due to changes in lifestyle have become a worldwide problem, especially in developed countries. Obesity and overweight have increased the prevalence of insulin resistance, diabetes mellitus and the metabolic syndrome. Moreover, nonalcoholic fatty liver disease (NAFLD), the hepatic manifestation of the metabolic syndrome, has become the leading chronic liver disease. Alterations in life style may be required for patients with liver diseases.

LIFESTYLE RECOMMENDATION FOR PATIENTS WITH LIVER INJURY (TABLE 1)

Most patients with acute hepatitis are asymptomatic, although some, mostly those with serious condition with jaundice, experience general malaise. Bed rest has

*Corresponding author Kazuto Tajiri: The Third Department of Internal Medicine, University of Toyama, Toyama, Japan; Email: tajikazu@med.u-toyama.ac.jp

Yukihiro Shimizu (Ed)

been traditionally recommended for patients with acute liver injury until the patient is free of jaundice. If the patient is young and previously healthy, less restrictive behavior, consisting only of rest after each meal, may be sufficient. Rest is needed until the patient becomes symptom-free, the liver is no longer tender, and serum bilirubin level is less than 1.5 mg/dL.

Table 1. Life style recommendation for patients with liver injury.

General recommendation
Avoid excessive calorie intake
Ensure a well-balanced diet
Quit smoking
Cease drinking alcohol
For symptomatic patients
Adequate resting may be required.
For asymptomatic patients
Adequate exercise should be recommended.

Treatment of chronic hepatitis, which previously consisted mainly of rest and supplementation, has been changed to active treatment, such as interferon or anti-viral drugs. Most patients with chronic hepatitis show no definitive symptoms and their clinical course will last for a long period of time. Recommendations are now for a more active lifestyle rather than to restrict their daily activities too much, with no restriction in housekeeping required. Physical fitness is encouraged by gradually more strenuous exercises. Recent findings that hepatic steatosis or obesity contributes to disease progression [2, 3] indicates the importance of exercise in the management of chronic viral hepatitis. More recently, weight loss was reported to improve disease progression in patients with chronic HCV infection [4], and moderate exercise alone was found to reduce serum ALT levels in the absence of any other pharmacological treatments including anti-viral agents [5]. Experimental evidence showing that protein synthesis in the liver is not unchanged after intense exercise [6] supports the validity of exercise therapy in the management of chronic hepatitis.

The importance of exercise therapy has been especially highlighted in the treatment of patients with nonalcoholic fatty liver disease. Moderate exercise (walking or jogging for 30 to 60 min/day. 3-5 times/week) has been associated with body weight reduction, improved insulin resistance, and improved ALT levels [7, 8]. Obese patients with chronic liver injury should perform physical exercises for weight loss, as shown in Table **2**. Other, life style modifications, such as adequate sleep and rest after meals, may improve chronic liver injury. Alcohol consumption is a definite risk factor for liver disease progression, and cessation of alcohol drinking in patients with chronic viral hepatitis may be particularly required. Tobacco smoking is also associated with elevated ALT levels and disease progression among HCV-seropositive, but not among HBsAg-seropositive, individuals [9]. Therefore, cessation of smoking is recommended for patients with chronic hepatitis C. Since alcohol consumption and tobacco smoking cannot be easily reduced [10], these patients should be repeatedly advised about the importance of these lifestyle changes.

The absence of symptoms in patients with chronic hepatitis suggests that they should be monitored by pre-planned liver function test, as well as viral monitoring in patients with viral hepatitis. Treatment with interferon has been associated with various side effects, including fever, arthralgia, headache, appetite loss, hair loss, decreased blood cell counts, depression, and pneumonia. Patients should therefore be told about the possibilities of those symptoms and the need for early management.

Table 2. Physical exercise recommendations in weight loss programs.

Engage in moderate-to-vigorous exercise for at least 60 minutes per day (at least 5 days per week)
Walking may be the preferred exercise
Check the baseline number of steps by a pedometer, then add 500 steps at 3-day intervals to a target value of 10,000-12,000 steps per day.
Jogging (20-40 min/day), biking or swimming (45-60 min/day) may replace walking. Physical exercise is intended to produce a calorie consumption of at least 400kcal/day, favoring weight loss, maintaining muscle mass and preventing weight cycling.

Although patients with early phase cirrhosis show no specific symptoms, disease progression is accompanied by various symptoms. Life style changes that should be recommended to these patients, particularly those with advanced cirrhosis, include avoidance of alcohol. Moreover, patients should be monitored for hepatic failure, fluid retention, encephalopathy, and the prevention of variceal hemorrhage (Table **3**). Initial manifestations of symptoms in patients with advanced cirrhosis include hematemesis and tarry stool, both indicators of the rupture of esophageal varices; body weight gain and leg edema, both indicators of ascites; oral bleeding or petechia due to thrombocytopenia, or sleep disturbance due to minimal hepatic encephalopathy. Constipation is a risk factor for hepatic coma, and patients with cirrhosis may be required to have at least one bowel movement per day.

Table 3. Clinical manifestations for early detection of hepatic failure.

Jaundice: yellowing of skin or conjunctiva. dark urine
Ascites : abdominal fullness, body weight gain, leg edema
Coagulation disorder: bleeding tendency
Encephalopathy: sleep disturbance, flapping tremor

In addition, psychosocial stress contributes to the progression and outcome of liver diseases. This stress may be due to immune cell dysfunction caused by glucocorticoids and/or catecholamines. Psychosocial conditions should also be considered in managing patients with liver diseases.

DIET THERAPY FOR PATIENTS WITH ACUTE LIVER INJURY

Low-fat and high-carbohydrate diets have been traditionally recommended for patients with acute liver injury because these diets are suitable for anorexic patients. If diet cannot provide adequate calorie intake, intravenous supplementation should be considered. As shown in Table **4**, a low-fat diet may be desirable for anorexic patients, in that these diets reduce the load for digestion and absorption. When the appetite recovers, a high protein diet is recommended [1]. There is no clear evidence for strict dietary restrictions, and supplementary vitamins and amino acids are not necessarily recommended. The diet usually recommended to patients with acute hepatitis is a diet that stimulates patient appetite. Thus, a well-balanced diet containing vitamins and minerals may be desirable.

DIET THERAPY FOR PATIENTS WITH CHRONIC LIVER INJURY (TABLE 4)

Patients with chronic hepatitis may require a protein-rich diet to supplement protein production in the liver. The diet should be well-balanced and include vitamins and minerals. Sodium restriction is necessary for prophylaxis of ascites retention, with severe sodium restriction required for decompensated patients. Strict restriction of water intake may be unnecessary, but over intake of water should be avoided. Patients at risk for developing hyperammonemia or hepatic coma require a low protein diet. However, protein-energy malnutrition has been reported in 30% to 90% of patients with liver cirrhosis [11]. Malnutrition is associated with poor survival and surgical outcomes in cirrhotic patients, and nutritional supplementation with branched-chain amino acids (BCAA) may improve the quality of life and prognosis of these patients [12, 13].

Administration of BCAA, as a treatment for malnutrition in patients with liver cirrhosis, has been reported to improve liver function, energy metabolism, and quality of life in these patients [14-16]. In contrast, a high caloric load may be harmful as cirrhotic livers frequently show glucose intolerance [17]. A combination of BCAA and an α-glucosidase inhibitor may improve glucose intolerability [18]. Moreover, hepatic glycogen stores are found to be decreased in patients with liver cirrhosis, leading to a severe catabolic state during fasting. Late evening snacks with BCAA are effective to avoid such nocturnal starvation and improved nutritional status [15, 16].

Table 4. Prefered diet composition for liver diseases.

	Acute hepatitis / Acute on chronic hepatitis	Chronic hepatitis / Compensated cirrhosis	Decompensated cirrhosis / Hepatic failure	Fatty liver / Obesity
Energy (kcal/kg)	27-30	30-33	30	15-25
Protein (g/kg)	1.1-1.2	1.2-1.3	0.7-1.0	1.1-1.3
Lipid (g/kg)	0.6	0.85-0.9	0.85	0.3-0.6
Carbohydrate (g/kg)	4.5	4.5-5.0	4.8-5.0	2.0-3.5
Protein energy ratio (%)	15	15	9-12	20-30
Lipid energy ratio (%)	20	25	25	20-25
Carbohydrate energy ratio (%)	65	60	63-66	50-55
P/S ratio	1.0	1.0-1.5	1.0-1.5	1.0-1.5
NaCl (g)	6-7	8	4-5	4-6

PROPHYLAXIS FOR PATIENTS WITH LIVER DISEASES

Liver diseases often lead to chronic liver injury and sometimes to advanced liver diseases or hepatocellular carcinoma. Efforts to prevent the progression of liver disease should include not only medical treatment but promoting life style modifications. In managing viral hepatitis, for example, prevention of transmission is important. Prevention of transmission of hepatitis A virus (HAV) should include protection against transmission through the fecal-oral route or person-to-person contact (including sexual activity). Vaccination should be considered for travelers to endemic areas (Table **5**).

In endemic areas, intake of fresh water and fresh vegetables may be a cause of infection with hepatitis A. In addition, the feces of infected patients contains HAV and can transmit the infection. We should advise both the patient and his/her family that intra-family transmission can be prevented by avoiding fecal transmission.

Table 5. Endemic areas of hepatitis virus.

Hepatitis A virus
Africa, Asia, South and Central America, Middle East
Hepatitis B virus
High prevalence: sub-Saharan Africa, Asia, South Pacific region
Intermediate prevalence: North Africa, Southern and Eastern Europe, Indian subcontinent, Amazon basin
Low prevalence: Western Europe, United States
Hepatitis D virus
Mediterranean, Eastern European, Africa, South America
Hepatitis E virus
India, Southeast and Central Asia, Africa

Patients infected with HBV should be informed that HBV is found in blood and in other body fluids, including saliva, vomit, semen and vaginal secretions, which could be the sources of transmission of HBV. In particular, the highest concentrations of HBV can be found in blood and serous exudates. Furthermore, HBV is found to be viable and infectious for 7 days on environmental surfaces at room temperature. Perinatal infection occurs in 70% to 90% of children born to HBeAg-positive mothers but in <15% of those born to HBeAg-negative mothers. Administration of hepatitis B immunoglobulin and HBsAg vaccine (3 times over 180 days) has been found to prevent 95% of mother-to-child transmissions. However, despite vaccination at birth, 5% of these babies will still become HBV carriers [19-21]. The precise mechanism is unclear, but HBV infection should be assessed even after vaccination. Percutaneous and permucosal contact, especially sexual contact, are the major sources of HBV transmission. Patients and their partners should therefore be advised to avoid risks of HBV-infection (Table **6**).

Universal immunization with the HBV-vaccine has been recommended by the World Health Organization. Adequate prophylaxis for HBV-infection, including vaccination, should be considered.

Prophylaxis for HCV infection should address transmission through blood and blood products. HCV is ten-fold less transmissible from parent to child than HBV (1% to 10% for those born to HCV-RNA positive mothers). Unsafe injections of drugs of abuse are the main sources of HCV-infection, including needle-stick exposure of health-care workers, sharing a razor or toothbrush, and unsafe piercing and tattooing.

Table 6. Subjects with high risk of HBV infection.

Needle stick injury
Drug injection
Sexual contacts
Mucous membrane pollution in health-care setting
Tattooing
Piercing
Sharing razors
Sharing tooth brushes
Bites, breaks in the skin, dermatologic lesions or skin ulcers may increase the risk of HBV infection.

MESSAGES FROM HEPATOLOGISTS TO GENERAL PHYSICIANS

1. Rest is preferable in patients with liver disease for retaining blood flow to the liver, and serum transaminase levels are somewhat decreased by resting alone in patients with high activity. However, strict resting is not recommended except in patients with liver failure or extreme water retention.

2. As excess nutrition may exacerbate liver diseases, diet therapy and adequate exercise should be considered in the management of various liver diseases. Exercise has also been shown to improve muscular insulin sensitivity, leading to improvement of hyperinsulinemia found in patients with various liver diseases. Moreover, as muscle metabolizes NH_3 or amino acids, adequate exercise in cirrhotic patients is recommended to maintain the muscle volume.

ACKNOWLEDGEMENTS

We are very thankful to Ms. Asma Ahmed, manager publications, Bentham Science Publishers, for her patience and long-term assistance.

CONFLICT OF INTEREST

The author confirms that he has no conflict of interest to declare for this publication.

REFERENCES

[1]   Sherlock S, Dooley J. Diseases of the liver and biliary system. 11th ed. Oxford, UK ; Malden, MA: Blackwell Science 2002: xvi, pp. 706.

[2]   Perumalswami P, Kleiner DE, Lutchman G, *et al.* Steatosis and progression of fibrosis in untreated patients with chronic hepatitis C infection. Hepatology 2006;43:780-787.

[3]   Leandro G, Mangia A, Hui J, Fabris P, Rubbia-Brandt L, Colloredo G, Adinolfi LE, *et al.* Relationship between steatosis, inflammation, and fibrosis in chronic hepatitis C: a meta-analysis of individual patient data. Gastroenterology 2006;130:1636-1642.

[4]   Everhart JE, Lok AS, Kim HY, Morgan TR, Lindsay KL, Chung RT, Bonkovsky HL, *et al.* Weight-related effects on disease progression in the hepatitis C antiviral long-term treatment against cirrhosis trial. Gastroenterology 2009;137:549-557.

[5]   Vazquez-Vandyck M, Roman S, Vazquez JL, Huacuja L, Khalsa G, Troyo-Sanroman R, Panduro A. Effect of Breathwalk on body composition, metabolic and mood state in chronic hepatitis C patients with insulin resistance syndrome. World J Gastroenterol 2007;13:6213-6218.

[6]   De Feo P, Lucidi P. Liver protein synthesis in physiology and in disease states. Curr Opin Clin Nutr Metab Care 2002;5:47-50.

[7]   Harrison SA, Day CP. Benefits of lifestyle modification in NAFLD. Gut 2007;56:1760-1769.

[8]   Bellentani S, Dalle Grave R, Suppini A, Marchesini G. Behavior therapy for nonalcoholic fatty liver disease: The need for a multidisciplinary approach. Hepatology 2008;47:746-754.

[9]   Wang CS, Wang ST, Chang TT, Yao WJ, Chou P. Smoking and alanine aminotransferase levels in hepatitis C virus infection: implications for prevention of hepatitis C virus progression. Arch Intern Med 2002;162:811-815.

[10]   Zani C, Donato F, Chiesa M, Baiguera C, Gelatti U, Covolo L, Antonini MG, *et al.* Alcohol and coffee drinking and smoking habit among subjects with HCV infection. Dig Liver Dis 2009;41:599-604.

[11]   Muller MJ. Malnutrition in cirrhosis. J Hepatol 1995;23 Suppl 1:31-35.

[12]   Merli M, Riggio O, Dally L. Does malnutrition affect survival in cirrhosis? PINC (Policentrica Italiana Nutrizione Cirrosi). Hepatology 1996;23:1041-1046.

[13]   Fan ST, Lo CM, Lai EC, Chu KM, Liu CL, Wong J. Perioperative nutritional support in patients undergoing hepatectomy for hepatocellular carcinoma. N Engl J Med 1994;331:1547-1552.

[14]   Moriwaki H, Miwa Y, Tajika M, Kato M, Fukushima H, Shiraki M. Branched-chain amino acids as a protein- and energy-source in liver cirrhosis. Biochem Biophys Res Commun 2004;313:405-409.

[15]   Nakaya Y, Okita K, Suzuki K, Moriwaki H, Kato A, Miwa Y, Shiraishi K, *et al.* BCAA-enriched snack improves nutritional state of cirrhosis. Nutrition 2007;23:113-120.

[16]   Marchesini G, Bianchi G, Merli M, Amodio P, Panella C, Loguercio C, Rossi Fanelli F, *et al.* Nutritional supplementation with branched-chain amino acids in advanced cirrhosis: a double-blind, randomized trial. Gastroenterology 2003;124:1792-1801.

[17]   Garcia-Compean D, Jaquez-Quintana JO, Gonzalez-Gonzalez JA, Maldonado-Garza H. Liver cirrhosis and diabetes: risk factors, pathophysiology, clinical implications and management. World J Gastroenterol 2009;15:280-288.

[18]   Korenaga K, Korenaga M, Uchida K, Yamasaki T, Sakaida I. Effects of a late evening snack combined with alpha-glucosidase inhibitor on liver cirrhosis. Hepatol Res 2008;38:1087-1097.

[19]   Stramer SL, Wend U, Candotti D, Foster GA, Hollinger FB, Dodd RY, Allain JP, *et al.* Nucleic acid testing to detect HBV infection in blood donors. N Engl J Med 2011;364:236-247.

[20]   Lai MW, Lin TY, Tsao KC, Huang CG, Hsiao MJ, Liang KH, Yeh CT. Increased seroprevalence of HBV with mutations in the s gene among individuals greater than 18 years old after complete vaccination. Gastroenterology 2012;143:400-407.

[21]   Wu TW, Lin HH, Wang LY. Chronic hepatitis B infection in adolescents who received primary infantile vaccination. Hepatology 2013;57:37-45.

Medical Management of Patients Following Liver Transplantation

Yasuhiro Nakayama[1,*] and Yukihiro Shimizu[2]

[1]The First Department of Internal Medicine, University of Yamanashi, Toyama, Japan and [2]Gastroenterology Center, Nanto Municipal Hospital, Japan

Abstract: Patients with fulminant hepatic failure, decompensated cirrhosis, or hepatocellular carcinoma defined according to the Milan criteria (no single lesion greater than 5 cm or no more than three lesions, the largest ≤ 3 cm) are potential candidates for liver transplantation. The 5-year survival rate after liver transplantation is 70% to 80%.

Keywords: Ascites, decompensated liver cirrhosis, encephalopathy, esophageal varices, fulminant hepatic failure, hepatocellular carcinoma, liver transplantation, MELD score, Milan criteria.

KEY POINTS

1. Long-term survival after liver transplantation is excellent. However, there is a shortage of appropriate organ donors.

2. Any patient with documented fulminant hepatic failure, decompensated cirrhosis, or hepatocellular carcinoma defined according to the Milan criteria (no single lesion greater than 5 cm or no more than three lesions, the largest ≤ 3 cm) is a potential candidate for liver transplantation [1].

3. Any patient with one of the defined complications of end-stage liver disease (ascites, variceal bleeding, encephalopathy, or hepatocellular carcinoma) and/or MELD score of 10 to 15 should be considered for referral to a transplant center [2].

4. It is important to monitor hypertension, diabetes, hyperlipidemia, and renal function as well as perform cancer surveillance after liver transplantation.

Corresponding author Yasuhiro Nakayama: The First Department of Internal Medicine, University of Yamanashi, Toyama, Japan; Email: ynakayama@yamanashi.ac.jp

BACKGROUND OF LIVER TRANSPLANTATION

The first successful liver transplant was performed in the USA by Thomas Starzl in 1967 [3]. Although liver transplant was performed during the 1970s on a limited basis, the 1-year survival rate remained below 20% [4]. The introduction of immunosuppression with cyclosporine in the early 1980s significantly improved the survival rate at 1 year to over 50% [5], and the introduction of immunosuppression with FK506 in the early 1990s significantly reduced acute rejection and improved the 1-year survival rate to over 80% [6]. These advances led to the gradual adoption of liver transplantation worldwide, with 1- and 5-year survival rates improving to 85% to 90%, and 70%, respectively, over the past 10 years. However, the number of cases of liver transplantation has decreased after 2006 due to a shortage of organ donors in the USA (Fig. **1**).

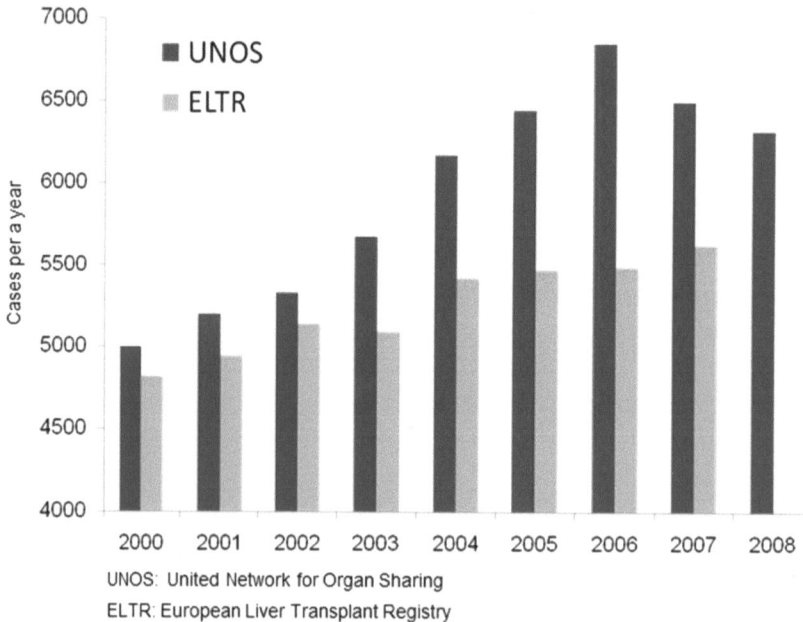

UNOS: United Network for Organ Sharing
ELTR: European Liver Transplant Registry

Figure 1: Changes in the number of liver transplantation cases.

With the current shortage of donor organs, about 5% to 10% of patients in the USA listed for liver transplantation will die without receiving a transplant [7]. Broelsch *et al*. reported the first successful series of living-donor liver transplantation (LDLT) to children in 1990 [8]. Based on their experience, Hashikura *et al*. extended the indications for LDLT to adult patients in 1994 [9].

The majority of livers are procured from deceased donors. The effort to expand the donor pool has provided alternative means of organ supply, including living donors, split-liver transplantation, and utilization of expanded criteria donors (ECD). In Asian countries, approximately 90% of donor-organs for liver transplantation are obtained from live donors, as the deceased donor rate is low due to social and religious factors [10, 11]. The peak of adult LDLT was in 2001 in the USA, but the sudden death of a living donor postoperatively in New York led to a continual decline in the number of LDLT. Split-liver transplantation is two allografts that have been created from a single deceased donor liver allograft. Left lateral segment or left split grafts have mainly been transplanted into children and right split or right tri-segment graft into adult, both show excellent outcomes [12].

ALGORITHM OF LIVER TRANSPLANTATION

An algorithm of the determination of a candidate for liver transplantation is shown in Fig. (**2**).

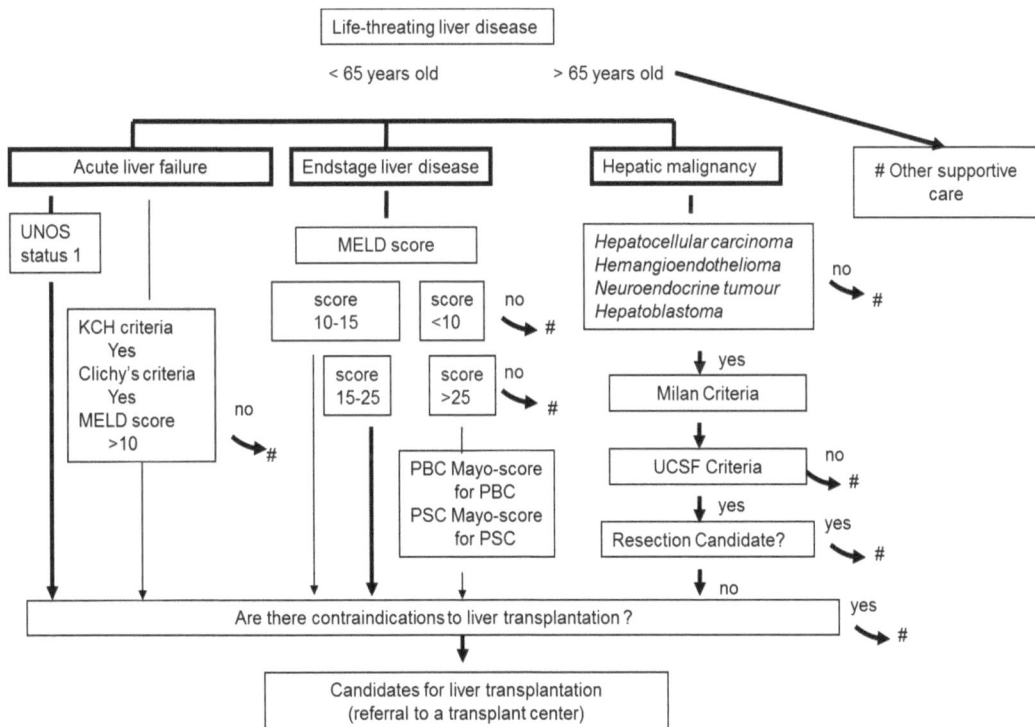

Figure 2: Algorithm for selection of candidates for liver transplantation.

Any patient with fulminant hepatic failure, decompensated cirrhosis, or hepatocellular carcinoma (HCC) is a potential candidate for liver transplantation. There are various underlying liver diseases (Table **1**).

Table 1. Underlying indications that can lead to transplantation.

Child	Adult
Congenital cholestatic disease	Acute Liver failure
Biliary atresia	Drug-induced (ex. Paracetamol)
Alagille's syndrome	Viral hepatitis
Byler disease	Cryptogenic acute Liver failure
Caroli's disease	Malignancy
Congenital Metabolic disease	Hepatocellular carcinoma
α-1 antitrypsin deficiency	Hemangioendothelioma
Wilson's diseasene	Neuroendocrine tumour
OTC deficiency	Chronic Liver failure (usually underlying cirrhosis)
Tyrosinemia	Chronic Viral hepatitis(HBV, HCV)
Neonatal Haemochromatosis	PBC and cystic fibrosis
Glycogen storage disease	PSC and IgG4-associated sclerosing cholangitis
Gaucher's disease	Alcohol-related liver disease
Crigler-Najjar type 1	AIH (acute/chronic)
Acute Liver failure	Cryptogenic cirrhosis
Acute Wilson's disease	Sarcoidosis
Cryptogenic acute Liver failure	Budd-Chiari syndrome (acute/chronic)
Malignancy	Congenital Metabolic disease
Hepatoblastoma	α-1 antitrypsin deficiency
Haemangioendothelioma	Familial amyloid polyneuropathy
Chronic Liver failure	Citrulinemia
Cryptogenic cirrhosis	Wilson's disease (acute/chronic)
	Haemochromatosis
	Familial intrahepatic cholestasis
	Congenital cholestatic disease
	Biliary atresia
	Miscellaneous
	Polycystic liver disease
	Congenital hepatic fibrosis
	Portopulmonary hypertension
	Hepatopulmonary syndrome
OTC: Ornithin transcarbamylase	Nodular regenerative hyperplasia

In adults, chronic active hepatitis and cirrhosis, due to viral hepatitis, autoimmune liver disease, or biliary diseases, are the most common conditions requiring transplantation [13], while the most common cause of liver transplantation is biliary atresia in children and adolescents less than 18 years old [14]. Contraindications for transplantation include severe cardiopulmonary disease, malignancy outside of the liver within 5 years, alcohol consumption, and drug use. The first step in deciding the timing of referral is to determine whether there have been complications of end-stage liver disease (ascites, variceal bleeding, or hepatic encephalopathy). This is followed by determination of the severity of illness using the Model for End-Stage Liver Disease (MELD) score system in patients aged 18 years or older (Table **2**) or the Pediatric End-Stage Liver Disease (PELD) scoring system in those younger than 18 years old (Table **3**). Patients with a Child–Turcotte–Pugh (CTP) score > 7 and MELD score > 10 should be considered for referral to a transplant center. Patients with acute liver failure or decompensated cirrhosis with MELD scores > 15 are given higher priority for donor organs [15]. The addition of serum Na concentration to the MELD score, in the form of the MELD-Na score, has been shown to be a more effective model for risk prediction in patients awaiting liver transplantation, particularly in those with low MELD scores [16] (Tables **2**, **3**). Patients with HCC according to the Milan criteria are candidates for transplantation. A donor with compatible_blood type, normal liver functions, and similar body weight, and without fatty liver is suitable. In the USA, approximately 10% of all listed patients die or are considered too sick before a suitable organ becomes available for transplantation [7]. Surveillance for varices and HCC should continue while patients are on the waiting list.

Table 2. Estimation of the severity of liver disease using the MELD score and MELD-Na score.

MELD= 3.8 log[serum bilirubin (mg/dL)]
+ 11.2 log[INR]
+ 9.6 log[serum creatinine (mg/dL)]
+ 6.4 [etiology (0 or 1)]

Etiologic score
0 = cholestatic or alcoholic
1 = other etiologies

On-line calculators are now available:
(www.unos.org/resources/MeldPeldCalculator.asp?index=98)

MELD-Na = MELD
− [serum Na (mEq/l)]
− [0.025 × MELD × (140 − serum Na (mEq/l)]
+ 140

On-line calculators are now available:
http://www.mayoclinic.org/medical-professionals/model-end-stage-liver-disease/meld-na-model

CONTRAINDICATION FOR LIVER TRANSPLANTATION

Liver transplantation should be avoided in patients incapable of enduring the procedure due to mental, physical, or social problems (Table **4**). Severe cardiopulmonary disease prevents a transplanted liver from surviving. Active infections are a serious threat to a successful procedure. Irreversible encephalopathy due to acute hepatic failure accompanied by associated brain injury caused by increased fluid in the brain tissue precludes liver transplantation. Malignancy outside the liver within the past 5 years is associated with a high risk of recurrence due to immunosuppressive agents.

Table 3. Estimation of the severity of pediatric liver disease using the PELD score.

$$
\begin{aligned}
\text{PELD Score} = \quad & 0.480 \log[\text{bilirubin (mg/dL)}] \\
+ & 1.857 \log[\text{INR}] \\
- & 0.687 \log[\text{albumin (g/dL)}] \\
+ & 0.436 \quad [\text{Age factor (0 or 1)}] \\
+ & 0.667 \quad [\text{growth factor (0 or 1)}]
\end{aligned}
$$

Age score
0= more than 1 year old
1= less than 1 year old

Growth score
0= no growth failure
1= growth failure (<-2 SD)

On-line calculators are now available:
(http://www.unos.org/resources/MeldPeldCalculator.asp?index=99)

Table 4. Contraindications for liver transplantation.

Severe cardiopulmonary diseases
Active infection
Irreversible encephalopathy due to acute hepatic failure
Malignancy outside of the liver within the past five years
Acquired immunodeficiency syndrome/HIV infection
Drug/Alcohol abuse (must abstain for >6 months)
Incapable of understanding transplantation due to brain
    disease, mental disease or dementia

Underlying HIV infection may induce severe immunodeficiency. Patients with active alcohol or drug abuse must abstain for at least 6 months prior to transplantation. Liver transplantation should be avoided in patients who are incapable of understanding the operation due to brain injury, mental disease, or dementia. In addition, patients with several other conditions, including prior hepatobiliary surgery, HIV infection, old age (≥ 65 years old), portosystemic shunt, portal vein thrombosis, re-transplant, multiple organ transplantation, or obesity, have been reported to show elevated risk in liver transplantation [17, 18]. Each transplant center has different criteria for determining whether liver transplantation is or is not indicated in such cases.

TIMING OF LIVER TRANSPLANTATION

Fulminant Hepatic Failure

The indications for liver transplantation in cases of acute liver failure are judged according to the degree of decrease in coagulation factors, progress of hepatic encephalopathy, and the level of cerebral edema. Kings College Hospital's (KCH) criteria are the standard and the most commonly used prognostic criteria for acute liver failure [19]. Age (≤ 11 years old or ≥ 40 years old), etiology of fulminant hepatic failure (non-A – E hepatitis or drug toxicity), prothrombin time (≥ 50 s), time from icterus to coma (≥ 7 days), and serum bilirubin level (≥ 18 mg/dL) are poor prognostic factors for acute liver failure without liver transplantation. Patients with fulminant liver failure with a life expectancy of less than 7 days without a liver transplantation should be given priority for the operation. However, transplantation should be avoided in cases in which neurological damage caused by severe cerebral edema due to acute hepatic failure is not expected to recover or if there are other contraindications, such as active infection [20]. The details are described in Chapter 3.

End-Stage Liver Disease (Decompensated Liver Cirrhosis)

Any patient with one of the complications of end-stage liver disease, such as ascites, variceal bleeding, encephalopathy, or HCC, should be considered for referral to a transplant center [2]. Two models are often used to measure the severity of chronic liver disease, *i.e.*, the CTP score and the MELD score (Table **2**). A MELD score of ≥ 10 points or CTP score of ≥ 7 points is suitable for consideration of liver transplant. Prior to 2002, the severity of liver disease and suitability for liver allocation were based on the CTP classification system. The CTP classification and its variations have also been used to stratify patients with chronic liver disease to predict mortality and morbidity. However, as it relies on many subjective criteria, CTP has been superseded by the MELD and PELD scores. Organ Allocation based on MELD, which gives priority to sicker patients on the waiting list, has led to an increased mean MELD score at LT, decreased number of patients on the waiting list, decreased waiting time, and decreased mortality rate of patients on the waiting list. To make it as objective as possible, the MELD score is calculated using only laboratory data, *i.e.*, serum creatinine, bilirubin, and international normalized ratio (INR). A patient's score can range from 6 to 40. The mortality rate within 3 months was reported to be 8% for patients with MELD score < 10, 26% for a score of 10 – 19, 56% for a score of 20 – 29, 66% for a score of 30 – 39, and 100% for those with the maximum score of 40 [21]. Merion *et al.* reported that deceased donor transplant recipients had a 79% lower mortality risk than comparable candidates that did not on undergo a transplant [15]. However, at lower MELD scores, recipient mortality risk during the first year posttransplantation was much higher than that for comparable candidates (Hazard ratio (HR) = 3.64 at MELD 6 – 11; HR = 2.35 at MELD 12 – 14). On the other hand, at MELD 18 – 20, mortality risk was 38% lower among transplant recipients compared to comparable candidates that did not on undergo a transplant. Therefore, survival benefit increased with increasing MELD score; at the maximum score of 40, transplant recipient mortality risk was 96% lower than that for candidates [15]. However, the intraoperative requirements of transfusion, vasopressors, ventilator, and dialysis were significantly increased in patients with high MELD scores (> 30) compared to those with low MELD scores (≤ 30) [22]. A suitable MELD score for liver transplantation is thus considered to be between 18 and 30.

Primary Biliary Cirrhosis (PBC) and Primary Sclerosing Cholangitis (PSC)

Primary biliary cirrhosis (PBC) accounts for about 5% of liver transplants, but this number has gradually declined in recent years [23]. Primary sclerosing cholangitis (PSC) accounts for about 5% of all transplants. In cases of PBC or PSC, the survival rate could be calculated from various clinical data, and the timing of the liver transplant is decided based on these forecasts. In PBC, patients with repeated ruptured esophageal varices, refractory itching, refractory ascites, refractory hepatic encephalopathy, serum bilirubin level ≥ 5 mg/dL, and serum albumin level ≤ 2.8 g/dL should be considered for liver transplantation. A MELD score of 15 points or Mayo risk score of 5.9 – 7.8 points suggests a recommendation for liver transplantation (Table **5**) [24].

Table 5. Mayo scoring system for predicting the need for transplantation in PBC.

R= 0.871 log[serum bilirubin (mg/dL)]
   -2.53 log[serum albumin (g/dL)]
   +0.039   [age (year)]
   +2.38 log[PT time (s)]
   +0.859   [edema score]

Edema score
  0 = no edema
  0.5 = diuretic-controlled edema
  1 = diuretic-uncontrolled edema

On-line calculators are available:
(http://www.mayoclinic.org/gi-rst/mayomodel2.html)

The average recurrence rate of PBC after the transplant operation is 9% to 35%, and ursodeoxycholic acid (UDCA) is not effective to prevent relapse after transplantation in PBC [25]. Although PBC transplant recipients receiving cyclosporine have a lower risk of disease recurrence, the development of recurrent PBC had no impact on long-term survival [26].

In PSC, persistent icterus and repeated severe cholangitis lead to consideration of liver transplantation. Patients with Mayo risk score ≥ 2 points (high-risk group) should be considered as candidates for liver transplantation (Table **6**) [27]. The prognosis is predicted from several factors, *i.e.*, age, prothrombin time, serum albumin value, serum bilirubin value, serum aminotransferase levels, history of esophageal variceal hemorrhage, presence of ascites, and diuretic use. However, attention should be paid to the development of cancer, especially in the bile duct and colon, in patients with PSC. There is debate regarding the incidence of recurrent PSC posttransplantation but it may occur in 15% to 20% of patients [28]. Therefore, an early transplant is not recommended in PSC because re-transplantation is difficult.

Table 6. Mayo scoring system for predicting the need for transplantation in PSC.

$$R = 0.03 \; [age(y)]$$
$$+ 0.54 \log [bilirubin \; (mg/dL)]$$
$$+ 0.54 \log [aspartate \; aminotransferase \; (U/L)]$$
$$+ 1.24 \; [variceal \; bleeding \; (0 \; or \; 1)]$$
$$- 0.84 \; [albumin(g/dL)].$$

History of variceal bleeding score
0= no history
1= past history

On-line calculators are now available:
(http://www.mayoclinic.org/gi-rst/mayomodel3.html)

Hepatitis B Virus (HBV) Infection

The process to determine the timing of liver transplantation is the same as that described for acute liver failure and decompensated cirrhosis of other etiologies. There are two problems associated with HBV infection-related liver transplantation: 1) relapse of HBV infection after transplantation in acute liver failure, chronic hepatitis, and cirrhosis; and 2) relapse of HBV infection after transplantation in anti-HBc antibody-positive donors.

When a diagnosis of fulminant hepatitis B is confirmed, it is necessary to consider the use of antiviral drugs, such as lamivudine, entecavir or tenofovir, because they can be used safely and have been suggested to improve the prognosis. In fulminant hepatitis B, the re-infection rate of HBV after liver transplantation is 17%, which is lower than those for chronic hepatitis B and liver cirrhosis B [29]. Re-infection could be prevented by long-term administration of hepatitis B immune globulin (HBIG). In chronic hepatitis and cirrhosis caused by HBV infection, the re-infection rate of HBV after liver transplantation is 33% under long-term HBIG administration alone

[30], and rate of recurrence is 16% to 41% with antiviral drug administration, such as lamivudine alone [31]. Recently, the re-infection rate was reported to become 10% or less with combination therapy consisting of lamivudine and a large amount of HBIG 3 months before transplantation, and liver transplantation in HBV infection can be performed relatively safely [32, 33]. Use of HBIG continues based on the level of the antibody levels so that the value of anti-HBs antibody can be maintained at 500 mIU/mL for the first 6 months and 200 mIU/mL afterwards. The problem with this treatment is that HBIG is a blood product and is therefore very expensive. Various methods, including vaccination, have been tried in patients to reduce the total amounts of HBIG needed in this method. However, because almost all patients are treated with immunosuppressive agents to prevent graft rejection, antibody acquisition by vaccination is generally difficult. HBV infection was reported to occur in 50% and 78% of liver transplant recipients from anti-HBc antibody-positive donors in Spain [34] and the USA [35], respectively. Administration of large amounts of HBIG after transplant operation has been performed in an attempt to prevent re-infection by HBV in grafts from anti-HBc antibody-positive donors [36]. Oral antiviral agents with greater potency and a higher barrier to resistance, such as tenofovir and entecavir, have recently been approved for the use in patients with decompensated cirrhosis and are the first-line therapy in this setting. These drugs have been used successfully in such patients [37].

Hepatitis C Virus (HCV) Infection

Hepatitis C virus (HCV)-related chronic liver disease is the most frequent indication for liver transplantation in the USA. The process used to determine the timing of liver transplantation is the same as that described for acute liver failure and decompensated cirrhosis of other etiologies. Although it was initially thought in the 1990s that prognosis was not different between HCV-positive transplant recipients and other transplant recipients, it has since been reported that the survival period of HCV-positive transplant recipients was shorter than those of other transplant recipients. Analysis performed by the United Network for Organ Sharing (UNOS) in 2002 indicated that the 5-year survival rates were 76.6% and 69.9%, and the graft survival rates were 67.7% and 56.8% in HCV-negative and HCV-positive liver transplant recipients, respectively [38]. Ninety-five percent of HCV-positive transplant recipients cannot avoid re-infection with HCV after liver transplantation [39]. Necroinflammatory changes in the liver appear in 50% of HCV-positive transplant recipients within 1 year after liver transplantation, and in 90% within 10 years [40]. Fibrosis deposition is accelerated in liver transplant recipients with recurrent HCV infection compared with non-immunosuppressed patients; 20% to 30% of transplant recipients develop graft cirrhosis within 5 years after liver transplantation [41]. A small proportion of patients (5%) experience a rapid and aggressive form of recurrence (fibrosing cholestatic hepatitis). Old donor age and female transplant recipient are higher risk factors for developing severe recurrence of hepatitis C [42]. No definitive treatment to prevent re-infection by HCV has yet been developed. The sustained virological response (SVR) rate is only 30% in patients treated with combination therapy consisting of pegylated interferon (PEG-IFN) and ribavirin (RBV) [43]. The low SVR rate is possibly because 80% of patients cannot be administered a sufficient dose of IFN. Splenectomy has been performed at transplantation in an attempt to increase platelet numbers [44]. However, triple therapy (PEG-IFN+ribavirin+teraprevir/boceprevir) may be useful, and IFN-free regimens that combine two or three different directly acting antiviral agents (with or without ribavirin) could soon become the standard of care for HCV-infected patients awaiting liver transplant [37]. Although it has been reported that cyclosporine A showed a preventive effect against HCV proliferation *in vitro*, most studies comparing cyclosporine A with FK506 did not find significant differences in survival of grafts or patients *in vivo* [45, 46].

Hepatic Malignancy

Liver transplantation is considered in patients with liver cancer when their liver function is decreased. The Milan criteria—number and diameter of tumors ≤ 3 and ≤ 3 cm, or 1 and ≤ 5 cm, represent the gold standard for indication for liver transplantation in patients with HCC (Table 7) [1].

Table 7. Milan and UCSF criteria for the indication for liver transplantation in patients with HCC.

Milan criteria

1. Single tumor ≤ 5 cm in size
2. More than 3 tumors each ≤ 3 cm in size
3. No macrovascular invasion
4. No extrahepatic and LN metastasis

UCSF criteria

1. Single tumor ≤ 6.5 m in size
2. More than three tumors each ≤ 3 cm in size
3. Total tumor diameter ≤ 8 cm,
4. No macrovascular invasion
5. No extrahepatic and LN metastasis

The relapse rate was shown to be significantly higher in cases outside the Milan criteria. However, the University of California, San Francisco (UCSF) criteria (Table 7) have recently shown good results with a 2-year survival rate of 86% in cases deviating from the Milan criteria [47]. Opinion is divided regarding whether adjuvant chemotherapy is effective for HCC. It is uncertain whether rapamycin is superior to other immunosuppressive agents [48]. There is no indication for liver transplantation in intrahepatic cholangiocarcinoma and metastatic liver tumor except for carcinoid and neuroendocrine tumors.

Alcoholic Liver Disease

Alcoholic liver disease accounts for 10% to 12% cases of liver transplantation in the USA, and the survival rate during the first 1 year after liver transplantation is similar to those in other diseases. However, survival rates in patients with alcoholic liver disease are lower than those in other diseases 2 years after transplantation. This reduction in survival rate is due to recurrence of alcohol dependence, poor compliance with medications, and comorbidities of other alcohol-induced diseases. Liver transplantation for alcoholic liver disease should be discussed carefully, and may be considered in the following cases: patients that will have employment after the operation, that do not have other severe alcohol-induced diseases, that can stop drinking for 6 months, and that are both socially and economically stable [49]. Acute alcoholic hepatitis is a contraindication for liver transplantation due to the lack of the required period of abstinence.

INDICATION CRITERIA FOR LIVER TRANSPLANTATION

It is important to judge the indication or lack of indication of donors to improve patient survival, and inappropriate donors should be excluded (Table 8).

Table 8. Contraindications for organ donation.

Severe untreated systemic sepsis
Acquired immunodeficiency syndrome
Active viral hepatitis B or C, cytomegalovirus
Viral encephalitis
Active extracranial malignancy
Risk of rare viral or prion protein illness, viz. Creutzfeldt-Jakob disease
Recipients of cadaver human pituitary growth hormone
Undiagnosed acute or progressive neurological disorder with or without dementia
Active West Nile virus or Rabies
Active disseminated tuberculosis

The ideal, general donor criteria include age ≤ 50 years, normal liver functions, hemodynamic stability, and no systematic infections or cancers [50]. Patients with visceral tumors other than primary brain tumors are contraindicated as liver transplantation donors, and cerebral peritoneal shunt in primary brain tumor is also a contraindication. The presence of anti-HIV antibody is also a contraindication. It is favorable for the donor and recipient to have the same blood type to improve recipient survival rate, and a similar body size is also suitable. As the liver from older donors cannot tolerate ischemia or long-term preservation, the cold ischemic period should be kept as short as possible. Sex is also an important factor in liver transplantation, and transplantation from a female donor to a male recipient shows significantly reduced 10-year survival and 10-year graft survival rates [51]. Fat infiltration in the donor liver over 50% is a contraindication for transplantation. Although it has been shown that ABO mismatch causes graft loss, it is difficult to determine how to treat such marginal donors in each facility due to organ shortages. Recently, the graft survival rate has greatly improved in liver transplantation with ABO mismatch with the use of rituximab, prostaglandin E1, and splenectomy [52]. The definition of expanded criteria donor (ECD) liver allograft is not universal and somewhat center-based. An ECD liver may be considered but not limited to the following: donor age > 65, steatosis $> 30\%$ of graft volume, peak donor serum sodium level > 155 mEq/L, use of high-dose or multiple vasopressor agents, prolonged intensive care unit stay, and long cold ischemic time (> 12 h) [50]. Donation after cardiac death [53], HCV-positive donor to HCV-positive recipient, and HBV-positive donor will be new possibilities for donor selection.

PEDIATRIC LIVER TRANSPLANTATION

Cholestatic diseases such as biliary atresia, Alagille syndrome, and Byler diseases are the major diseases necessitating liver transplantation in infants, followed by acute liver failure and metabolic diseases (Table **1**). PELD score has been introduced for decision making regarding the priority of infant liver transplantation in the USA (Table **3**) [54]. Age, INR, serum albumin, serum total bilirubin, and growth factor are used for evaluation of patient prognosis. A calculated score < 6 is associated with a 3-month survival rate of 92% [54], while calculated scores of $7 - 15$ and > 25 have rates of 85% and 76%, respectively [54]. There is a serious problem in cases of fulminant hepatic failure in that the etiology in infants is often uncertain. Therefore, the prognosis is difficult to predict, and clarification of the cause will lead to selection of the appropriate treatment for each patient, resulting in improvement of the prognosis in future. The most frequent metabolic diseases associated with liver transplantation are α1-antitrypsin deficiency and Wilson disease. These metabolic diseases often have a good prognosis compared with other diseases, and close examination may be required to decide on the optimal timing of transplantation [55]. Indications for transplantation in cases of Wilson disease are Wilsonsian fulminant hepatitis, non-compensatory cirrhosis, uncontrollable hemorrhage due to portal hypertension, advanced neurological disease, and medication-refractory cases. A prognostic score has been proposed, and a score $\geq$ 12 points is thought to be suitable for liver transplantation according to the index of mortality (Table **9**) [56].

Table 9. Prognostic index for predicting mortality in Wilson disease.

a) Prognostic index in fulminant Wilson hepatitis (WPI)

Score	Bilirubin (mmol/L)	AST (IU/L)	PT(seconds)
0	0-100	0-100	<4
1	101-150	101-150	4-8
2	151-200	151-300	9-12
3	201-300	301-400	13-20
4	>301	>401	>20

b) Revised Wilson prognostic index (RWPI)

Score	Bilirubin (mmol/L)	INR	AST (IU/L)	WBC (10^9/L)	Albumin (g/L)
0	0-100	0-1.29	0-100	0-6.7	>45
1	101-150	1.3-1.6	101-150	6.8-8.3	34-44
2	151-200	1.7-1.9	151-300	8.4-10.3	25-33
3	201-300	2.0-2.4	301-400	10.4-15.3	21-24
4	>301	>2.5	>401	>15.4	<20

COMPLICATIONS AFTER LIVER TRANSPLANTATION

Postoperative complications can be divided into surgical and medical complications (Table **10**). Surgical complications after liver transplantation are further categorized as vascular, biliary, and others. There are three major types of medical complications after liver transplantation: 1) early acute graft failure (day 1-2); 2) acute (between 2 weeks and 2 months) or chronic (between 2 months and 2 years) rejection; and 3) infections. The medical complications are outlined below.

Early Acute Graft Failure/Primary Non-Function (Day 1-2)

Early acute graft failure occurs 24-48 hours after transplantation in 3% to 4% of cases and is mainly due to graft insufficiency [57]. Excessive organ storage time, long ischemic period, rejection in the super-acute stage, or shock in the recipient may be responsible for early acute graft failure. The condition is serious when the liver function does not improve or general conditions gradually worsen with circulatory failure or progression of renal acidosis. In addition, thrombosis of the hepatic artery or the portal vein, and hepatic venous obstruction may be seen. Re-transplantation is necessary in such cases.

Rejection

Acute Cellular Rejection

Acute cellular rejection usually occurs within the first 2 weeks to 2 months after transplantation, and is found in 50% of transplant recipients [58]. It is usually asymptomatic and identified by abnormal blood tests, such as raised liver enzyme or bilirubin levels. Nonspecific symptoms, such as low-grade fever, may be seen. The bile ducts and hepatic vascular endothelial cells are usually involved, and liver biopsy is needed for the diagnosis [59] and to exclude alternative etiologies, such as sepsis, recurrent diseases, ischemia, or drug toxicity. This form of rejection is often reversible, either spontaneously or by additional immunosuppressive therapy with methylprednisolone, and can be graded as mild, moderate, and severe rejection, associated with 37%, 48%, and 75% unfavorable short-term and 1%, 12%, and 14% unfavorable long-term outcomes, respectively [60].

Table 10. Complications after liver transplantation.

Surgical complications
Rejection (Acute, chronic)*
Infection
Biliary complications (e.g. anastomotic, rejection, ischemia, ABO mismatch etc)
Immunosuppression-related drug toxicity*
Hypertension
Diabetes
Obesity
Hyperlipidemia
Renal dysfunction
Hyperuricemia
Osteoporosis
Malignancies
Disease recurrence*

* Diagnostic liver biopsy should be considered.

Chronic Rejection (Vanishing Bile Duct Syndrome)

Chronic rejection usually occurs several months to years after liver transplantation, and is an uncommon complication occurring in an estimated 5%

to 10% of transplant recipients. It is also referred to as "vanishing bile duct syndrome" because intrahepatic bile ducts progressively disappear [61]. Chronic rejection is usually identified by abnormal blood test results, such as elevated liver enzymes, bilirubin, and ALP, and the patients may show jaundice with pruritus. The most common risk factor is a recent change in immunosuppressive agents. Liver biopsy is usually needed for diagnosis, and biopsy specimens can be used to determine the severity of disease [59]. Histological tests often demonstrate vasculopathy in the main branches of the hepatic artery and disappearance of the bile ducts. In the early stages of chronic rejection, immunosuppression should be applied to restore graft function, but this is not always successful. Increased tacrolimus [62], steroid pulse therapy, and rapamycin [63] may be effective for chronic rejection in the early stages. However, immunosuppression is ineffective after the bile ducts have vanished, and re-transplantation may be required.

Infection

Bacterial, fungal, or viral (cytomegalovirus, Epstein–Barr virus, herpes simplex virus) infections usually occur within the first 2 days to 2 weeks after transplantation, and are relatively common occurring in roughly 50% of transplant recipients [64, 65]. The possibility of sepsis should always be considered in patients with infection. The chest, urine, blood, abdomen, and indwelling cannula should first be examined as possible sources of infection. Immunosuppressive agents may mask common signs of infection, such as fever or leukocytosis.

FOLLOW-UP AFTER LIVER TRANSPLANTATION

Non-hepatic causes of death from 1 year after liver transplantation include malignancy (22%), cardiovascular disease (11%), infection (9%), and renal failure (6%), whereas liver allograft failure accounts for less than one third of such deaths [66]. It is important to monitor patients for hypertension, diabetes, hyperlipidemia, and renal function as well as perform cancer surveillance after liver transplantation (Table **10**) [67]. Close cooperation between the family doctor and the transplantation center may be required [67, 68]. To obtain sufficient immunosuppression, patients may need to take several drugs and the interactions between these immunosuppressants and other drugs should be monitored carefully (Table **11**) [67]. The ultimate goal is to use the lowest dose of immunosuppressants possible to maintain the graft in a good condition.

Immunosuppressive therapy is usually started with a combination of calcineurin inhibitor, such as cyclosporine or tacrolimus and corticosteroids, or triple-drug protocols including calcineurin inhibitor, corticosteroids, and antimetabolite such as azathioprine or mycophenolate mofetil [69]. Patients are then weaned off corticosteroids often by the 6th week after transplantation, although it may be avoided in patients with hepatitis C. A randomized controlled trial performed in the UK concluded that tacrolimus was associated with a better clinical outcome at 1 year compared with cyclosporine [70].

Table 11. Interactions of immunosuppressants, tacrolimus, cyclosporine, and rapamycin, with other drugs.

Inhibitors of the cytochrome P-450 system that can increase blood levels of immunosuppressants:
erythromycin, clarithromycin, clotrimazole, fluconazole, ketoconazole, grapefruit juice, diltiazem, verapamil, nicardipine, metoclopramide, ranitidine
Inducers of the cytochrome P-450 system that can decrease blood levels of immunosuppressants:
warfarin, carbamazepine, phenytoin, phenobarbital, rifampin, rifabutin

Routine monitoring should include assessment of complete blood count, renal function, and liver biochemistry, and the frequency of the tests should be determined according to the time after transplant and clinical course. To monitor the degree of immunosuppression, serum levels of drugs such as tacrolimus, cyclosporine, and rapamycin should be measured in the morning before drug administration, and the target levels should be determined by the transplant unit [71]. For metabolic risk surveillance, fasting lipids, glucose, uric acid, and blood pressure should be monitored [71]. Drugs usually needed in patients with metabolic risk include pravastatin, calcium channel blockers, and angiotensin-converting enzyme (ACE) inhibitors. Exercise, cessation of smoking, and a low fat diet should be emphasized in such cases. Drug interactions should always be considered. Unlike other statins, pravastatin does not interact with calcineurin inhibitors and is therefore recommended for the treatment of hyperlipidemia. Transplant induces substantial increases in the incidence rates of almost all carcinomas [72]. Surveillance should therefore be performed for colon, uterine cervix, breast, and skin cancer depending on the sex and age of the patient. Vaccination for influenza and pneumococci is considered necessary, but the use of live vaccines must be avoided. Psychosocial support should be provided for alcohol or drug abuse, and some patients may require counseling or drug treatment for depression after transplantation [73]. Renal impairment is common, and care should therefore be taken to avoid dehydration and to consider potential drug toxicities (*e.g.,* calcineurin inhibitors and nonsteroidal antiinflammatory drugs). The possibilities of rejection in patients presenting with liver dysfunction should be considered and discussed with the transplant team [68]. Close collaboration among primary care physicians and the transplant center is required for optimal care of orthotopic liver transplantation recipients. The transplant center should be notified for further work-up in cases with: (1) difficulty in controlling metabolic complications (diabetes, hypertension, hyperlipidemia, chronic kidney disease); (2) development of new malignancy, including skin cancers, in liver transplant recipients; (3) introduction of new long-term medications with potential to interact with calcineurin inhibitors; (4) pregnancy after liver transplant; or (5) new elevation of liver enzymes or function test results [67].

MESSAGES FROM HEPATOLOGISTS TO GENERAL PHYSICIANS

1. Patients with possible transition to fulminant hepatic failure and those with advanced liver cirrhosis or hepatocellular carcinomas are candidates for liver transplantation. In contrast to HCC, it should be noted that cholangiocarcinomas are not indicated for liver transplantation.

2. Early identification of candidacy for liver transplantation is an important role of general physician, and the candidates should be referred to hepatologists as soon as possible to avoid missing an opportunity for liver transplantation.

3. Prognosis of patients undergoing ABO-mismatch liver transplantation has improved markedly in recent years.

4. In living donor liver transplantation, a candidate donor is mandatory, and should be explored simultaneously with the identification of a candidate for the recipient.

5. Graft rejection and infection under immunosuppression are the most common causes of poor prognosis of liver transplant recipients.

6. Monitoring of the blood levels of immunosuppressive agents should be performed regularly by hepatologists to control graft rejection and infection.

ACKNOWLEDGEMENTS

We are very thankful to Ms. Asma Ahmed, manager publications, Bentham Science Publishers, for her patience and long-term assistance.

CONFLICT OF INTEREST

The author confirms that he has no conflict of interest to declare for this publication.

REFERENCES

[1] Mazzaferro V, Regalia E, Doci R, Andreola S, Pulvirenti A, Bozzetti F, Montalto F, Ammatuna M, Morabito A, Gennari L. Liver transplantation for the treatment of small hepatocellular carcinomas in patients with cirrhosis. N Engl J Med 1996;334:693-699.

[2] UpToDate: Patient selection for liver transplantation, Last literature review version 17.1: January 2009

[3] Starzl TE, Groth CG, Brettschneider L, Penn I, Fulginiti VA, Moon JB, Blanchard H, Martin AJ Jr, Porter KA. Orthotopic homotransplantation of the human liver. Ann Surg 1968;168:392-415

[4] Dienstag JL, Cosimi AB. Liver transplantation--a vision realized. N Engl J Med 2012;367:1483-1485

[5] Calne RY, Rolles K, White DJ, Thiru S, Evans DB, McMaster P, Dunn DC, Craddock GN, Henderson RG, Aziz S, Lewis P. Cyclosporin A initially as the only immunosuppressant in 34 recipients of cadaveric organs: 32 kidneys, 2 pancreases, and 2 livers. Lancet 1979;2:1033-1036.

[6] Multicenter FK506 Liver Study Group. A comparison of tacrolimus (FK 506) and cyclosporine for immunosuppression in liver transplantation. The U.S. N Engl J Med 1994;331:1110-1115.

[7] Alqahtani SA, Larson AM. Adult liver transplantation in the USA.Curr Opin Gastroenterol 2011;27:240-247.

[8] Broelsch CE, Whitington PF, Emond JC, Heffron TG, Thistlethwaite JR, Stevens L, Piper J, Whitington SH, Lichtor JL. Liver transplantation in children from living related donors. Surgical techniques and results. Ann Surg 1991;214:428-437

[9] Hashikura Y, Makuuchi M, Kawasaki S, *et al.* Successful living related partial liver transplantation to an adult patient. Lancet1994;343:1233-1234.

[10] Chen CL, Kabiling CS, Concejero AM. Why does living donor liver transplantation flourish in Asia? Nat Rev Gastroenterol Hepatol 2013;10:746-751.

[11] Ng KK, Lo CM. Liver transplantation in Asia: past, present and future. Ann Acad Med Singapore 2009;38:322-331.

[12] Rogiers X, Malagó M, Gawad K, Jauch KW, Olausson M, Knoefel WT, Gundlach M, Bassas A, Fischer L, Sterneck M, Burdelski M, Broelsch CE. *In situ* splitting of cadaveric livers. The ultimate expansion of a limited donor pool. Ann Surg 1996;224:331-339

[13] Murray KF, Carithers RL Jr; AASLD. AASLD practice guidelines: Evaluation of the patient for liver transplantation. Hepatology 2005;41:1407-1432.

[14] Spada M, Riva S, Maggiore G, Cintorino D, Gridelli B. Pediatric liver transplantation. World J Gastroenterol 2009;15:648-674.

[15] Merion RM, Schaubel DE, Dykstra DM, Freeman RB, Port FK, Wolfe RA. The survival benefit of liver transplantation. Am J Transplant 2005;5:307-313.

[16] Kim WR, Biggins SW, Kremers WK, Wiesner RH, Kamath PS, Benson JT, Edwards E, Therneau TM.Hyponatremia and mortality among patients on the liver-transplant waiting list. N Engl J Med 2008;359:1018-26

[17] O'Leary JG, Lepe R, Davis GL. Indications for liver transplantation. Gastroenterology 2008;134:1764-1776.

[18]   Varma V, Mehta N, Kumaran V, Nundy S.Indications and contraindications for liver transplantation. Int J Hepatol 2011;2011:121862.

[19]   O'Grady JG, Alexander GJ, Hayllar KM, Williams R. Early indicators of prognosis in fulminant hepatic failure. Gastroenterology 1989;97:439-445.

[20]   Polson J, Lee WM; American Association for the Study of Liver Disease. AASLD position paper: the management of acute liver failure. Hepatology 2005;41:1179-1197.

[21]   Wiesner RH, McDiarmid SV, Kamath PS, Edwards EB, Malinchoc M, Kremers WK, Krom RA, Kim WR. MELD and PELD: application of survival models to liver allocation. Liver Transpl 2001;7:567-580.

[22]   Xia VW, Du B, Braunfeld M, Neelakanta G, Hu KQ, Nourmand H, Levin P, Enriquez R, Hiatt JR, Ghobrial RM, Farmer DG, Busuttil RW, Steadman RH. Preoperative characteristics and intraoperative transfusion and vasopressor requirements in patients with low *vs.* high MELD scores. Liver Transpl 2006 Apr;12(4):614-620.

[23]   Lee J, Belanger A, Doucette JT, Stanca C, Friedman S, Bach N. Transplantation trends in primary biliary cirrhosis. Clin Gastroenterol Hepatol 2007;5:1313-1315.

[24]   Murtaugh PA, Dickson ER, Van Dam GM, Malinchoc M, Grambsch PM, Langworthy AL, Gips CH. Primary biliary cirrhosis: prediction of short-term survival based on repeated patient visits. Hepatology 1994;20:126-134.

[25]   Silveira MG, Talwalkar JA, Lindor KD, Wiesner RH. Recurrent primary biliary cirrhosis after liver transplantation. Am J Transplant 2010;10:720-726.

[26]   Montano-Loza AJ, Wasilenko S, Bintner J, Mason AL. Cyclosporine A protects against primary biliary cirrhosis recurrence after liver transplantation. Am J Transplant 2010;10:852-858.

[27]   Kim WR *et al.* A revised natural history model for primary sclerosing cholangitis. Mayo Clinic Proceedings 2000;75:688-694

[28]   Graziadei IW, Wiesner RH, Batts KP, *et al.* Recurrence of primary sclerosing cholangitis following liver transplantation. Hepatology 1999;29:1050–1056.

[29]   Samuel D, Muller R, Alexander G, Fassati L, Ducot B, Benhamou JP, Bismuth H. Liver transplantation in European patients with the hepatitis B surface antigen. N Engl J Med 1993;329:1842-1847.

[30]   Samuel D, Muller R, Alexander G, *et al.* Liver transplantation in European patients with the hepatitis B surface antigen. N Engl J Med 1993;329:1842–1847.

[31]   Villamil F. New approaches in prevention of HBV recurrence. In: Ginès P, Forns X, Abraldes G, *et al*, eds. Therapy in liver diseases. Barcelona, Spain: Elsevier Doyma, 2011:343–352.

[32]   Markowitz JS, Martin P, Conrad AJ, *et al.* Prophylaxis against hepatitis B recurrence following liver transplantation using combination lamivudine and hepatitis B immune globulin. Hepatology 1998;28:585–589.

[33]   Dumortier J, Chevallier P, Scoazec JY, *et al.* Combined lamivudine and hepatitis B immunoglobulin for the prevention of hepatitis B recurrence after liver transplantation: long-term results. Am J Transplant 2003;3:999–1002.

[34]   Prieto M, Gomez MD, Berenguer M, Cordoba J, Rayon JM, Pastor M. *et al. De novo* hepatitis B after liver transplantation from hepatitis B core antibody-positive donors in an area with high prevalence of anti-HBc positivity in the donor population. Liver Transpl 2001;7:51-58

[35]   Dickson RC, Everhart JE, Lake JR, Wei Y, Seaberg EC, Wiesner RH. *et al.* Transmission of hepatitis B by transplantation of livers from donors positive for antibody to hepatitis B core antigen. The National Institute of Diabetes and Digestive and Kidney Diseases Liver Transplantation Database. Gastroenterology 1997;113:1668-1674

[36]   Cholongitas E, Papatheodoridis GV, Burroughs AK. Liver grafts from anti-hepatitis B core positive donors: a systematic review. J Hepatol 2010;52:272-9.

[37]   Crespo G, Mariño Z, Navasa M, Forns X. Viral hepatitis in liver transplantation. Gastroenterology 2012;142:1373-1383.

[38]   Forman LM, Lewis JD, Berlin JA, *et al.* The association between hepatitis C infection and survival after orthotopic liver transplantation. Gastroenterology 2002; 122:889-896.

[39]   Gane EJ, Portmann BC, Naoumov NV, Smith HM, Underhill JA, Donaldson PT, *et al.* Long-term outcome of hepatitis C infection after liver transplantation. N Engl J Med 1996;334:815–820

[40]   Prieto M, Berenguer M, Rayon JM, *et al.* High incidence of allograft cirrhosis in hepatitis C virus genotype 1b infection following transplantation: relationship with rejection episodes. Hepatology 1999;29:250–256.

[41]   Berenguer M, Prieto M, San Juan F, Rayón JM, Martinez F, Carrasco D, Moya A, Orbis F, Mir J, Berenguer J. Contribution of donor age to the recent decrease in patient survival among HCV-infected liver transplant recipients. Hepatology 2002;36:202-210.

[42]   Belli LS, Burroughs AK, Burra P, Alberti AB, Samonakis D, Cammà C, De Carlis L, Minola E, Quaglia A, Zavaglia C, Vangeli M, Patch D, Dhillon A, Cillo U, Guido M, Fagiuoli S, Giacomoni A, Slim OA, Airoldi A, Boninsegna S, Davidson BR, Rolles K, Pinzello G. Liver transplantation for HCV cirrhosis: improved survival in recent years and increased severity of recurrent disease in female recipients: results of a long term retrospective study. Liver Transpl 2007;13:733-740.

[43]   Angelico M, Petrolati A, Lionetti R, Lenci I, Burra P, Donato MF, Merli M, Strazzabosco M, Tisone G. A randomized study on Peg-interferon alfa-2a with or without ribavirin in liver transplant recipients with recurrent hepatitis C. J Hepatol 2007;46:1009-1017.

[44]   Ikegami T, Toshima T, Takeishi K, Soejima Y, Kawanaka H, Yoshizumi T, Taketomi A, Maehara Y. Bloodless splenectomy during liver transplantation for terminal liver diseases with portal hypertension. J Am Coll Surg 2009;208:e1-4.

[45]   Berenguer M, Royuela A, Zamora J. Immunosuppression with calcineurin inhibitors with respect to the outcome of HCV recurrence after liver transplantation: results of a meta-analysis. Liver Transpl 2007;13:21-29.

[46]   Berenguer M, Aguilera V, San Juan F, Benlloch S, Rubin A, López-Andujar R, Moya A, Pareja E, Montalva E, Yago M, de Juan M, Mir J, Prieto M. Effect of calcineurin inhibitors in the outcome of liver transplantation in hepatitis C virus-positive recipients. Transplantation 2010;90:1204-1209.

[47]   Yao FY, Ferrell L, Bass NM, Bacchetti P, Ascher NL, Roberts JP. Liver transplantation for hepatocellular carcinoma: comparison of the proposed UCSF criteria with the Milan criteria and the Pittsburgh modified TNM criteria. Liver Transpl 2002;8:765-774.

[48]   Gomez-Martin C, Bustamante J, Castroagudin JF, Salcedo M, Garralda E, Testillano M, Herrero I, Matilla A, Sangro B. Efficacy and safety of sorafenib in combination with mammalian target of rapamycin inhibitors for recurrent hepatocellular carcinoma after liver transplantation. Liver Transpl 2012;18:45-52.

[49]   Neuberger J, Schulz KH, Day C, Fleig W, Berlakovich GA, Berenguer M, Pageaux GP, Lucey M, Horsmans Y, Burroughs A, Hockerstedt K. Transplantation for alcoholic liver disease. J Hepatol 2002;36:130-137.

[50]   Saidi RF.Current status of liver transplantation. Arch Iran Med. 2012;15:772-776.

[51]   Candinas D, Gunson BK, Nightingale P, Hubscher S, McMaster P, Neuberger JM. Sex mismatch as a risk factor for chronic rejection of liver allografts. Lancet 1995;346:1117-1121.

[52]   Takada Y. Some aspects of adult living donor liver transplantation: small-for-size graft and ABO mismatch. Hepatobiliary Pancreat Dis Int 2009;8:121-123.

[53]   Monbaliu D, Pirenne J, Talbot D. Liver transplantation using Donation after Cardiac Death donors. J Hepatol 2012;56:474-485.

[54]   Freeman RB Jr, Wiesner RH, Roberts JP, McDiarmid S, Dykstra DM, Merion RM. Improving liver allocation: MELD and PELD. Am J Transplant 2004;4:114-131.

[55]   Hansen K, Horslen S. Metabolic liver disease in children. Liver Transpl 2008;14:391-411.

[56]   Dhawan A, Taylor RM, Cheeseman P, De Silva P, Katsiyiannakis L, Mieli-Vergani G. Wilson's disease in children: 37-year experience and revised King's for liver transplantation. Liver Transplantation 2005;11:441–448.

[57]   Johnson SR, Alexopoulos S, Curry M, Hanto DW. Primary nonfunction (PNF) in the MELD Era: An SRTR database analysis. Am J Transplant 2007;7:1003-1009.

[58]   Wiesner RH, Demetris AJ, Belle SH, Seaberg EC, Lake JR, Zetterman RK, Everhart J, Detre KM. Acute hepatic allograft rejection: incidence, risk factors, and impact on outcome. Hepatology 1998;28:638-645.

[59]   Demetris AJ, Seaberg EC, Batts KP, Ferrell LD, Ludwig J, Markin RS, Belle SH, Detre K. Reliability and predictive value of the National Institute of Diabetes and Digestive and Kidney

        Diseases Liver Transplantation Database nomenclature and grading system for cellular rejection of liver allografts. Hepatology 1995;21:408-416.

[60]   Batts KP. Acute and chronic hepatic allograft rejection: pathology and classification. Liver Transpl Surg 1999;5:S21-29.

[61]   Wiesner RH, Ludwig J, van Hoek B, Krom RA. Current concepts in cell-mediated hepatic allograft rejection leading to ductopenia and liver failure. Hepatology 1991;14:721-729.

[62]   Wiesner RH, Batts KP, Krom RA. Evolving concepts in the diagnosis, pathogenesis, and treatment of chronic hepatic allograft rejection. Liver Transpl Surg 1999;5:388-400.

[63]   Neff GW, Montalbano M, Slapak-Green G, Berney T, Bejarano PA, Joshi A, Icardi M, Nery J, Seigo N, Levi D, Weppler D, Pappas P, Ruiz J, Schiff ER, Tzakis AG. A retrospective review of sirolimus (Rapamune) therapy in orthotopic liver transplant recipients diagnosed with chronic rejection. Liver Transpl 2003;9:477-483.

[64]   Hadley S, Samore MH, Lewis WD, Jenkins RL, Karchmer AW, Hammer SM. Major infectious complications after orthotopic liver transplantation and comparison of outcomes in patients receiving cyclosporine or FK506 as primary immunosuppression. Transplantation 1995;59:851-859.

[65]   Fishman JA. Infection in solid-organ transplant recipients. N Engl J Med 2007;357:2601-2614.

[66]   Watt KD, Pedersen RA, Kremers WK, Heimbach JK, Charlton MR. Evolution of causes and risk factors for mortality post-liver transplant: results of the NIDDK long-term follow-up study. Am J Transplant 2010;10:1420-1427.

[67]   Singh S, Watt KD. Long-term medical management of the liver transplant recipient: what the primary care physician needs to know. Mayo Clin Proc 2012;87:779-790.

[68]   McCashland TM. Posttransplantation care: role of the primary care physician *versus* transplant center. Liver Transpl 2001;7:S2-12.

[69]   Woodroffe R, Yao GL, Meads C, Bayliss S, Ready A, Raftery J, Taylor RS. Clinical and cost-effectiveness of newer immunosuppressive regimens in renal transplantation: a systematic review and modelling study. Health Technol Assess 2005;9:1-179, iii-iv.

[70]   O'Grady JG, Burroughs A, Hardy P, Elbourne D, Truesdale A; UK and Republic of Ireland Liver Transplant Study Group. Tacrolimus *versus* microemulsified ciclosporin in liver transplantation: the TMC randomised controlled trial. Lancet 2002;360:1119-1125.

[71]   Lucey MR, Terrault N, Ojo L, Hay JE, Neuberger J, Blumberg E, Teperman LW. Long-term management of the successful adult liver transplant: 2012 practice guideline by the American Association for the Study of Liver Diseases and the American Society of Transplantation. Liver Transpl 2013;19:3-26.

[72]   Vallejo GH, Romero CJ, de Vicente JC. Incidence and risk factors for cancer after liver transplantation. Crit Rev Oncol Hematol 2005;56:87-99.

[73]   Krahn LE, DiMartini A. Psychiatric and psychosocial aspects of liver transplantation. Liver Transpl 2005;11:1157-1168.

Subject Index

www.ingramcontent.com/pod-product-compliance
Lightning Source LLC
Chambersburg PA
CBHW050821220326
41598CB00006B/278